10 LOOK POUNDS THINNER, 10 YEARS YOUNGER— INSTANTLY

Books by Barbara Coffey

Beauty Begins at 40

Glamour's Success Book

Glamour's Health and Beauty Book

Look 10 Pounds Thinner, 10 Years Younger—Instantly

10 LOOK 10 POUNDS THINNER, 10 YEARS YOUNGER— INSTANTLY

A NO-DIET, NO-EXERCISE PLAN

Barbara Coffey

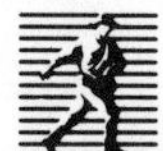

PRENTICE HALL PRESS
New York London Toronto Sydney Tokyo

Published by Prentice Hall Press
A Division of Simon & Schuster, Inc.
Gulf + Western Building
One Gulf + Western Plaza
New York, NY 10023

PRENTICE HALL PRESS is a registered trademark of
Simon & Schuster, Inc.

Library of Congress Cataloging-in-Publication Data

Coffey, Barbara.
Look 10 pounds thinner, 10 years younger—instantly: a no-diet, no exercise plan / Barbara Coffey.—1st ed.
pp. cm.
ISBN 0-13-416975-1
1. Clothing and dress. 2. Beauty, Personal. I. Title.
II. Title: Look ten pounds thinner, ten years younger—instantly.
TT507.C645 1988
646.7′2—dc 19 87-29285
CIP

Design by Stanley S. Drate/Folio Graphics Co., Inc.

Illustrations by Durell Godfrey

Manufactured in the United States of America

10 9 8 7 6 5 4 3 2 1

First Edition

This book is dedicated to all those women who lament an extra ten pounds every time they weigh themselves and wish they could turn the clock back about ten years when they look in the mirror. Take heart. Help is here.

ACKNOWLEDGMENTS

After more than twenty years in the fashion and beauty business, you absorb a great deal. I am grateful for all the good minds I've been stimulated by, especially those of my friends and co-workers over the years at *Glamour*. Special thanks also go to Edward Tricomi and Bob Prestiani at Pipino Buccheri Salon in New York. Their know-how and enthusiasm are always stimulating and a pleasure.

CONTENTS

INTRODUCTION

Looking good—slim and pretty, that is—has become a national preoccupation. Every woman wants to look better, and in particular, every woman over thirty wants to look *younger* and slimmer. If you have thumbed through your share of beauty and diet books and have been disappointed or disillusioned because you don't have the time, energy, or money to follow the various "look good" plans, this book is just what you've always wanted. It will tell you how to look both younger *and* thinner without dieting and without spending a lot of time and money on beauty plans that either don't work or are too time-consuming or expensive. In short, what you're going to get in the next sixteen chapters are instant results. Nothing worthwhile is accomplished without some effort, but there is one very special secret in this book; and that is something that, once learned, will become habit and will work for a lifetime. Part of the success of the technique you're going to learn is based on a frame of mind, on the way you feel about yourself. The other part is based on solid, sound information that can take off years and pounds. For example, your hair style can make you look ten years older or ten years younger than you are! It can make you look uptight and unapproachable or warm and appealing.

My friend Susan is a perfect example of how hair can change your looks for the better, and how attitude can spoil the change. For years, Susan had worn her pale blond hair in a shoulder length pageboy. When she was twenty-five, her hair flashed sexily around her shoulders and looked wonderful. When she was thirty, it still looked pretty terrific, but when she was thirty-eight, not only had shoulder-length pageboys become as obsolete as waist cinchers but Susan's pageboy made her look as though she were a throwback to waist-cincher days. Her friends kept urging her to cut her hair and finally, reluctantly, she went in for a "little trim." Her savvy hairdresser suggested he restyle Susan's hair slightly. Since she had been going to the same stylist for years, Susan trusted him. What she got was a lovely new cut that framed her face with wispy bangs. Everyone told her how becoming the new look was and how much younger it made her appear. Susan agreed, but as her hair grew out from the new cut, she began to urge it back into the same old style. In spite of the encouragement of friends and the reinforcement of her own mirror, she felt more comfortable with her old style. What she needed, in addition to a change in hair style, was a change in her point of view, a nudge in her attitude toward herself. What this book will give you is a gentle nudge in many directions. It will give you the courage to make changes and to live happily with them.

Hair can and does make one of the most striking impacts on a woman's appearance, but it is far from the whole story. Makeup counts, too. Too much makeup defeats your purpose and adds years rather than subtracts them. Clothes and their color count. Black *is* slimming, for example, and it *is* chic and sophisticated, but it can also be dull and unflattering. Red can be slimming, even white can take off the pounds—if you know how to wear it. When it comes to clothes, cut can be more important than fit and you can learn the secret of the right cut in one trip to any good department store.

You *can* learn how to look thinnner, younger, better than ever—now. It's all here. Just turn the page and start reading.

1 MIND OVER BODY

Have you ever awakened in the morning and for some inexplicable reason felt terrific? The feeling lasted all day and you felt a sense of something special about yourself. Luckily, we all have days like this. Sometimes it's because our hair looks terrific after a new cut or just happens to fall in place perfectly after a styling. Sometimes it's because something good has happened in our lives—a raise at work, a thoughtful gift from a lover or spouse. Dozens of things can make us feel good about ourselves. The point is—remember the feeling. You sail through the day feeling good and that sense of well-being will almost always result in some compliments. More than one person will tell you how good you look that day. Chances are, what people are responding to has more to do with your attitude than the way you look. You feel good, so you radiate confidence, a glow, a sense of well-being.

A woman I know recently told me this story. She was newly divorced and had moved into a new apartment that was all her own. At first, the responsibility of the apartment overwhelmed her and tension showed in her face and the way she carried herself. But as she got used to the idea of being on her own, she began to enjoy her new home and took special pleasure in coming home every night to a place that brought her happiness. She began to feel as though she had a special little secret all her own. The pleasure of this thought and the way the thought changed her attitude began to be reflected in her looks. Tension slipped away and was replaced with a glow. She felt good about herself and it was easy to see, because her entire demeanor changed.

Most of us don't have something as dramatic as this to cause a steady change in our basic attitude about ourselves. We swing back and forth from day to day, sometimes feeling terrific, sometimes feeling mediocre. We allow ourselves to become preoccupied with supposed flaws and to dwell on them continually. It is hard indeed for the average woman to feel good about herself most of the time. We are surrounded by media images of slim, perfect beauty, and we feel pressure to match the ideal. Clearly, most of us can't. Why must we match some impossible ideal in order to feel good about ourselves? The answer lies deep within our socialization as women. After so many years of liberating ourselves from ideas and behavior patterns that hold us back, we are still being brought up to feel that if our looks don't conform to some impossible image, we won't get our share of the good things in life. Looking objectively we can easily see that this is nonsense, but the idea makes a deep impression nonetheless. For a woman, her ticket to success is often based largely on how closely she matches the image of the "perfect" woman.

All this may seem strange to read in a book about instant beauty results. It is . . . and it isn't. There is no doubt that the better looking a woman is, the more easily she can achieve many things in life—getting and keeping the man she wants, getting and keeping the job she wants, being regarded positively by her friends. But the women who achieve many of these things are not necessarily great beauties. They are women who have learned to make themselves as attractive as they can be, to do this effortlessly every day, and then forget about the whole thing. Knowing that they look their best, they are free to get on with the other things that matter in their lives.

What you can learn from this book is how to look *your* best. You can learn that most of us, try as we might, are probably always going to weigh five or ten pounds more than we'd like. We are going to be stuck with fine hair or hair that is too curly or a nose that's a bit too big or lips that are too thin. And, as we get older, we're going to see some of the inevitable signs of aging appear in our faces and bodies. I suggest that instead of focusing on these negatives as so many women do, you learn to counteract the negatives with little tricks of dress and makeup, then forget them. Get on with your life. You'll discover that once you've done whatever is realistically possible about the things that bother you, it will make you feel good about yourself and you'll project a sense of well-being that will be perceived as attractiveness.

The goal of this book is to teach you how to counteract the things that befall all of us simply because very few of us are perfect. Once you've done this and you see the positive results, let the good feeling it engenders be your most important beauty asset.

I can best explain all this by telling you about Helen. Helen is considered a beauty by her friends. She's one of those women who would seem to have it all—great looks and a good body. I had lunch with Helen recently and told her how marvelous she looked. She acknowledged that she did receive many compliments from her friends, but since she knew I was writing this book, she asked me to take a good look at her. Helen looks years younger than she is.

She knows how to pick the right clothes to give her a youthful, ageless look. She's not a great beauty, feature by feature. She has extremely fine hair that she says she struggled with for years. Then one day a smart hairdresser told her to cut it very short and wear it wispy and framing her face. She did and she also had it lightened a bit because a lighter color was more flattering and alive than her "mousey" brown hair. Careful makeup made the most of her best feature—great cheekbones. But when she pointed it out, I noticed that she had very thin lips, not the sultry pout of TV and magazine beauties. Her hips were, at best, womanly, certainly not slender. She did have good legs, which she made the most of by collecting wonderful, sexy shoes.

The point is, Helen is far from perfect, yet most people think she's pretty terrific looking. She has learned to put herself together well, to focus on her good points, then forget about looks and get on with enjoying her life. Because she's learned to make the best of her looks, she enjoys the enormous benefit of feeling good about herself, which communicates a sense of special looks and presence.

There's no reason any woman—even you—can't learn to be a Helen. In knowing you've made the best of whatever you have and in not constantly focusing on negatives, you'll develop techniques and an attitude that will be perceived as beauty—you own special kind of beauty.

FINDING YOUR BEST FEATURE

One of the things that can help you feel good about yourself is learning that you have some good features and playing them up. Take a few minutes to think back about what you've been most complimented for. Is it your hair, your legs, your eyes? If many people have singled out some particular feature, it must be because it's outstanding. Tuck that knowledge away for now and then remember it as you read some of the specific tips in this book. There are ideas here to play up all kinds of good points in addition to hiding bad ones.

If you can't come up with anything, try this little experiment: Try to see yourself as another person. How, you might ask, can you possibly do that? The easiest way to do it is to sneak up on yourself. Try to catch a glimpse of your reflection in a shop window. Think of the reflection not as yourself but as someone else. Because you can often catch a quick glimpse of yourself as you walk on the street, it's much easier to gain a perspective different from the one you get standing in front of a mirror. You are only too familiar with your image in a mirror. Your glance will instinctively go to what you like least about yourself. But if you try to capture a quick, fleeting look, then think back to what you remember, you're likely to gain some new perspective. If you are walking with a friend and your attention is focused on your conversation, this is the perfect time to catch a quick, off-guard look at yourself. You might notice a warm smile or a figure that's a lot better than you thought, or perhaps you might simply realize that you carry yourself with dignity and presence. Tuck these perceptions away to focus on when you're learning how to make the best of what you have.

HOW REALISTIC IS YOUR VIEW OF YOU?

A few years ago, *Glamour* magazine did a major survey of its readers to determine how realistic their attitudes about their bodies were. Of the almost thirty-five thousand young women surveyed—women who, because of their youth, were most likely to have good bodies—over 75 percent felt they were overweight! The survey asked the women for their height and weight. By any reliable height-weight figures, only 25 percent of those women could possibly be considered overweight. What this says is that an overwhelming number of women have totally unrealistic views of their bodies. We think we're fat. We feel fat; we probably act as though we're fat by hiding our bodies or at least by not feeling proud of them, when by any normal standard we are not at all overweight. Thus the American preoccupation with fatness.

This is not to say that many of us would not look and feel better five or ten pounds thinner. It is to say that most of us are harder on ourselves than we need to be. You might start off your new "feeling good" campaign by checking your weight against the chart here to see by how much you are actually overweight. If you realize the situation is not as bad as you think, you will feel better about yourself, and that will make you more adventuresome with the clothes you wear and how you wear them.

HEIGHT	SMALL FRAME	MEDIUM FRAME	LARGE FRAME
4′10″	102–111	109–121	118–131
4′11″	103–113	111–123	120–134
5′0″	104–115	113–126	122–137
5′1″	106–118	115–129	125–140
5′2″	108–121	118–132	128–143
5′3″	111–124	121–135	131–147
5′4″	114–127	124–138	134–151
5′5″	117–130	127–141	137–155
5′6″	120–133	130–144	140–159
5′7″	123–136	133–147	143–163
5′8″	126–139	136–150	146–167
5′9″	129–142	139–153	149–170
5′10″	132–145	142–156	152–173

SOURCE: Metropolitan Life Insurance Company.

2 WHAT'S KEEPING *YOU* FROM LOOKING YOUR BEST?

In addition to the psychological attitudes that are at work in all of us, there are other things that keep us from looking our best. After you've conquered mind over matter, focus on your style and see if you can relate to any of the following stories. Find your counterpart and decide to make room for improvement now!

Linda is a perfect example of a modern woman groping to find a way to make the image in her head and the one in her mirror correspond. But her struggle is more than that. It is also a struggle with her life style. She is thirty years old and lives in a beautiful one-bedroom apartment in Chicago. The apartment, she knows, is far too expensive for her budget, but its open, sunny vistas are important to her well-being, since she lives in a big city and has a demanding job in a brokerage house. The moment Linda saw the apartment, she knew she had to have it. Every morning when she awakens to the sun streaming in her bedroom windows, she is glad she made the choice she did. She doesn't mind forgoing the movie or dinner out a couple of times a week. She doesn't have time for it anyway. She does mind that her clothes closet seems to hold nothing but dress-for-success suits and that tonight, when she has one of her rare dinner dates, she feels she has nothing to wear. She knows vaguely that she should be able to do something with her old navy blue suit to make it sexier, prettier for after work. She also knows she'd like to have more casual weekend clothes than she has, but her budget just won't permit it.

As though this weren't enough, Linda is beginning to be unhappy with her face as well as her wardrobe. She doesn't like the tiny lines forming around her mouth and the crinkles at the corners of her eyes. The fact that her dark brown hair is becoming lightly laced with gray doesn't please her. It's nothing very serious now, Linda realizes, but it makes her sense acutely the passing of time and her inability to find a way to put herself together so that she doesn't always feel she comes up short. An honest look at her body in her bedroom mirror as she undresses for bed each night also reveals that she has put on ten pounds since she left college—the result of too many client lunches and rushed meals at fast-food restaurants.

Linda is a perfectly normal young woman with the kinds of problems thousands of other women her age have. She's focused on getting ahead in her career for the past seven years and her looks and her social life show the effects. Now, having just had her thirtieth birthday, she's beginning to feel the first twinges of dissatisfaction. If she doesn't learn to deal with them now, they will increase as time goes by.

Linda needs to learn to shop on her limited budget in a way that gives her some off-hours clothes, as well as those she needs for her career. She needs to organize her shopping techniques so that she can get the most from the time she has to shop. She also knows that as long as she has to put up with the time pressures of her career now, she won't be able to diet or exercise seriously, yet she wants to look slimmer.

There's help for Linda here and for all the other women who share her life style. This book can help her learn to shop successfully, to find the right clothes at the best prices. Linda can learn new strategies and use them effortlessly for years to come. She can learn how to take care of her looks instantly so that she won't have to worry constantly about the passage of time. She can and will be happier with herself if she learns the easy-to-use techniques outlined in this book.

Susan is thirty-six, married, and the mother of two children. She works as a substitute teacher to bring in extra income while still staying home with her family as much as possible. She is happy with her life, but she's not happy with her looks. The demands of a young family and a part-time job leave her little time to spend on herself. Moreover she, like so many other young and not so young women, feels the pressure of trying to match some perfect image she carries in her head. Susan, too, has budget problems. She'd like to be able to spend more on clothes. Susan's biggest problem, however, is her body. Raising and cooking for two children, and eating essentially the same foods they eat as they grow up, Susan is growing, too, but she's growing out, not up. She's gained fifteen pounds in the past ten years. She has neither the time nor the inclination to diet and exercise very much, but she's acutely unhappy with the way she looks in her clothes. She is so single-mindedly focused on her body that she hasn't really paid attention to how out of date her hair style is, or to the fact that she's been using the same makeup routine for five years.

Susan wants to change, she just doesn't know how. When she starts to read all the involved diet plans around, her eyes glaze over and the thought of exercising for half an hour several times a week seems impossible. She doesn't have an extra hour and a half each week. Not now. Susan, too, and all the women who have similar problems can benefit from this book. She can learn to camouflage much of her excess weight through smart clothing choices, and she can learn to get more quality for her money when she shops. She'll also learn techniques that will help her identify her beauty problems so that she won't look out of date. Having a fresh contemporary beauty look can help compensate for other problems such as excess weight.

Rachel has different problems, but they are typical of those many women have today. She is forty-five and divorced. Back in the dating world at midlife, she feels overwhelmed by her competition. Her years of experience in living seem nothing compared to the trim bodies and fresh faces of the women ten years younger. The best help this book can give Rachel is a psychological lift. Feeling more positive will make her feel more able to accomplish the things that are important to her in her new life style, such as an improved social life and just plain fun.

Lila is fifty-two. She is a beauty, but her fifty-two years are apparent on her face and body. There's nothing wrong with that. If more of us wore our ages proudly, we'd all feel better about ourselves, but the reality is that society puts a great deal of pressure on us to look young. Lila has also just gone through menopause and that has diminished her sense of feminity. Always slender, she has gained almost ten pounds during her menopausal years. Lila needs the boost in her self-image that learning to look her best can give her. She'll find that boost in the pages that follow, and so will all the women who share Lila's problems.

This book will give you concrete, instant help in looking younger, fresher, trimmer. That's a lot, but more than that, it will also give you psychological help, which can be even more important. If you learn to be a realist about the image problems all women face, you won't be so hard on yourself. You can come to the realization that you probably have a lot more going for you than you think, and you can come to see that some of the women you think look so marvelous are actually working with raw material no better than yours.

3 SHOPPING SMART

There is a lot more to shopping than just walking into a store, picking something out, paying, and leaving. Anyone can do that, but not anyone can shop smart. Everyone can, however, *learn* to shop smart.

Being a smart shopper involves two things. The first is understanding the choice of stores available to you and what each store offers. The second is shopping technique, the tricks that get you the most for your time and money.

WHAT STORES ARE BEST FOR WHAT

Walk into any shopping mall and you'll see a fairly standard choice of stores. First you'll notice a branch of the big downtown department store anchoring the mall. Then, scattered around, you'll find a clutch of discount and "off-price" stores. What does each of these stores have to offer you?

The Department Store

A department store, whether in a mall or in the heart of downtown, has the largest selection of all kinds and prices of clothes. You'll find the name brands, the store's private labels, and a lot of sale merchandise, depending on the time of year.

You will probably pay top dollar in a department store because much of the merchandise is brand name and therefore priced pretty much the same wherever it is sold. All department stores, however, have sale policies. Keep shopping in your favorite one and you will figure out just how and when the store puts clothes on sale. Also watch your local newspaper for advertised sales. Certain standard times of year—around Columbus Day, after the Fourth of July, and after the Christmas holidays—are sale times almost everywhere. You can, however, usually get great buys on designer clothes if you're not the first to buy. Most well-known designers' clothes arrive in department and specialty stores early in the season—the end of July and during August for fall and beginning in January and into March for spring. If you must have that gorgeous designer skirt to hang in *your* closet in August you'll pay top dollar. But if you can cool it until the temperature drops in early fall, reductions will begin to appear. Many designer departments in large department stores have special racks of marked-down clothes year round. When you're buying expensive designer clothes, remember that the store actually figures the initial reduction into its selling policy. It follows, as night follows day, that Brand X designer pants, for example, will start out at $200, but in only a month, the same pants may be reduced to $150 or even less depending on how well they sold at $200.

For a shopper, the main advantage of a department store is the quantity of merchandise available. You can see what is new in many price ranges. The other thing worth noting about department stores is a trend that's definitely on the increase: private-label merchandise. Most department stores have manufacturers with whom they work to create a line of merchandise sold only in that store that is priced very appealingly. In the case of very large stores with many branches across the country, the store may actually manufacture its own private-label merchandise in factories in countries where labor is cheap. The store passes on the savings to its customers in this privately labeled merchandise. The trendiest styles are not usually represented in this kind of merchandise, but the clothes are of good quality and well styled.

The Specialty Store

The specialty store or boutique doesn't have the vast array of merchandise a department store has, but it does have a very definite image. If you browse in a particular boutique, you'll very quickly be able to tell what kind of clothes you'll find there and whether they suit you. You'll also get good personal service, because sales help will get to know you and be good about finding styles you'll like. You will usually find the latest styles in most boutiques.

The "Off-Price" Store

This is the store that buys up "odd" merchandise. The merchandise is odd in the sense that it consists of styles made by well-known designers that didn't sell well, thus resulting in a surplus; groups of sweaters, blouses, shirts, and so forth, that arrived from the manufacturers too late to sell at the desired time; or perhaps even clothes with slight defects. Sometimes labels will be cut out because a designer doesn't want it known that his or her clothes are being sold in the store. Merchandising today is so complex and clothes are manufactured in so many distant countries that it's common for large quantities of clothes to arrive too late in a season for a department or specialty store; the off-price store is one way to dispose of these perfectly good clothes.

You must be a savvy shopper to shop here. You won't get much help from the sales personnel, even if you can locate them. The atmosphere will be bare bones, but the prices will be right and you can often find great buys. Off-price stores are not "quick shops." It takes time to browse through the racks to see what is there, whether it's first run or damaged, and whether it's right for you.

Discount Stores

There are many kinds of discount stores around, but basically what's meant here is a store that sells merchandise of lesser quality. You will not usually find national brands here. There will be some quality merchandise if it's an upscale discount store, but you must know quality and examine what you're buying. Styles will be conservative, not trendy, and sales help minimal. This is a good place to fill in on basics and leisure clothes.

SHOPPING STRATEGIES

Now that you know what the various kinds of stores have to offer you, you need to develop strategies to make the most of each.

Time-saving Strategies

Although you may think these suggestions sound time-consuming, in the long run, you will find they make you a better shopper and a faster one.

At least twice a year, in spring and fall, save a chunk of time and visit the best, largest department store in your area. Don't plan to shop. You're "just looking." What you're looking for is what's new. What do you see the store featuring on mannequins and displays? What are they promoting? Go from department to department, making notes on a piece of paper. Since many department stores now have special designer boutiques, you can cover a lot of territory within the confines of one store. Don't be afraid to look into the very expensive designer departments. You're not buying, only investigating what is available and what is new. If you can possibly spare the time, spend a few hours browsing through the boutiques that you find carrying your kind of clothes, too. The purpose of this shopping adventure is to see what is new this season so that you can keep your wardrobe as up to date as possible.

Now, spend a little time at home with the notes you've made and select what works for you from what is available, according to the techniques of dressing young and slim in the following chapters. Then have a look at your closet. Where are the holes? What needs to be added? Replaced? Here, too, you should make some notes. Don't count on remembering that you have very few good-looking sweaters or blouses or that your skirts all look pretty dowdy. Write down what you want to buy.

You should also canvas the off-price and discount stores in your neighborhood so you know where you're likely to find the basic things you need. You needn't do this every season, because this kind of merchandise doesn't reflect fashion trends.

If you are the kind of shopper that must have help when you shop, head for a department or specialty store, the only place where you'll find the help you need. It is worth befriending a salesperson who knows your likes and dislikes so that helping you will become quick and easy. Ask to be called when a sale is scheduled. Ask to be notified if something you especially like goes on sale.

If your department store has a personal shopper, and most do, don't be afraid to use this service—it can be a great help. Surprisingly, you don't have to buy an armload

THE TIP-OFFS TO QUALITY

- *Fabric.* Learn to identify quality fabrics. Natural fabrics such as wool, linen, silk, and cotton tend to be used more in high-quality clothes. Synthetic fabrics are not usually found in quality clothes. Sometimes a fabric blend (part natural fiber, part synthetic) will be more durable. If you buy a blend, the higher percentage should be natural fiber. It will drape and tailor better than an all-synthetic fiber.
- *Detail.* Look at such little details as tucks, darts, and hems. Are they generous or stingy? Poor-quality clothes skimp on fabric and detail.
- *Finishing.* Look at the inside of a garment. Are the seams finished carefully or are they frayed or raveled? Are the buttonholes clean or frayed?
- *Cut.* Quality clothes almost always have good cuts (see page 22). The cut is part of the quality of any good garment, and makes the garment look better on you.
- *Style.* Believe it or not, the finest quality is usually conservatively styled. Women have learned to invest in traditionally styled high-quality clothes because they last a long time. If you pay a bit more, you'll more than make up for the price in the number of years you'll feel good wearing the clothes.

of clothes to use this service. It's usually free and the shopper will be cooperative if you appear serious about buying.

If you are a confident shopper, you can take on off-price or discount stores. With your list of "needs" in hand, scan the racks for what you want and don't allow yourself to be distracted by the things you don't need. Try to see if the store organizes merchandise in any particular way. Are the "big" buys all together? Are designer buys all assembled together? Are slightly damaged clothes all together? Any sense of organization you can discover will save you time, but your biggest time saver now is knowing exactly what you want and need.

Money-saving Strategies

As you've already learned, buying early in the season at a department store is *not* the way to get a bargain. Head to a department or specialty store later in the season when quality merchandise begins to go on sale. Watch your local newspaper for sales.

Learn to be a quality shopper. If you can teach yourself to identify quality, you can take advantage of bargains in discount and off-price stores.

Shopping Pitfalls

If you follow the strategies set forth here, you should avoid many of the common pitfalls. Still, it's a good idea to run through the most common errors and how to avoid them.

I don't really need it, but it's such a bargain. Stores are in business to sell, and they have very good ways of luring you in. In a department store, there are many impulse-buy items on the first floor, especially near escalators and elevators. You'll see signs for special purchases or very elaborate displays all geared to convince you to buy.

Don't—unless you really need the item. Learn to have a purpose when you're in a store and you won't be so tempted. If you buy something you don't need or won't use, it's no bargain no matter how cheap it is.

I'll diet into it. Never buy something that is too small and think you'll lose weight. Chances are whatever you buy will just end up hanging in your closet. Even if you do manage to squeeze into it, it's not going to do much to flatter you.

I love the style, not the color. How often have you bought something in a style you adored but in a color you really didn't find flattering or that didn't work with most of what you owned? We all fall victim to this shopping error from time to time, but you can learn to limit your mistakes. Walk away if you don't like both the style and the color.

I'll find something to wear with it. If you find a top (shirt, sweater) or a bottom (pants, skirt) or even a pair of

TO THE RESCUE

- Don't overlook the wealth of fast, good shopping you can do through the mail. Find catalogues that feature clothes, and sizes, that work for you.
- If you lack shopping confidence, shop with a friend who knows you well and whose taste you respect. Bounce your ideas off your friend.
- Window shop. Check out windows of good stores for current style trends. You don't have to go inside the store, so you can do it on your time, whenever you just happen by an interesting shop.
- Use your telephone to save time. Making a few well–thought-out calls to favorite stores to find out if they have something close to what you are looking for will save you hours of walking around.

shoes that you love, but you can't imagine what you'll wear with it, don't buy it! You'll end up just letting the item take up space in your closet or spend more time and money trying to find something to go with it.

I don't really like it, but it will do. You're really looking for a pair of beautifully cut, light gray flannel trousers but all you find are a pair of dark gray ones that aren't so well cut. You're not in love, but you want to get out of the store. Don't buy those pants! You probably won't wear them and you'll eventually end up finding the right ones at some point and spending more money for them. Hold out for what you really want.

4 POUND-PARING STRATEGIES

Sara is thirty-six, five foot four, and weighs 130 pounds. She wishes she weighed 120 and were twenty-nine again. Wishing won't make it so. Because she knows how to pick fresh, young, flattering styles, Sara looks young, slender, and radiantly attractive—and a good ten pounds thinner than she really is. When I saw her last, she was wearing a shrimp-colored oversize sweater and a slim, short, rust leather skirt. She matched her stockings to the color of her skirt and wore shoes that were just a shade darker. She looked wonderful! Sara is a smart woman who has mastered all the pound-paring strategies; she looks terrific now and will still look terrific for years to come.

There's a difference between pound-paring strategies and pound-paring clothes. Of course, some strategies require certain kinds of clothes, but before you actually get to the clothes, you must learn the strategies.

If you shop for hours, try on countless numbers of clothes and leave stores feeling that *slim* is a word about as likely to be applied to you as, say, *Wonderwoman,* take heart. It's not your body that's the problem; it's the kind of clothes you've been trying on. The right dress can't replace a diet, but if you're like most of us and just carrying ten extra pounds or so, clothes *can* make you look as though you've just finished a successful diet. Here are some strategies to keep in mind.

LEARN HOW TO SPOT A GOOD CUT

Make no mistake; cut does *not* mean fit. Something that fits you can be poorly cut. Cut is subtle, tricky, and immensely important. It is what many, but unfortunately not all, expensive clothes have.

The best way to learn to identify a good cut is to go shopping. Have a ball: Go to the best, most expensive stores in your town and try on all the clothes that appeal to you. Focus especially on pants, jumpsuits, slim skirts, and anything that has a definitely defined waistline. Notice how these clothes "hang" on your body. Notice that well-cut pants are generously cut; pleats are full and fall gracefully, the better to hide an ample tummy or a generous derrière. Dresses with definite waists don't pull or bind and the waist lies at your waist. After you've spent some time carefully looking at the way some of these clothes look on your body, move on to the stores or departments with less expensive clothes. Try on the same types of clothes. Notice the difference in cut. If you still think cut is fit, try on a pair of pants that is supposedly your size (be honest about what your size *is*). Now try on the next larger size. You'll probably notice that instead of looking better, the next size is just plain too big. The waistband will be too large, the seat will stick out, etc. One word to the wise, however. Sometimes, you can move up a size and get the *look* of a better cut. It's a trick that some women use to make inexpensive clothes look better. Once you've learned to identify the right kind of cut, you'll easily be able to tell whether moving up a size results in a better look—or just a bigger one.

THINK LONG, THINK SLIM, THINK VERTICAL

You don't have to be a genius to understand that a long line is going to elongate your body and make you look slimmer. Think of the effect of a V-neck, of vertical seaming, what you might find, for example, in a princess-style dress or a wrap dress. Think of any detail in styling that elongates the body. Think, too, of a pattern that elongates the body, a vertical stripe, for example.

LEARN THE ONE-COLOR, ONE-TONE THEORY

Separates are a great all-American look, but you must know how to wear them. Never wear sharply contrasting colors on top and bottom. One color—or much more interesting, tones of one color—are more flattering, more slimming. Think of a beige top moving into a deeper fawn-colored skirt or pants. Think of a soft green sweater and a deeper bottle-green skirt or a pale gray silk blouse and a slate gray skirt. Don't stop here. You've got legs and feet, too! Soft gray stockings worn with a gray skirt will continue the long line, take off pounds. A gray or black shoe will help even more. Soft sea-foam green stockings and deeper green shoes will work magic with the bottle-green skirt. If you think it sounds expensive to have a wardrobe of stocking colors instead of a drawer full of standard beige, ask yourself if it's any more expensive than buying clothes you don't wear because you're not happy with the way you look in them . . . or constantly buying yourself little presents to cheer yourself up because you're not happy with your looks. A wardrobe of stocking colors and a couple of pairs of shoes in different colors are two of the best fashion investments you can make. You can, however, minimize the expense of all this and create a more sophisticated wardrobe while doing so. *Limit your clothes color choices to two or three basic colors that are flattering to you.* If you look good in beiges or browns, buy most of your new major pieces in shades of beige or brown. This way you won't find yourself needing dozens of pairs of stockings and shoes and your clothes will coordinate with each other more easily. If, for example, you pick major pieces in beiges and browns, your jackets, skirts, and pants will all work well together. If you simply buy what strikes you at the time (something we all tend to do), you'll end up with green jackets, navy pants, and brown skirts. Try making that mix into a polished, coordinated wardrobe! When you buy major pieces in only two or three colors, you can add color and variety with accessories such as belts and scarves or even jewelry. Another good wardrobe color choice might be navy and wine, if these colors look good on you, or gray and deep blues. The idea is to avoid buying pieces in any color that strikes your fancy. If you practice the one-color, one-tone strategy, you'll always look slimmer because the single tone elongates and slims your body.

To help you get the hang of this kind of dressing, have a look at the chart below. The colors on top are basics, the ones you should choose for major pieces such as pants, jackets, and skirts. The colors below are accent colors that will add variety and spice to your basic colors. You should buy basics in no more than three colors, and they should work together so that when you combine a top and bottom you have a tone-on-tone look that gives you the illusion of length and slimness. Don't forget to carry out the idea in shoes and stockings, too.

You don't always have to duplicate an exact tone-on-tone look. If, for example, you are wearing a navy jacket, sweater, or blouse, and a gray or wine skirt, you will get the same slimming illusion because there is no sharp color contrast, top and bottom. *Always tone stockings and shoes to your skirt or pants.*

Basic Colors	Brown/beige/tan	Taupe/gray/navy	Black/gray/navy	Taupe/military green
Accent Colors	coral rust shrimp tangerine apricot cognac amber	red sapphire blue soft blues mauve	emerald green sapphire blue violet gold	moss greens sea-foam greens white gold

DON'T WEAR TENTS

Who is that woman walking down the street in a big, dark blue "tent"? A tent is any kind of dress or separates that hangs as though Omar the tentmaker had done the draping. It has all the sex appeal of a pine tree. It doesn't fool a soul into thinking you're thin. Why do women wear tents? Unfortunately, most of us assume that we can hide a few too many curves or all-out bulges by wearing loose styles. Don't get caught up in this philosophy. It doesn't fool anyone. Even if you're quite overweight, you'll look much better by taking the trouble to find clothes that fit well and are well cut. Leave the tents for campers and uninformed fashion victims.

DON'T THINK YOU CAN'T WEAR KNITS

A great many women simply bypass knits out of habit. These days a knit isn't just a knit. Walking around in the trendiest tweedy knit or in something ultraclingy is definitely not going to make you look slimmer, but many knits can pare pounds. There is so much variety in knits today that any woman can and should wear them. They are durable, flattering, and extremely comfortable, and they have enormous fashion impact. Knits to avoid are the thick nubby ones and the very inexpensive ones, which almost always cling unappealingly. Look for flat knits such as jersey, quality double knit, anything that doesn't hug the body too tightly. The cut of a knit is extremely important. Find a knit with a good cut in a flattering color and you'll have a wonderful look. Don't forget to color match two-piece knits, top and bottom, and to keep stockings and shoes in the same color family. You can't miss looking great.

USE THE SLIMMING POWER OF STRIPES

You don't have to look for the biggest, boldest vertical stripe you can find. That's just doing the obvious, and many times, the obvious solution is not really the best one. In dresses, skirts, and pants, a narrow pin stripe looks crisp and slimming. Pin-stripe flannel pants paired with a sweater or shirt in the same color family are a wonderfully slimming look. In summer, you'll find more stripe variety in anything from dresses to bathing suits. Take advantage of the choices.

USE FABRIC TO SLIM

Heavy imported tweeds are beautiful, seductive, and usually very expensive. Resist their seductive powers. Nubby tweeds, velours, or heavy piles, as appealing as they may look in the store, won't do a thing for anyone but a beanpole. Learn to look for gabardines, silks, flat knits, or lightweight flannels. They have slimming power.

Looking slim and young can also mean looking sexy and more feminine. Fabric can help enormously here. There are times when you probably want to project a softer, more feminine image. For those times, picking the right fabric, as well as the right style and color, does the trick.

The chart below shows you which fabrics add to a feminine image and which create a more tailored, hard-edged look. You can, of course, look wonderful in crisp, tailored clothes. They are the most appropriate for many business occasions. But you should be aware of what images fabric can create, then pick accordingly.

Image	Soft, sexy, feminine	Crisp, tailored, businesslike
Fabric	suede velvet challis satin silk crepe soft knits soft leathers jersey	tweeds gabardine broadcloth double knit twills heavy leathers

CONCENTRATE FASHION INTEREST ON TOP

Most women find they are "bottom heavy." Just one stroll down the street should convince you of this. Take a look at the derrières in front of you. Chances are, most of them are what you'd have to call "generous." Weight tends to accumulate on the bottom half of the female body—hips, thighs, stomachs. If you look for clothes with some top interest, a pretty neckline, a shoulder detail—even fashionably large shoulder pads will do the trick—you'll take the emphasis away from the heaviest part of your body and transfer it to a slimmer part.

SLIM DOWN FROM THE INSIDE OUT

Take a look around you, in your office, on the street. Put everyone's underwear to the bulge test and see how many women pass. Many won't because their clothes will reveal telltale bulges and rolls around panty and bra lines. To test what you own: Try on all your bras and panties under a knit or jersey dress. Is there a bulge at the panty line? Is there a bulge under your arm at the top of your bra or in back, over or under your bra? If so, toss the underwear. Find the styles that fit you well and keep buying them. It's actually a good idea to buy in quantity—a dozen bras or panties at a time. You'll save shopping time and money (buy them on sale) and you'll always have the right underpinnings.

LEARN TO DRESS IN SEXY LAYERS

As you learned before, dressing younger and thinner means adding a certain amount of sensuality to your image. Dressing in layers can do just that. Avoid heavy layers (big tweedy sweater vests or heavy jackets) but do experiment with soft, silky knit vests over silky shirts. This combination looks wonderful over skirts or pants. An open vest falling softly around a silky shirt and a skirt or pants is another wonderful look. Usually a longer vest or jacket, one that hits well below the hips, is more flattering and sexy. Try it and you'll see.

PARE POUNDS WITH WRAPS

Because wrap-style dresses or tops create a V-line at the neck or sometimes all the way down the front of the dress, a wrap or surplice style is very flattering. Finding at least one top and one dress that wrap should be one of your pound-paring strategies. Part of your strategy should also be to make the most of the long, slimming V-line. To do this, you should pick a solid color. If you wear a wrap top and slim skirt, they should be very close to each other in color to make the most of the elongating line the wrap gives. The particular color you pick will depend on your likes and dislikes and what you have in your wardrobe. This is a strategy that should be easy to carry out because wrap clothes are always in style and always in the stores.

TO THE RESCUE

- Think bright colors. If you follow any of the pound-paring strategies mentioned in this chapter, you *can* wear bright colors. Just make sure the top and bottom of a separates look don't contrast too dramatically. A bright blue blouse with a navy skirt would look great, or a pumpkin-colored blouse with a rust skirt. Try a bright yellow wrap dress or a mustard-colored one—pick any upbeat color that flatters you for an instant, life-saving lift.
- When you're less than happy with something you're wearing, or even if you love it, add one wonderful piece of jewelry. This lifesaver works well when you are wearing clothes you already own—those you bought before you got pound-smart. The jewelry, if it's really a knockout piece, will take the focus away from a dress or pants that may not be as flattering as you'd like.
- Belt any dress or separates ensemble in the same color as the outfit. It's surprisingly slimming. A belt in a contrasting color only emphasizes waist and hips—not a great idea if you're trying to look thinner.
- Add a bright scarf at your neck to take the focus away from heavier areas such as hips and waist.

The Fit That's Too Tight

The fit of a pair of pants is probably more crucial than the fit of almost anything else. A poor fit shows up every figure flaw. It can, in fact, even create some you may not have. Here, the drawing shows a typical "bad fit." The pleats pull, causing the pockets to pull. The tight crotch creates the look of a "smiling crotch." The tightness through the crotch also emphasizes a hip bulge.

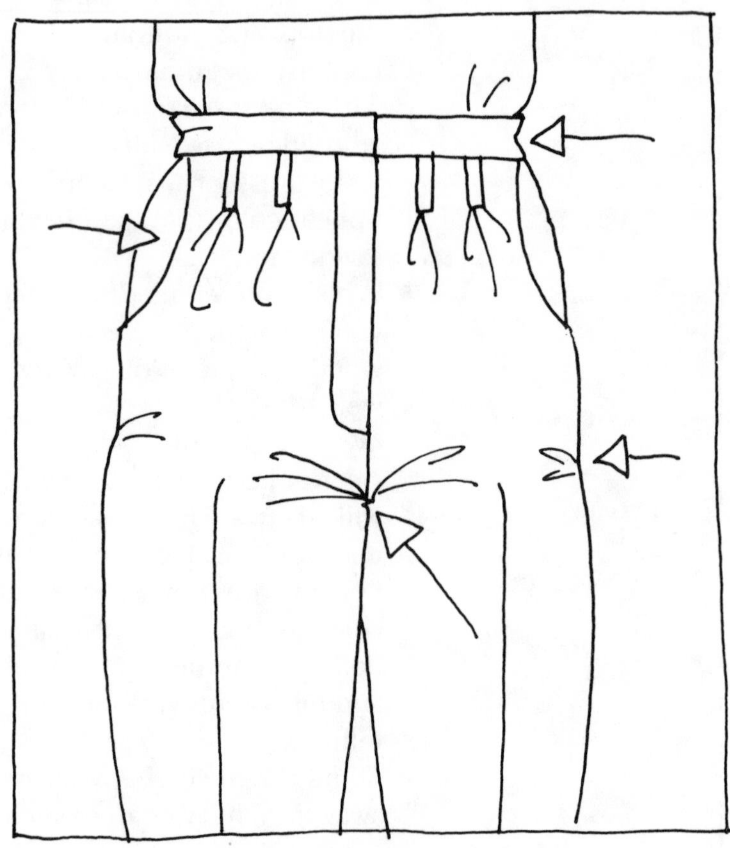

Too Big Is No Better than Too Tight

Pants that are too big are no more flattering than those that are too tight. Here, the waistband will never look trim and will allow a shirt or top of any kind to escape and bag at the waist. The pockets droop instead of lining up crisply. The crotch "frowns" because it also droops.

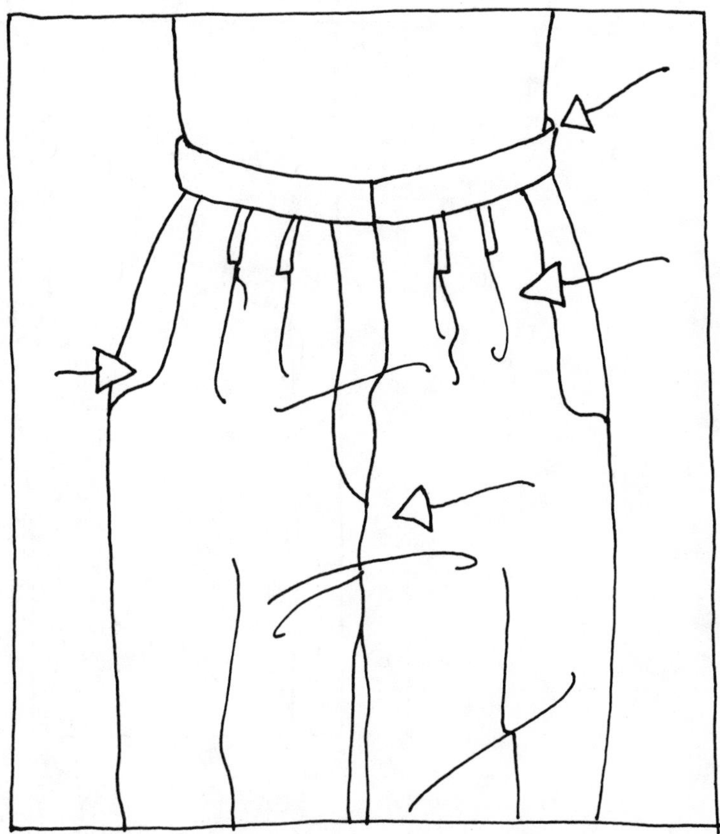

The Right Fit

Notice how much better the right fit looks. The waist fits properly, pockets are crisp and in line, pleats don't pull. The crotch hangs properly. It may take some effort to find a pair of pants that fits this well, but the effort is well worth it.

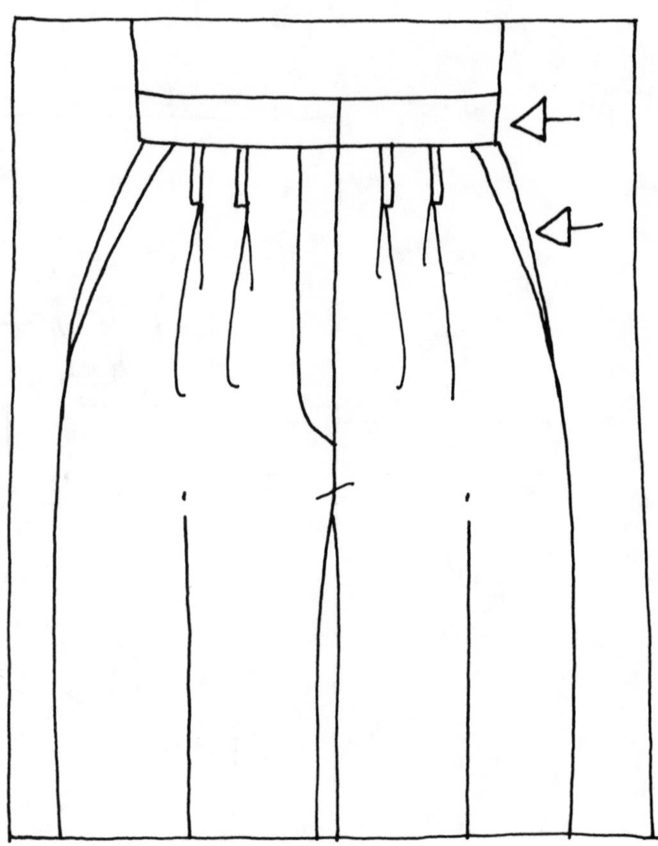

Too Tight Through the Rear

The worst view of a pair of poorly fitting pants is from the rear—a vantage point many of us miss by not looking in a "rearview mirror." Here, the waistband binds, causing a bulge, and the center seam pulls. The tightness through the hip causes a bulge and emphasizes "cheeks."

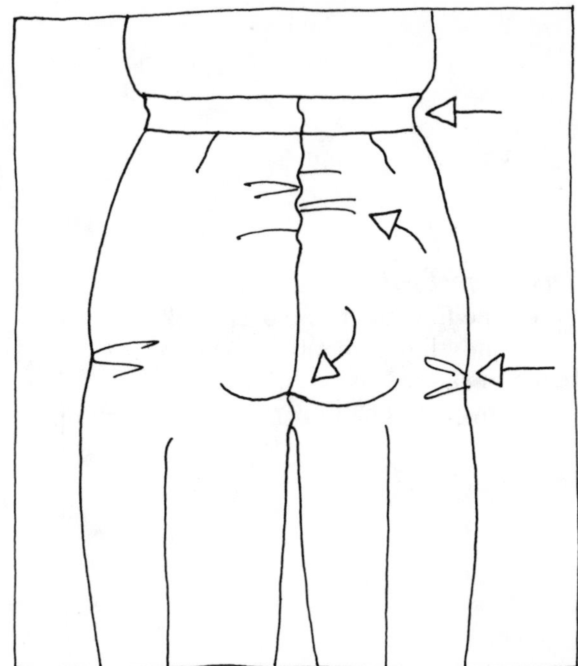

The Saggy Fit

A too-large waistband will gap in back as well as the front. Too much fullness through the hip will cause a sagging crotch—one of the most unfortunate aspects of a droopy rear view.

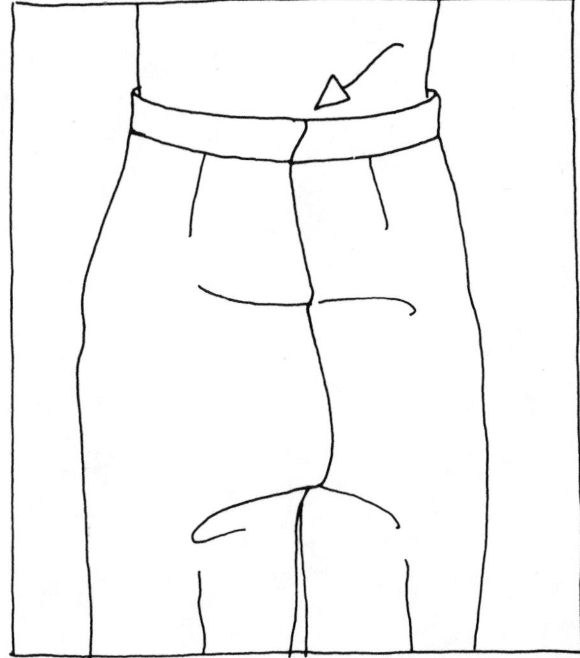

The Perfect Fit
When the fit is right, the back looks sleek and slim with not a bind or bulge in sight. This is the fit to aim for in any pair of pants.

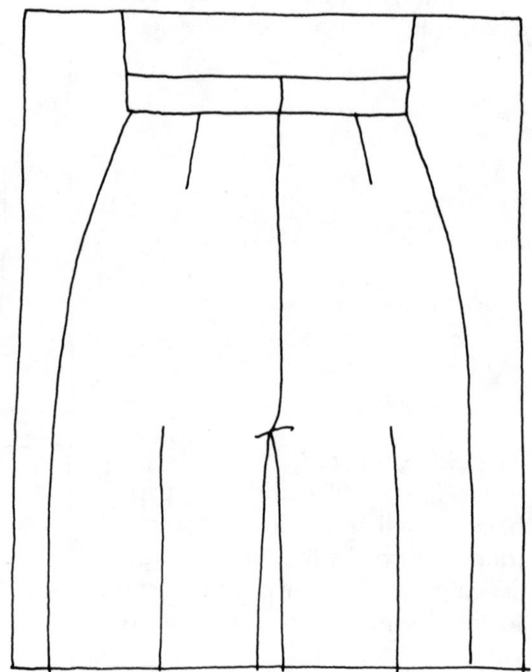

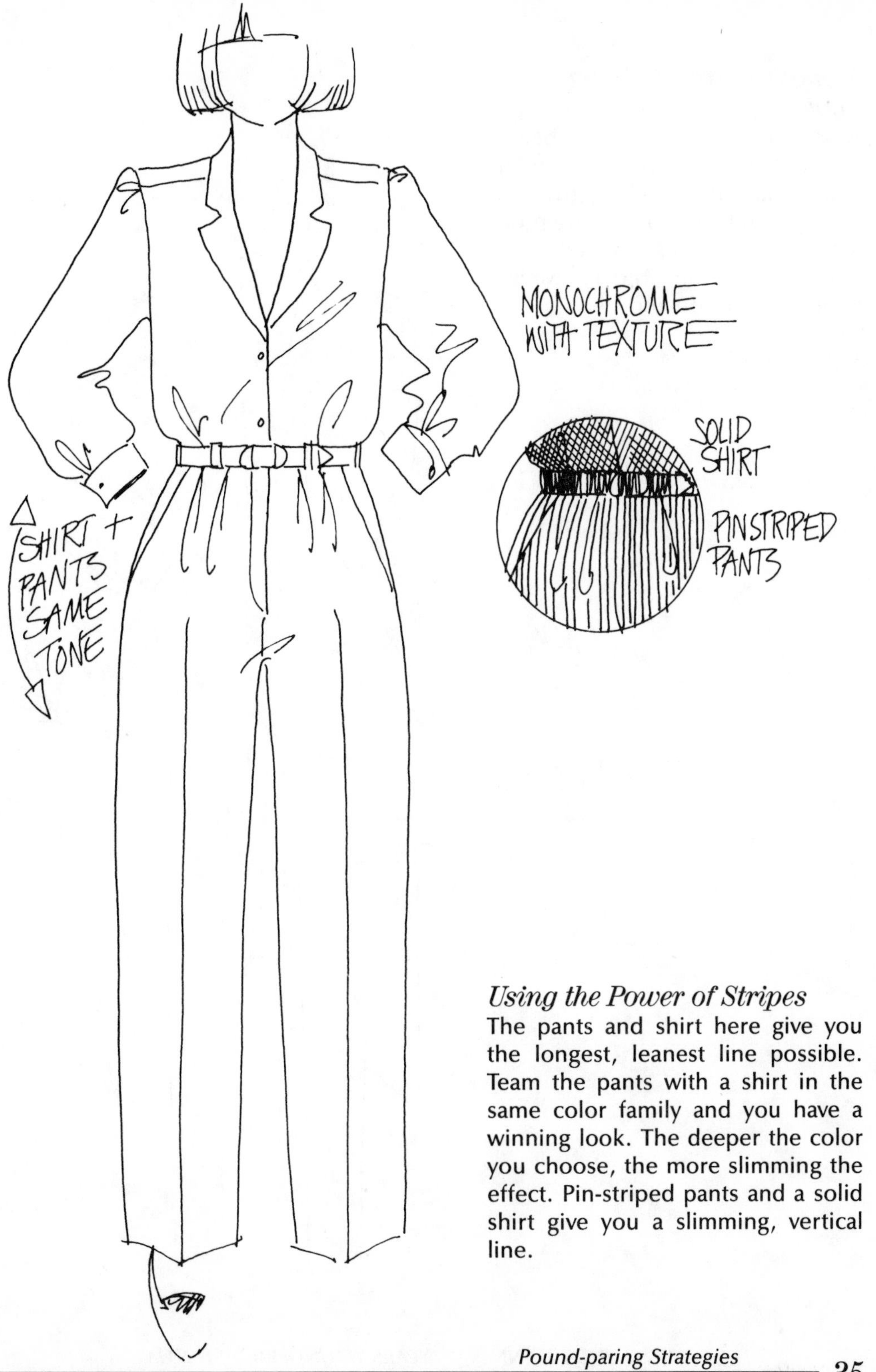

Using the Power of Stripes

The pants and shirt here give you the longest, leanest line possible. Team the pants with a shirt in the same color family and you have a winning look. The deeper the color you choose, the more slimming the effect. Pin-striped pants and a solid shirt give you a slimming, vertical line.

Elongated Lines, Slimming Look

Always think long! Here, a below-the-hip-length vest covers many hip and stomach flaws while it gives you a long, lean line. Worn over a pretty shirt and slim pants, you get a winning combination. The lightweight layers are also soft and sexy.

The Slimming Powers of a Wrap

The V-line that a wrap top or dress creates is very slendering. Here, a wrap top tucked into either pants or a skirt gives you a long line. Make wearing wraps part of your slimming strategy.

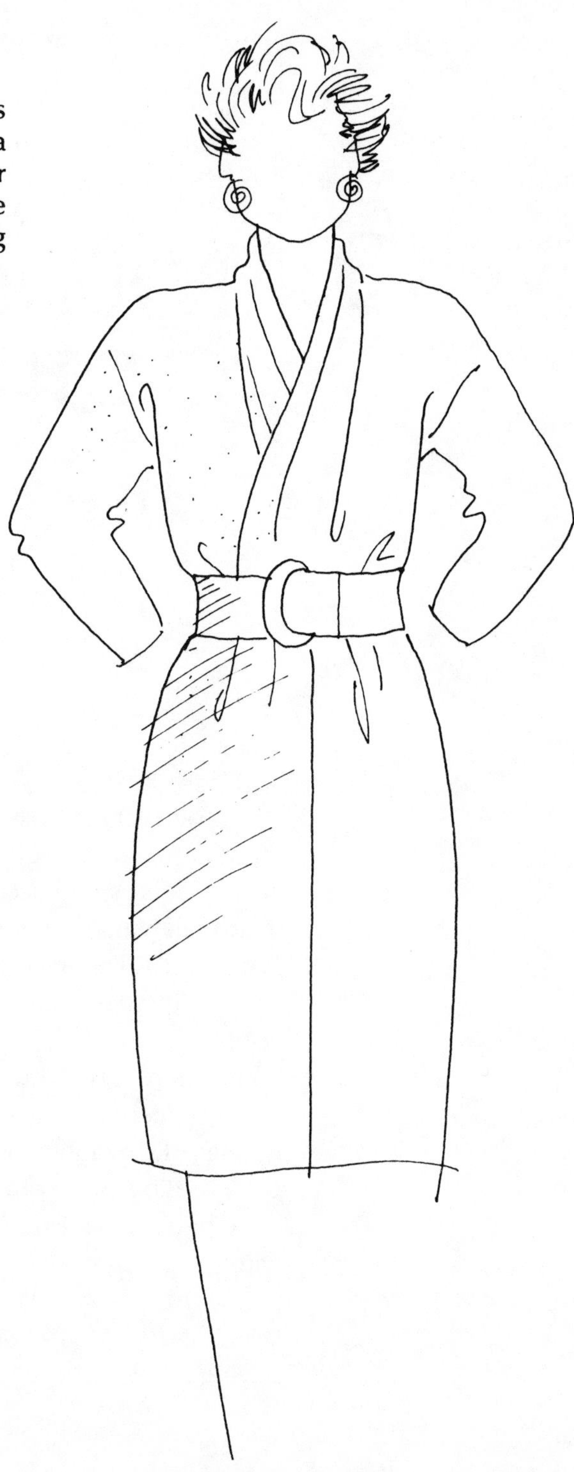

5 POUND-PARING CLOTHES

Consider this scenario. You're going shopping for some new spring or fall clothes. You go to your favorite stores and see racks and racks of this year's new colors and this year's trendy styles. You get hooked, you buy a rust silk shirt, which costs more than you can afford, and in another store, you buy a pair of navy pants, cut fashionably wide through the hip and slender at the ankle. Somewhere else you buy a wonderful tweedy sweater, mostly green, and a navy blue skirt with patch pockets at the hips. Everything you bought is new-looking in style and color . . . but hold on. How do these styles really look on *your* body? What do you have now or plan to buy to wear with the green sweater or the rust shirt?

If this sounds like you—and it probably sounds familiar to most of us—you're not shopping, you're grazing: buying a little here, a little there, with no real plan. Most of all, you're not thinking of your body and what will look right on it. Shopping for pound-paring clothes is a very special kind of shopping. It takes care and time, but it pays big dividends. And once you learn how to do it, you'll never again waste time or money buying things that will grace your closet, instead of your body. Shopping for pound-paring clothes means forgoing some of the newest, trendiest styles in favor of something more enduring, more flattering to your body. It means building a wardrobe of pound-paring clothes that you add to carefully each new season.

Though you can wear almost any style you really love if you follow the pound-paring strategies in the previous chapter, there are some clothes that take off pounds better than others. Learn what they are, how to wear them for maximum impact, and your friends will ask what diet you've been on!

SLIM SKIRTS

Yes, you read it right. A slim skirt is slimming. If you've been hiding in tents, A-line skirts and dresses, come out, come out, wherever you are. Naturally, just any slim skirt won't do. First you must pick ones that are well cut. By now you should be able to spot a good cut. This is the easy part. The next step is to find the best pound-paring slim skirt. The best ones are those with soft pleats at the waist or a few well-placed gathers. They skim the hips and thighs and never cup the buttocks. They are almost always lined. The lining helps them skim, but not hug the body. The worst choices have fly fronts or side closings with no pleats or gathers. Disastrous slim skirts are usually very inexpensive and, rather than falling straight down from the waist, they almost seem to curve inward and thus cup under the buttocks—very unflattering.

SLIT SKIRTS

Once you're comfortable with the idea that you can and should wear a slim skirt, try a slim one with a sexy slit. A slit at one or both sides elongates the leg, looks wonderful. A front slit, especially one that has an overlap so that a flash of leg shows when you walk, is exceedingly sexy. A back slit with an overlap makes for a very sexy exit. Words for the wise: Sit test any slit. A front slit that is merely an extension of the front seam doesn't sit well. It binds and usually exposes too much leg. Even one that has an overlap will not sit gracefully if the slit is too deep because it will fall open and expose too much leg. Beware of back or side slits that let your slip peek through—not at all sexy.

SOFT, WELL-TAILORED PANTS

Pants are undoubtedly the trickiest thing for anyone carrying even a few extra pounds to wear. They absolutely must be cut well, fit perfectly, and be the right style. Look for pants cut straight from the waist. Tapered styles or very full-hipped styles are not flattering to anyone but the thinnest among us. Look, too, for styles with generous front pleats that lie flat. If the pants aren't a perfect fit, the pleats will pull and look unattractive. Soft gathers also work nicely, providing the fabric is soft and drapable and there aren't too many gathers. Wrap-front pants are also good and provide some fashion interest, too. Never wear fly-front pants unless they also have front pleats. Never, never wear side-closed pants that have no pleats or softness across the front. They are death. If you're even slightly overweight, they emphasize every ounce; if you're thin, they make you look skeletal. Words to the wise: Always check the rear view. Pants that look terrific in front can look disastrous when making an exit. Watch that there is ease through the derrière, but avoid poorly cut pants that give you a "dropped seat" look because there is too much fabric in the seat.

TO THE RESCUE Help for problem body parts:

- Wear a slim skirt on the short side, just above or at the knee. It looks younger, sexier, slimmer on *any* body. Full skirts look more graceful worn longer, about midcalf. Wearing any skirt longer than midcalf makes you look dumpy and matronly. Tip for women with good legs: *Always* wear your skirts on the short side. Why hide a good thing?
- Balance an ample bottom with an oversize top. A fashionably big shirt or loosely cut, but well-styled sweater, or anything with fashionably large shoulder pads, will instantly broaden your shoulder line and minimize your lower body. Have a couple of these tops to pull over anything that tends to make you look hippy.
- Large breasts? Avoid dolman sleeves, cutaway armholes, clingy sweaters. Look for well-tailored set-in sleeves, style interest above the bustline.
- Tummy bulge? An oversize shirt or sweater will look instantly terrific over a slim skirt. Pants with generous pleats in front provide instant camouflage for a tummy.
- Saddle-bag thighs? Look for straight-leg pants in crisp fabrics like gabardine. Pick longer jackets, which are more flattering and more fashionable. Look for—surprise—a slim skirt, but be sure the cut is ample and that it skims, rather than clings to, hips and thighs. Balance this look with an oversize top.

BE A SOLDIER

Why does a well-tailored uniform always make a man look slim and terrific? Because it has a broad, well-cut shoulder line. You're not expected to go the uniform route, but you can take a lesson from one. When you pick a dress or top of any kind, pay special attention to the shoulder line. Any kind of extended shoulder—usually one that has a good set of shoulder pads—will give you a trim look and balance the proportion between hips and shoulders.

WRAP UP TO TAKE OFF POUNDS

One of the softest, prettiest looks in any fashion season is some sort of wrap top or dress, or a surplice neckline that looks as though it wraps. The V-neck and vertical line this style creates does a splendid job of making any woman look thinner. A particularly slimming and great-looking idea is a wrap or surplice top over a slim skirt. Watch this look take off the pounds!

Problem-free Slit

A slim skirt with a slit is a very sexy look, allowing a flash of leg to show when you walk and also giving you enough ease at the hem for a graceful walk. Look for a front overlap like the one sketched here. It will also look good when you sit because it won't expose too much leg. A slit that is merely an extension of a front or back seam *will* expose too much leg. A side slit, if it falls gracefully, need not have an overlap.

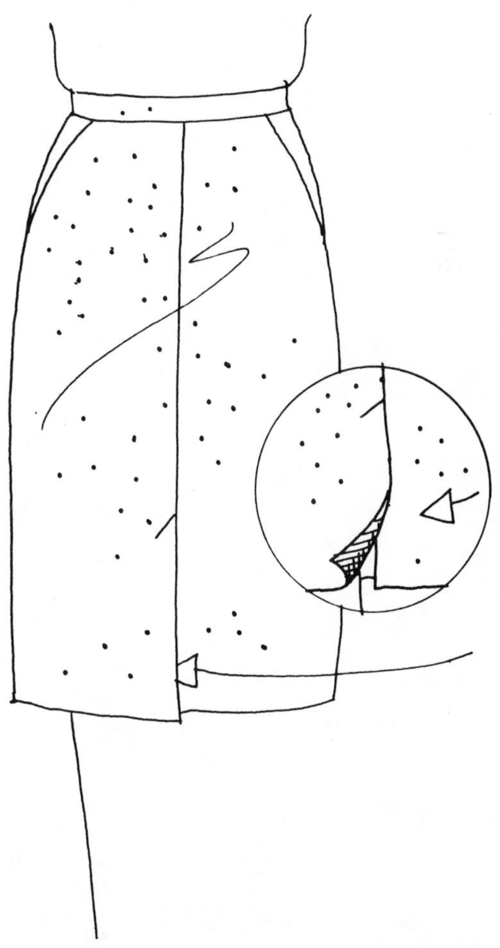

Sexy Pants

Wrap-front pants like the ones here are a flattering look. They are a wonderful evening or dress-up option in fabrics such as soft wool or silk. In cotton, they can be a casual weekend or play option that shows some imagination.

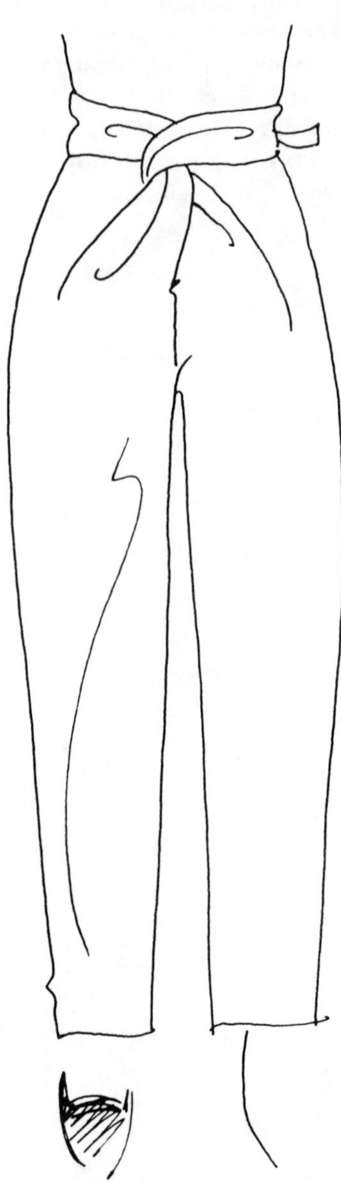

The Perfect Slim Skirt

The skirt here fits beautifully. It's slim and slimming thanks to a good cut and soft pleats in the front. Combine this with a wrap top for the leanest look possible. Don't underestimate the power good long, lean lines like these can have in creating the illusion of having fewer pounds and bulges.

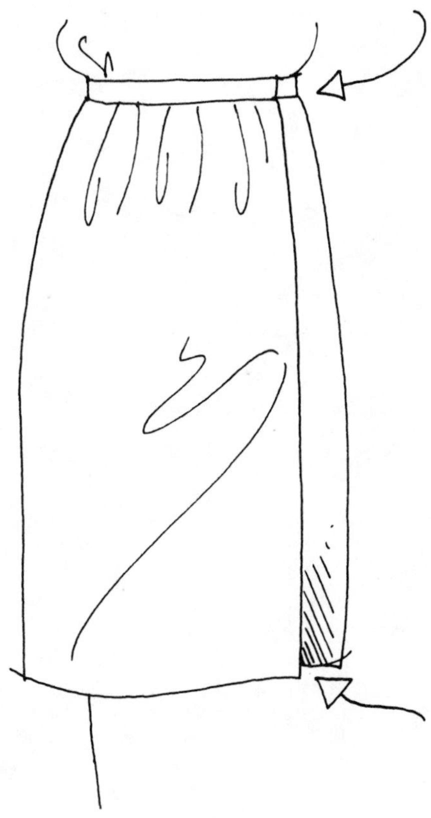

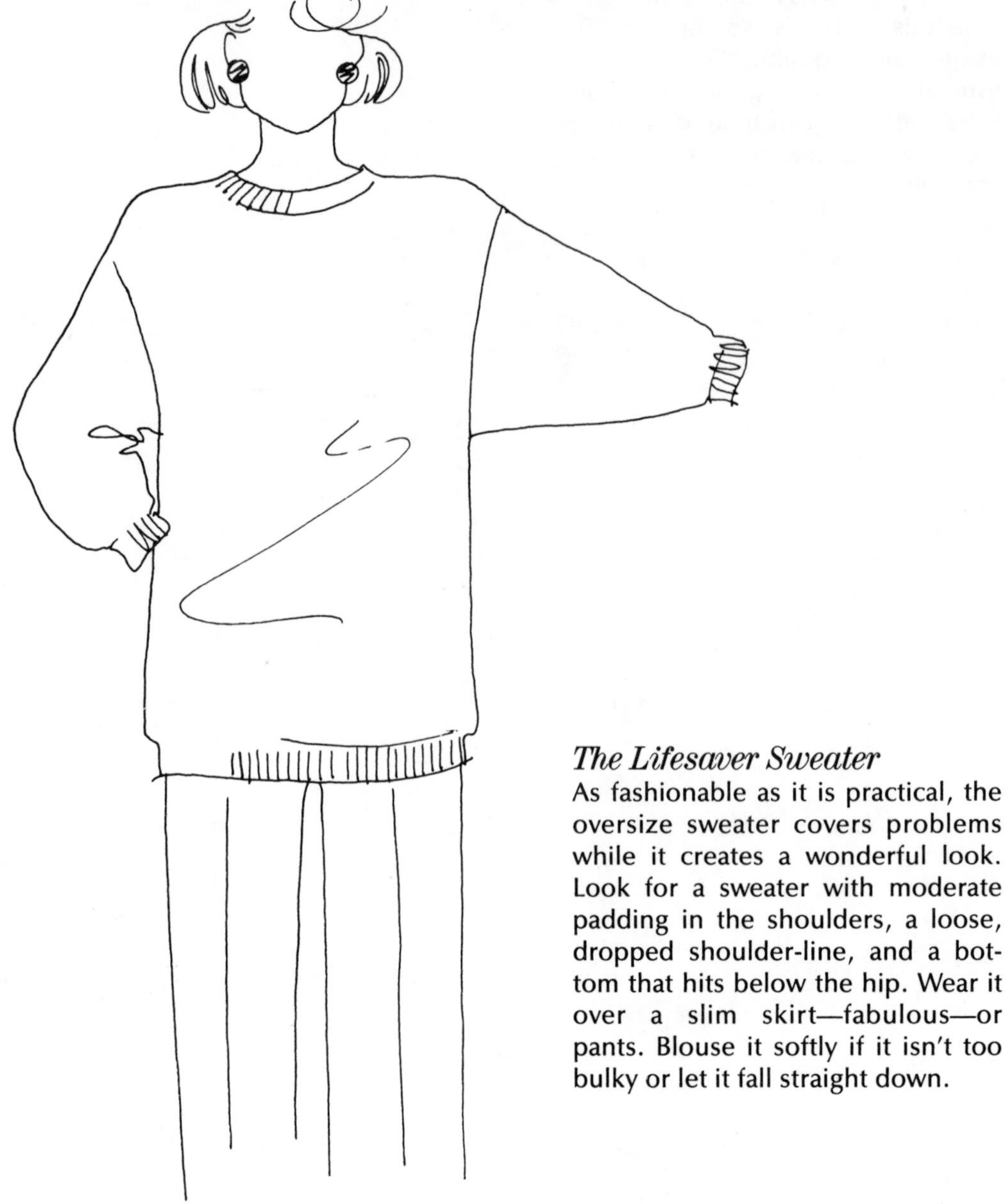

The Lifesaver Sweater
As fashionable as it is practical, the oversize sweater covers problems while it creates a wonderful look. Look for a sweater with moderate padding in the shoulders, a loose, dropped shoulder-line, and a bottom that hits below the hip. Wear it over a slim skirt—fabulous—or pants. Blouse it softly if it isn't too bulky or let it fall straight down.

6 SPECIAL STRATEGIES FOR SPECIAL PROBLEMS

What do most women consider worse than having to appear naked? Give up? Having to appear in a bathing suit. Most of us don't have to go naked in public, but almost everyone makes a public appearance in a bathing suit—on a crowded beach, at a pool, or just in the backyard with friends. Wherever it is, chances are it's definitely not what you'd call a fun event. Appearing in a bathing suit can make the most secure women feel neurotic. Next in line: the trauma of putting on a pair of shorts.

Bathing suits and shorts reveal more body than anything else we wear in public. They shake up and unearth all our insecure feelings about our bodies. The really unfortunate part of all this is that both bathing suits and shorts are worn at times that are supposed to be fun and we often spoil that fun by worrying about what we look like. No more. Here are strategies that can make any woman look her best in bare clothes. If looking *your* best isn't good enough, what you need isn't a new suit or pair of shorts, it's some kind of therapy to turn your head around! And what the therapy would do is teach you that no one can look perfect, so there's no point in trying or lamenting the fact that *you* can't look perfect. Instead, enjoy looking your best and have fun.

SHOPPING TECHNIQUES

Be prepared to spend some time shopping for a new bathing suit. The right one isn't likely to fall out of the sky like magic. Pick shops that have a large selection. This will cut down on the number of times you have to get dressed and undressed. It will also give you the best shot at finding your perfect suit.

THE RIGHT SUIT FOR THE FULL-BOSOMED WOMAN

Nature endowed you well, but too much of a good thing can be too much. You will always do best with one-piece suits. They allow for the coverage and construction that supports a full bust. This doesn't mean you can't wear a sexy suit. Many one-piece suits are extremely sexy, and, after almost disappearing for about a decade, the one-piece suit has been very popular for many seasons now. Look for a suit that has an inner bra, either a structured lining or a semblance of a real bra. If you can't find a suit you like with a built-in bra, look for one made in fabric that gives some support. Pick a more supportive, stretchable fabric rather than cotton. Watch the underarm area, where many suits allow breasts to spill out unattractively. A suit with a U-cut front and underarms that are cut high enough is the most flattering for a women with large breasts. A suit whose design incorporates some seaming under the bustline will also give more support.

In spite of your generous proportions, some suits will flatten your breasts unattractively. Many bikini tops and bandeau or strapless tops will do this. Watch out for them.

GREAT SUITS FOR THE WOMEN WITH SMALL BREASTS

Being small-breasted can be a great asset if you pick your suit carefully. You don't have to worry about exposing too much and support is not all-important. You have many more styles to choose from than your large-breasted sisters. You can wear either a one- or two-piece suit with equal ease. What you're looking for is a suit with some softness through the bosom. A bikini top with cups that slide on a band or are gathered on a band is ideal because the resulting gathers give softness and add fullness to a small bust. A one-piece suit with ruffles or a gathered top that is cut straight across the top is very flattering. Look, too, for a suit that has a design element that adds bust fullness.

The print in a suit can be a bust-enlarging asset. A suit with a big graphic design won't make you look as flat as a solid-colored suit. A deeply V'ed sexy neckline can also be good for you.

Watch out for suits that flatten you. Those made of very stretchy fabrics have too much elastic in them for you. Softer fabrics like cotton or silky, lightweight Lastex are a better choice.

There is another surprisingly good choice for the small-breasted woman. Surprising because these suits are actually made for a "matronly" figure, but if you're clever about picking a style and you shop in a store with a large selection, you can do well. Check out the suits with built in "ice-cream cone" cups. This is a very tricky business. Many of these suits can make you look as though you have a superstructure preceding you and there is often a shortage of small sizes. Some, however, can look terrific. The inner "cone" can add inches to your breasts without looking artificial. The only really helpful advice is to try on as many suits as you can to determine which are flattering to you. Look for those with high-cut legs—they are young looking—and rounded cups rather than pointed ones. Look, too, for suits with lower necklines and youthful prints or colors.

As a last resort, and to give you a choice from some of the really wonderful sexy suits around that just don't do a thing for your bosom, try sewing in a bra yourself. You can take apart an old fiberfill bra, trim the cups to size, and sew them in. You can also buy the "ice-cream cone" structure at some lingerie stores and sew it in yourself. Two cautions: If you're sewing in an old bra, wet-test the suit first to see how quickly the bra dries. You don't want to sit around forever in a suit with a wet top. If you're sewing in the cone-type bra, be prepared to cut this apart, too, and make the cups smaller. They'll be too large and artificial looking if you use them as is.

PERFECT CHOICES FOR TUMMY BULGES

A tummy bulge is almost a universal problem for a woman in a bathing suit. Surprisingly, it is one of the easiest problems to solve. First of all, always look for a suit made of a very stretchy fabric with a lot of elastic. It will help pull in your tummy. You can wear a two-piece suit if you're careful about where the bottom hits. Pick a two-piece with a bottom that hits below your bulge rather than one that cuts into it and makes an additional bulge over the top of the suit. If you have only a small bulge, a bikini with a tiny bottom can be quite sexy as long as the top of the bikini bottom hits *below* your tummy bulge.

Look for suits with design features that help conceal

your tummy. Big V'ed stripes with the apex of the V pointing down are great concealers. A big print is a good concealer, too. A solid-colored suit, especially in profile, will accent your tummy bulge.

SO YOU HAVE "SADDLE-BAG" THIGHS

For some perverse reason, nature seems to have made women prone to putting on weight in the thigh area, especially the upper thigh. The resulting bulge is not something most of us want to display on the beach. You have two choices here—to conceal or to reveal. Surprisingly, revealing is the better choice. The most flattering idea for this problem is a suit with a high French-cut leg that comes well above the bulge. This cut makes any leg look longer, slimmer, and sexier. It also won't bind your thigh bulge, making it look like a saddle bag wearing a belt! If you don't have the courage to reveal, you can of course, always conceal, but be careful here. Many suits that conceal a thigh bulge look as though they were made for eighty-year-olds. You don't want a dowdy suit. Look for one with a flirty leg ruffle, a short skirt, or a short short. The idea is to cover the bulge, but just barely. Don't choose any suit with a skirt or short that's longer than you need to cover the problem area.

THE NO-WAIST SYNDROME

In spite of what nature might have intended, some of us came off the assembly line with no real waist indentation. Create a waist! The easiest way to do this is to find a suit with a belt or a design that gives the illusion of a waist. Stripes will often do this. A suit that has a top in a different color from the bottom will also help create a waist.

COVER-UP STRATEGIES

Look for a cover-up that will work over *all* your suits. That means a neutral color unless your suits are a uniform color. Try on as many kinds of cover-ups as you can. Pay special attention to length. Where the garment hits your leg is terribly important. Some women will look best in a cover-up that is knee length, others can look sexy and great in something that's thigh length. Don't overlook the possibilities of a big oversize T-shirt or just an oversize button-front shirt. Don't, however, give up and wear any old shirt or T-shirt. The one you choose should be designed as a beach cover so that the fabric and proportion are correct. Read fabric and care labels carefully. You'll want to be certain a wet suit won't make your cover-up wrinkle badly or stay damp for hours. Be especially careful of terrycloth. It should have some synthetic in the terry or you'll stay a soggy, wet mass for hours. If you can find a cover-up that is made for your particular suit, you're in luck, but be cautious. Many cover-ups made to match suits look as though they belong either in a night club or hanging from a curtain rod. Often it's hard to find the in-between.

YES, THERE ARE SHORTS THAT WILL FLATTER YOU

Shorts also present a shopping problem. You must be prepared to spend some time shopping, although you can cut down on shopping time by discovering once and for all which length of shorts works best for your body, then stick to that length. To figure out what's best now, go to a department store or any shop that has a large selection of sizes and shapes. Try on everything from the shortest shorts to Bermudas. You may be surprised at what works best. In general, the heavier the leg, the longer the shorts should be. Bermuda or midthigh-length shorts usually look pretty terrible on thin legs. Very short shorts usually work best on thin legs. Watch the width of a leg as well as its length. Very wide shorts make thin legs look like little toothpicks poking out below them. A narrow leg can bind heavy thighs. Generally, a straight leg is most flattering and the same rules that apply to pleats and gathers for pants apply to shorts as well.

Color and fabric can also make a pair of shorts more flattering. Generally the more body the short fabric has, the better. A poplin or any kind of heavy cotton is usually more flattering than a lightweight cotton. The exception here is the shorts for thin legs. Too stiff a fabric is not flattering. You want something with some softness to drape the leg. Darker colors tend to be more slimming, but don't be afraid to try bright ones. Let your discerning eye guide you. In general, prints aren't flattering. Stay away from them unless you're very sure of yourself.

TO THE RESCUE

- Pick a bathing suit made of a sturdy fabric with a high elastic content. It will make almost any body look firmer, trimmer.
- When in doubt, buy a one-piece suit. It's less chancy than a two-piece.
- Look for a high-cut leg to slim and flatter any leg shape, especially short or heavy ones.
- Don't forget finishing touches with shorts or a bathing suit. Pretty but casual makeup, hair that is shiny clean, shorts or cover-up looking fresh and pressed. You need all the help you can get when you're baring this much.

If Your Breasts Are Large

The suit here offers many of the features that help a large bustline look terrific in a swimsuit. The U-shaped neckline is flattering in that it's low cut, but not so low that everything shows. The underarm area is cut high enough to support the breasts and keep them from pouring over the top of the suit. Underbreast seaming helps provide additional support.

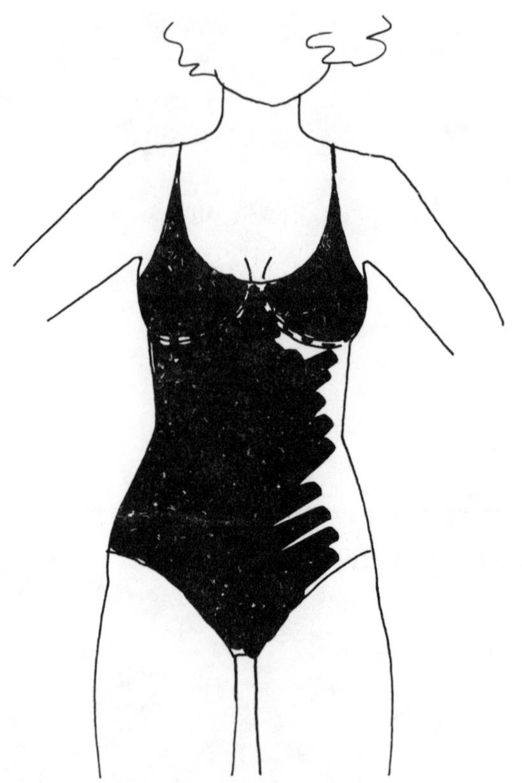

If Your Breasts Are Small

If you like a two-piece suit, consider one like this. The cups of the bra have softness at the base, giving the illusion of fullness. Look for cups with gathers or those that slide on a band allowing you to create the degree of fullness you want.

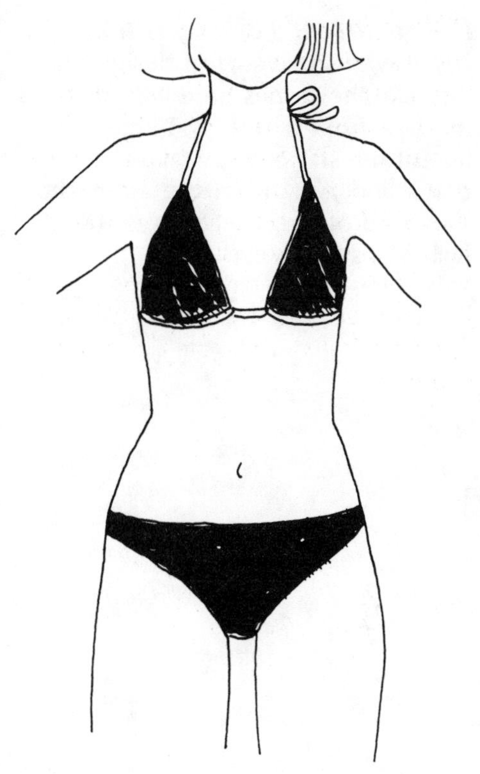

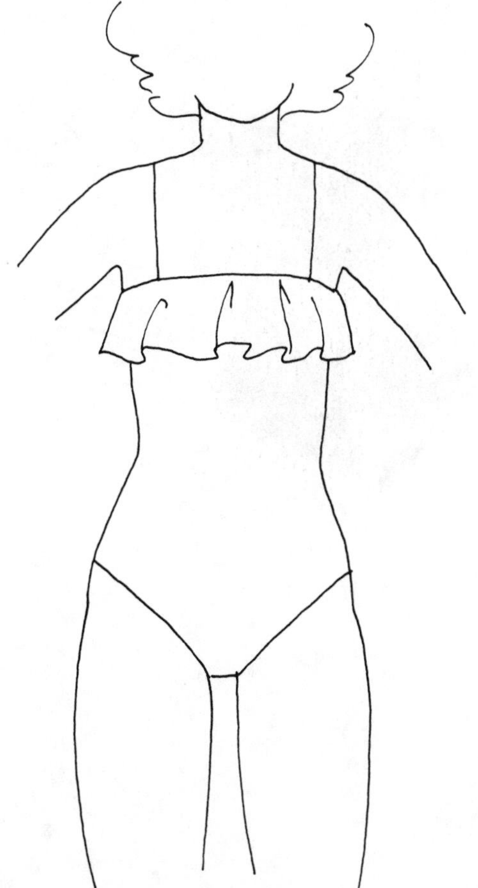

A one-piece suit like this with a softly ruffled top is flattering for a small bosom. It avoids looking cute, but it's feminine. The high-cut leg is flattering, too.

If You Have a Tummy Bulge

A suit with some sort of design feature like the stripes here help divert the eye from a tummy bulge. The line of the stripe helps take the eye down and away from the stomach. This kind of stripe also gives the illusion of a tiny waist.

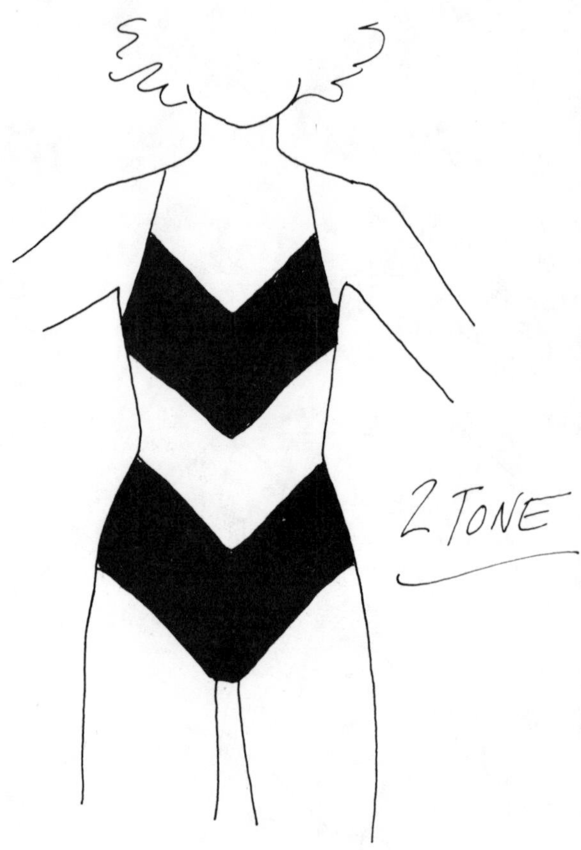

If Your Thighs Bulge

A suit like the one sketched here is wonderful flattery for a thigh bulge. The soft ruffle hides the bulge while giving the whole suit a feminine look. Another trick: Look for any suit with a very high-cut "French" leg like the one in the inset. The edge of the leg comes above the thigh bulge so it won't bind and creates the illusion of length and slenderness. Just what you want.

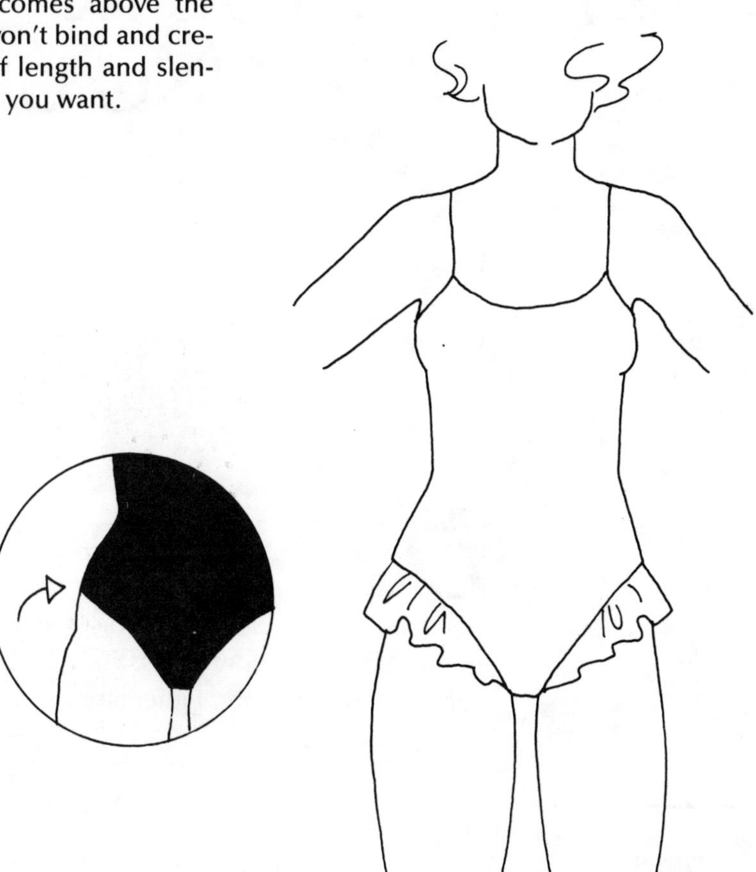

7 SO YOU'RE DRESSING UP!

Dress-up clothes tend to be barer, sexier, more revealing than most other clothes, which means that they are more threatening to most women. You can cover up—and be a stand-out in a sea of bare bodies—or you can learn to bare with care. Either strategy can work.

TRY A DRESS REHEARSAL

One of the reasons bare clothes of any kind are threatening to many women is our lack of acceptance of our bodies. You can become more familiar with and, more important, more accepting of your own bare body by simply looking at it more! This strategy works for any kind of bareness, whether it's created by a bathing suit or a bare evening dress. Start your new connection with your body by forcing yourself to take a good long look at it, preferably in a full-length mirror, whenever you can. When you're undressing for bed, really look at your body before you step into your nightie. Before you step into the shower, have a look at your body. Be aware of its feel as you soap and rinse yourself. Chances are, what you see and feel is better than you believe. You probably have some very nice assets that you usually let your eye—and your attitude—slide over. If there are things you simply can't learn to love, you can at least learn to get used to them. Forcing yourself to see your body as it is, rather than avoiding looking at it, should help keep you from magnifying faults in your mind.

After you've learned to be more accepting of your body, baring more of it won't seem so difficult. To pave the way, do a dress rehearsal of the next bare thing you have to wear. Do your makeup, wear the right accessories, and wear the dress for a couple of hours around your house. Get used to the feel of yourself in it when you sit, stand, move. Look at yourself in as many of these positions as you can. Much of the trauma of wearing bare clothes comes from fearing what you look like in varying positions and situations. Hold a drink, sit at the dinner table, become as familiar as you can with the way you'll wear a particular dress and you won't feel so self-conscious in it. You might try the same technique with a bathing suit or bare play clothes, too. Remember, however, the atmosphere these are worn in is more casual, less formal, and therefore sometimes not as threatening as more formal dress-up occasions. That's why I recommend the rehearsal, especially for dress-up clothes. In addition to all the body baring, you are usually in a more formal and more off-putting situation, and so becoming comfortable with your body is even more important.

STRATEGIES TO TRY

Earlier, I said you had the choice of covering up or baring. Actually, these are not the only options here. There are options between these two extremes, but let's start with covering up. This can often be a very clever strategy for several reasons. First of all, at most dressy events, the general inclination is to pick something bare because it follows traditional wisdom: To dress up means to bare. However, if you've ever noticed the impact of a good-looking woman with pale skin in the midst of a group of sun-tanned sun worshippers, you can get an idea of the impact covering up can have. While everyone else is baring it all, you can stand out in something smashing and completely covering. If the covered-up look also hides some things you don't feel comfortable with and don't want to bare, so much the better. Good-looking cover-up dresses often have a plain jewel neck or a soft cowl neck that shows a bit of skin at your throat, and long, slim sleeves. The look of long skinny sleeves is sexy and thinning. If your figure is good, go for a slim skirt with a sexy flounce or a deep slit. If you are hippy, go for something that is loose and skims the body. *Don't* fall into the trap of wearing something cute. Anything with a full, gathered skirt is probably going to fall into that category, although bias-cut full skirts usually look quite sophisticated. Something with too many ruffles or flounces will also end up looking too cute. Aim for as slim and sleek a line as you can find. One extremely pretty option is a cowl-necked, long-sleeved dress that just skims the body. It hints at the curves underneath, but doesn't cling to bulges. This can be found in a short or long version. It just takes a little shopping patience.

Black is probably the best, most useful color, but if you find something else you like and feel is flattering, by all means, buy it. Look for a cover-up dress in silk crepe, satin, velvet or perhaps a subtle, glittery fabric if you're doing something really festive. Be aware, however, that a fabric like this isn't as versatile as something less memorable. The same rationale holds for color. Although you should certainly consider any color that looks good on you, remember that the more striking the color, the more memorable. You can't, for example, wear the same red dress to several parties in one holiday season without being remembered for it. You could, however, get away with wearing a black dress numerous times.

Somewhere on the scale between covering up and baring all is a hedge that I think is particularly pretty and a smart choice if you want to give the illusion of baring yourself. Try a relatively simple, bare dress, say a slip dress that skims the body or a camisole-topped dress—or even a skirt and top that creates this effect—and slip a beautiful silk shirt over it. You can experiment with colors here. A very good idea is to make the dress black and the shirt a beautiful brilliant color. This way you can wear the same black dress and several different shirts over it for many parties, creating a really different look each time. The shirt should be a classic notched-collar shirt, and the more oversize, the better. The fabric should definitely be dressy—silk or silk looking is the best choice. Wear the shirt open down the front. This combination feels great as well as looks great. There is something sexy—both in looks and feel—about an open shirt and a bare dress. The shirt will cover a multitude of sins from flabby arms to a wide derrière. The only caution here is to be certain the shirt is generously cut and reaches below your hips. You want a look of luxury. A skimpy shirt won't give you that.

You can even try this strategy on a covered-up look. If the event you're going to isn't terribly dressy, you might wear a plain V-necked cashmere or other soft knit sweater with a slim skirt or even dressy pants. The pants or skirt and sweater should be the same color—black or white is a good choice. Then pop a beautiful shirt over it, leaving the shirt open down the front. Fabulous!

There are many great-looking dresses that fall somewhere in between bare and covered that you might try, depending on your figure. Most women can wear a dress that has a slightly bared neckline, say a deep V- or a U-neck. This can be a good combination with long sleeves if you feel your arms aren't your greatest asset. Sometimes a dress that's cut high in front but low in back can do the trick. So long as it doesn't bind anywhere in the back, this can be a great look.

Now, let's get to the really bare options. The barest, and a look that's having a revival now, is anything strapless. You can find strapless tops to pair with pants or a skirt. These are wonderful and sexy, but you must have a fairly small bosom and great arms to get away with this look. You can try this idea with a dressy jacket over it. The jacket helps cover some of the bareness while still giving the illusion of lots of bare skin. A dressy suit with a strapless top is a wonderful look that will take you to many kinds of occasions. The best bare options are a tank-topped dress, either long or short, or a slip-topped dress with narrow shoestring straps. Both of these can be found in loose, body-skimming cuts that are very pretty as long as your arms are not flabby or too plump. (Flabby upper arms are one of the easiest problems to fix: A *little* exercise can do wonders here.) Stay away from complicated styles with complicated necklines—keyhole varieties, V's that bare much too much, and anything that's very bare both front and back. A halter neckline is very pretty, just make sure it's comfortable. Some can make you feel as though your neck is caught in a vice.

FIVE THINGS TO REMEMBER ABOUT DRESS-UP LOOKS

- Don't pick a sequined, glittery, or sparkly dress unless you're going to wear it only once or twice. This kind of thing is so memorable, it will surely seem as though you have only one thing to wear.
- Don't opt for the barest dress unless you're gorgeous and have a really good figure. These looks are hard to

pull off and tend to make the wearer very self-conscious.

- Don't look for the cheapest thing you can find just because you aren't going to wear it often. Cheap looks cheap! Better to invest in something classic and handsome and wear it for years. You can always change its character with different jewelry.
- Don't combine a glittery fabric with glittery jewelry. Save the glitter for a simple dress. It makes the right impression here.
- Always look at the rear view. Bareness in back can make you look less than terrific if lingerie shows or bulges peek out. Check anything you buy in a three-way mirror while you're standing in a relaxed position.

FIVE POUND ADDERS

- Any dress, pants, or skirt that clings too closely will add pounds. Watch out for this because dressy clothes are often cut closer to the body than other styles.
- Any style that cuts into your body will add pounds. Whenever you bare a part of your body, be careful that the baring line of the garment doesn't cut into you. A dress that cuts under the arms makes you look heavy, one that binds in the waist does the same.
- A bulky sequin or brocade fabric will add pounds.
- A hemline that hits your leg at its heaviest part will add pounds. Watch especially for longer—not full-length—styles. A longish skirt that hits just above your ankles can be graceful, but not if your ankles are thick. One that hits midcalf can make calves look worse. Better to cover most of them.
- Watch that ruffles and flounces don't hit you at an unfortunate part of your body. They'll only accent flaws.

FIVE AGE ADDERS

- A dress that bares anything that you should keep covered will make you look older than you are.

- A dress that has a matronly cut will make you look older. Watch especially for inexpensive dressy clothes. They usually are not cut well.
- A dress in an unflattering color will make you look older. Many women end up with this problem because they liked the style, but not the color, or the color that worked wasn't available in their size. Have patience when you shop and you won't fall into this trap.
- A dress that is not dressy enough for the occasion it's worn for will make you look older. It makes people think you couldn't carry off something that was dressy enough.
- A dress whose hemline hits you at an unflattering spot will age you. Remember that the shorter you are, the more matronly you're likely to look in a midcalf or longer skirt—unless it's worn just above the ankle.

HOW TO COVER UP A DRESSY LOOK

Many women spoil a great look by putting the wrong coat over it. Never wear a street-length coat over a long dress. It looks absolutely terrible. If the event requires a long dress, chances are you're not going to be walking around much. Even if it's quite cold, you can probably get away with a wonderful stole wrapped around your shoulders. A soft mohair one is warm and gorgeous. A short dressy jacket is a handsome option. Sometimes you can get away with a relatively sporty fur jacket. A dressy one always works. If your jacket is trimmed with leather or suede or has a hood, chances are it's too sporty. Try your dress on with the fur jacket you're considering and decide whether you can get away with it. In warmer weather, a big silk shawl or even a huge silk scarf draped over your shoulders will probably get you from the car to wherever you're going.

TO THE RESCUE

- The right hair and makeup can take a dress-up look from so-so to sensational. Spend the extra time on both. Getting a free makeup consultation in a department store would be a good prelude to putting together festive makeup.
- *Never* try anything brand new in hair or makeup. Make sure you've done the makeup before or that you have a "dry run" of a new hair style.
- Consider the light you'll be seen in when making up. Candlelight is flattering, but calls for more makeup than regular light. So does any dim light.
- Fragrance will give you an extra shot of confidence for a special event. Here, you might try something new so long as you've adequately tested it in the store before you buy it. You're not as likely to be aware of your favorite fragrance because your nose has become accustomed to its scent. You'll enjoy and get some confidence from the fragrance of something wonderful and new.

Go Anywhere Cowl

The soft cowl-neck dress here is a wonderful dress-up choice. It can take you out to dinner, to the theater, to a reception, almost anywhere that a long dress isn't required. It works best in soft fabrics which will accent the drape of the neck. Matte jersey, panne velvet, or silky knits would be good choices. Keep accessories simple and your neckline clean. A pair of pretty earrings and possibly a bracelet are all you need. The beauty of this dress is the drape of the cowl neck, so don't gild the lily.

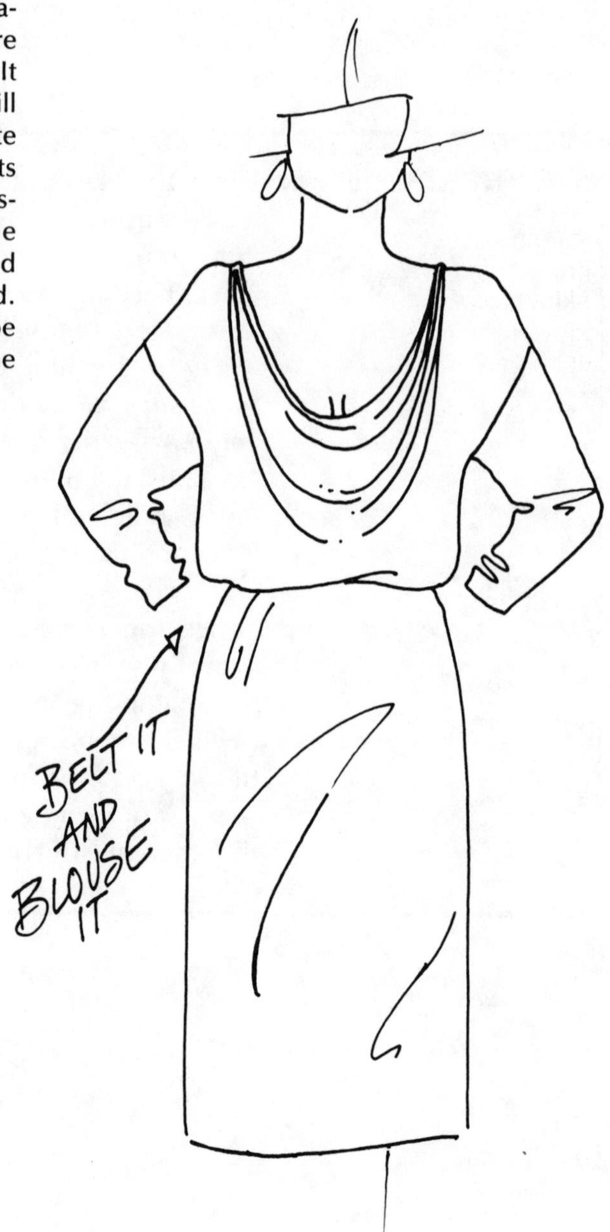

The Fabulous Jewel Neck

A jewel-neck dress like the one sketched here is another go-anywhere choice. In the short version, it will go to the theater, a concert, to dinner at a fine restaurant. The longer version, with a pretty flounce at the hem, will take you to more formal occasions such as a formal dinner party, a formal reception—anywhere that a ball gown isn't required. This dress works best when it skims, rather than clings, to the body under it. It can be a dressy knit, velvet, satin, or almost any dressy fabric.

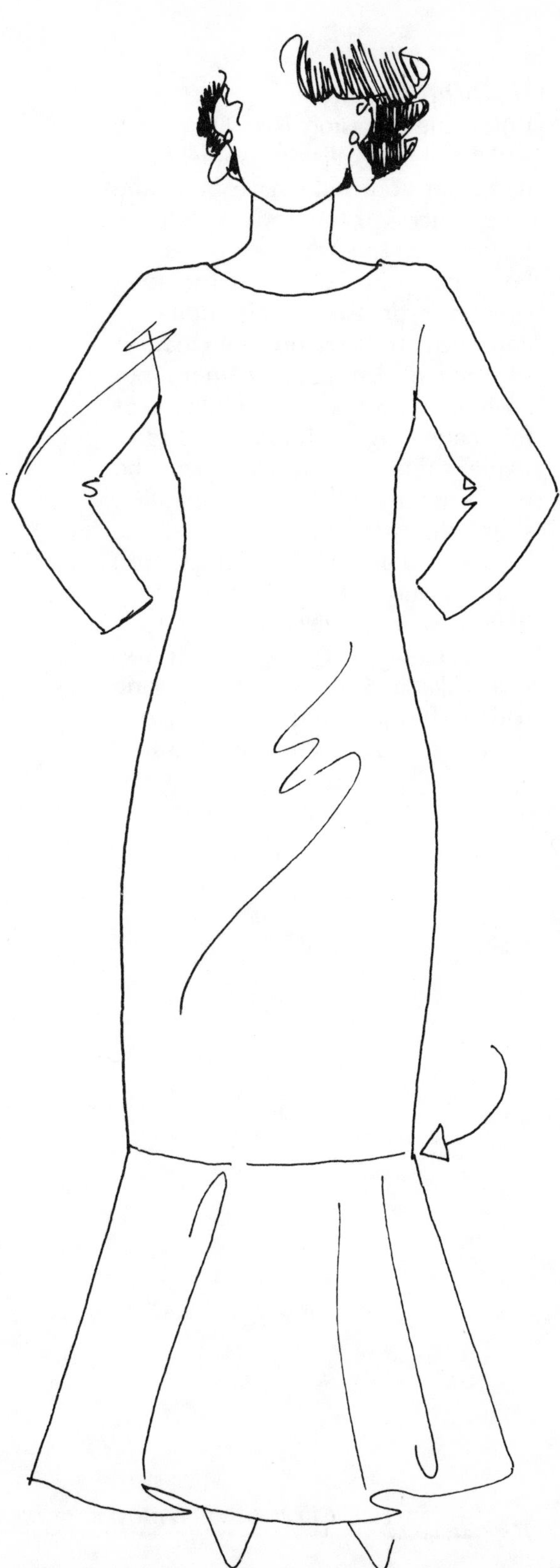

Hedging Bareness

When the occasion is really dressy and probably calls for some bareness, but you don't have quite the confidence—or the body—for it, try this hedge. This camisole dress can be either long or short. The long version is dressiest. The shoulders and neck are bare, but the cleavage is covered. For most women, not having an exposed cleavage gives them a feeling of confidence and of being somewhat covered. For the even less daring, add a beautiful shirt to cover up more. This is a better idea for a short dress. You must be very careful of proportions if you wear a shirt over the long dress. Choose a beautiful jewel-color classic shirt (don't pick one with a shirttail bottom) and wear it open over a black camisole dress.

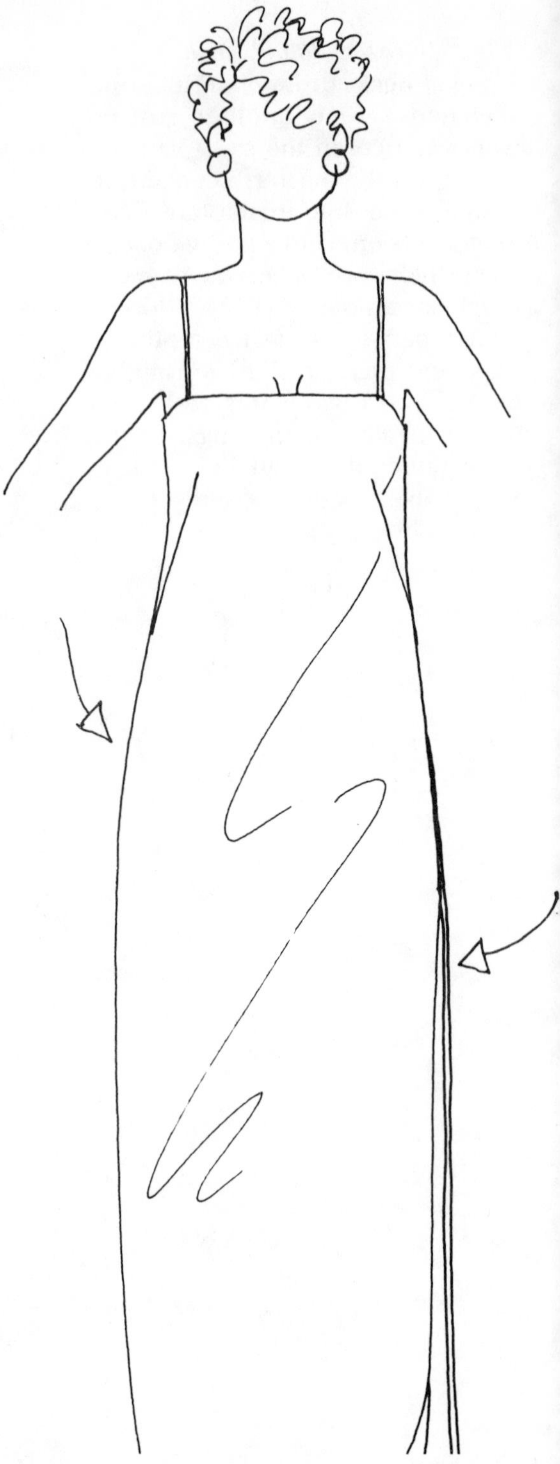

The Strapless Top

Coming back strong is the strapless top, direct from the fifties. It's a beautiful bare look, but should only be worn by a small-breasted woman who has shapely arms. It looks wonderful with a slim skirt or dressy pants, like the one here.

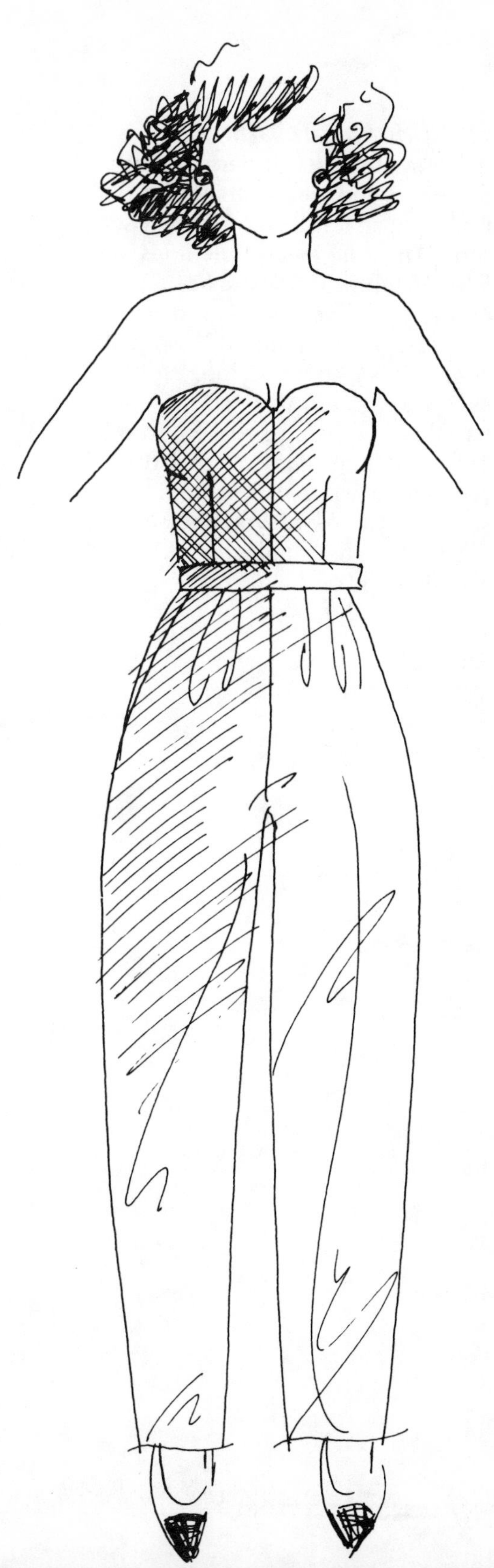

The Suit for Dressing Up

A dressy suit is a wonderful addition to a wardrobe. The simpler, the better, because it will endure many seasons. This one has simple lines and jeweled buttons for extra flash. Wool crepe or velvet are good fabric choices. A sensational idea with your suit is a strapless top. With the suit jacket open, you see flashes of bareness, yet you're really covered. This is a good choice for a dressy reception, a dressy business occasion, or whenever you feel in the mood for this "tailored" kind of dressing up.

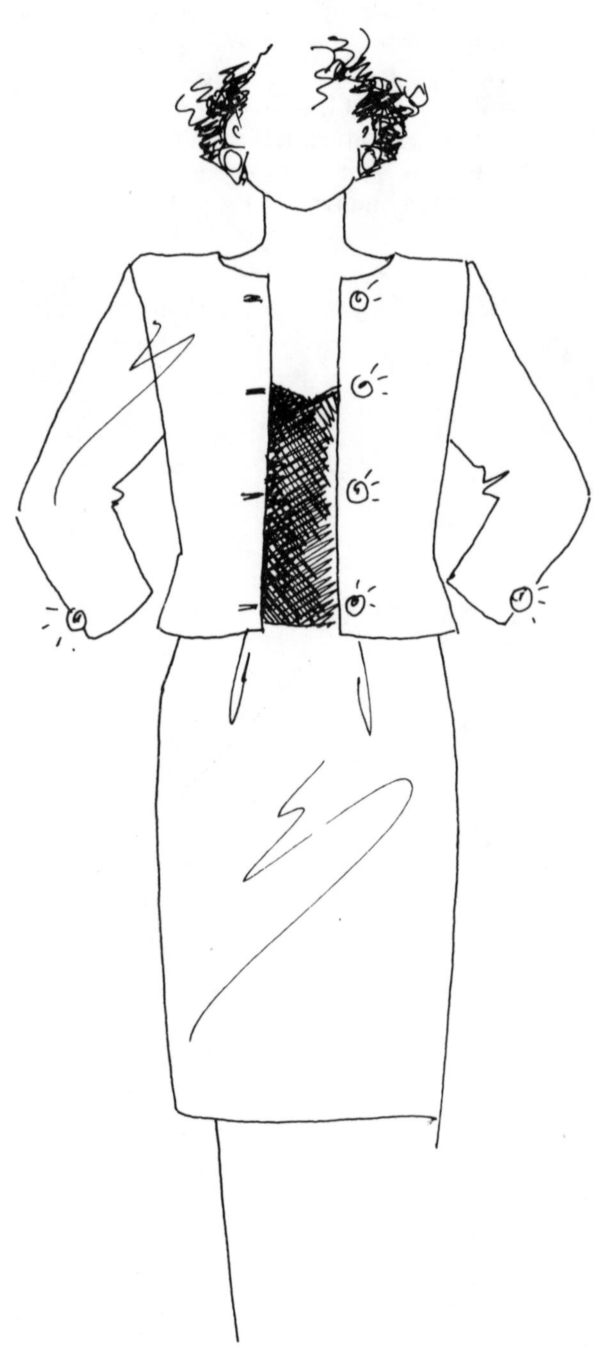

8 HOW TO DRESS 10 YEARS YOUNGER

You've been reading about the right clothes to make you look ten pounds thinner, now you're going to learn how to make your clothes take off years. What you will learn applies to a thirty-year-old woman as well as one who is fifty. When you have developed an eye for "ageless" clothes, you'll be able to spot the large number of women who don't use clothes to their fullest advantage. We all know or have seen countless young women, women only thirty or so, who look like forty-five-year-old matrons. Whether they dress out of an innate fear of femininity or because they work in a profession that calls for a conservative look, they have not yet learned the secret of ageless, feminine dressing. This kind of dressing works for any woman, no matter what her age. It works for a housewife or a career woman, even a career woman who works in an extremely conservative field such as banking or insurance.

Trying to achieve a fresh, contemporary look is really not difficult, but it certainly seems to trip up a great many women. The ones who make the worst mistakes are usually older women who have an exaggerated idea of what looking young is really about. I'd like to relate a favorite story of mine to prove the point. Although the woman in the anecdote is forty-five, I've seen women older, and a lot younger, make the same mistake. I have a male friend who adores his older sister. For years, I remember him telling me how great she looked and how young she appeared. She was ten years older than my friend and he said she looked ten years younger than he did. Finally, I met his sister on one of her trips to New York City. I looked forward to meeting this wonderful, young-looking woman—who was forty-five at the time. I was dumbfounded by the woman I met. She was with her daughter who was twenty and who looked wonderful, dressed in tweedy pants and a big oversize sweater. My friend's sister, on the other hand, looked absurd. She had on a tight black leather skirt which accentuated her ample hips. It was short enough to expose knees that would have looked better covered. The sweater she wore had huge, exaggerated shoulder pads and the bottom of the sweater hit her at her waist. The style didn't help conceal her thickening middle. Her idea of dressing young was clearly to look like a teenager. Her daughter, who was young, was wearing something that the older woman could also have worn successfully. The tweedy pants, provided they fit her properly, would have looked wonderful on a woman of any age, and the oversize sweater was a fashionable look that emphasized a slim figure while it could also conceal the faults of a not-so-slim one. The entire look was young, flattering, and appropriate for a woman of almost any age.

Fortunately, not too many women go as far off the track as this woman did. In an obviously frantic effort to look young, she had turned herself into a caricature of a trendy teenager. There is, however, one very common mistake made by many women. They tell themselves that since they are thirty-five or forty-five, they can't wear certain styles because these styles look too young. It's true that lacy, frilly, "little girl" styles do look too young for almost everyone—including teenagers. But a leather skirt that fits correctly, a stylish sweater with normal shoulder pads, cropped pants, and many other young-looking styles can be worn by women of all ages. They are what I call "ageless" clothes and most women would do well to learn to spot these kinds of clothes and to stick with them forever! You'll never go wrong with these clothes and you can vary them with the things that may be in fashion in any particular season.

DEVELOPING AN EYE FOR AGELESS CLOTHES

Ageless clothes can be worn by women of any age. They are neither cute nor matronly. They are never trendy, but they can be *fashionable.* Shoulder pads and oversize sweaters are fashionable now, for example, and as long as they are not carried to an extreme, a woman of twenty-five or a woman of fifty can take advantage of either style. Avoid anything fussy-looking: ruffles, bows, exaggerated looks of any kind. These are not ageless clothes. Slim skirts with slits or kick pleats are ageless. Pleated skirts, on the other hand, are not. The short ones, those that hit at about the knee, tend to look cute, and the longer ones, unless very well cut and probably very expensive, tend to look dowdy and matronly on many women. Gathered skirts are not ageless. Short ones are cute and longer ones tend to look matronly. Wrap skirts are ageless. The sarong wrap skirts around now are sexy and youthful without looking silly, even on a woman of fifty. The wrap gives a nice softness in front and if a flash of leg shows when you walk, so much the better, so long as the flash isn't an all-out exposure. A-line skirts are marginal. Many look matronly. If you're considering one, look at it carefully from the front and back and try it with both sweaters and blouses. Often a big, smashing belt can help an A-line pass the "ageless" test.

Most blouses that aren't too ruffly or bowed at the neck will pass the ageless test. A classic notched-collar silk shirt is a fabulous investment. If the quality is good, it will last for years and never go out of style. Cowl-necked blouses are soft and pretty and always ageless. High-necked blouses can look uptight and matronly. Buy carefully here. Make sure you're wearing one with something soft, such as beautiful, pleated-front trousers or a wrap skirt. Jewel-neck blouses usually pass the test, but they need help. Worn with a snappy skirt or pants and a handsome belt, they can look wonderful.

Good sweater looks, too, are relatively easy to spot. Classic round-necked styles always work in soft knits. Shetlands or Merino knits can look matronly unless you soften them with a silk shirt underneath or wear them with a very feminine skirt or pair of pants. Except for very casual wear, don't combine a Shetland-style sweater and an oxford cloth shirt. This looks terribly preppy and uptight. A well-cut oversize sweater worn with slim pants or a slim skirt, preferably one that hits just below the knee, is a wonderful, timeless look.

Dresses are trickier than separates. Many dress styles look matronly and nothing will help brighten them up. In this category, I will tick off some styles that may surprise you. Shirtwaist dresses are tough to wear. Most have very little style and are better avoided. Dresses with A-line skirts fall into the same category. Shirtwaist-type dresses with no defined waist, but a belt you tie to create a waist, are nowhere when it comes to style. If there is a rule about dresses, it's probably that two-piece ones are a safer bet than one-piece styles. A tunic dress, one with a long tunic top and a slim skirt, is a good bet. So is a wrap dress. Other exceptions are those dressy styles described in the chapter on dressing up.

Knits are usually a safe bet. Many are two-piece styles that actually look more like separates. Sweater-shaped knit dresses that you can belt usually work if you change the knit belt that usually comes with this kind of dress to a good-looking leather belt.

Suits are getting better all the time. We've moved from the stodgy, matronly "dress for success" suit to soft, feminine-looking versions. Unless you absolutely must wear one for business reasons, avoid the strictly tailored man's suit. Instead, look for suits with some softness: gathers in the skirt, a wrap skirt, a cardigan or Chanel-style jacket, a longer, oversize jacket. A classic blazer and a soft skirt will take the severity away from a suit look. Consider an unmatched suit. Some are bought this way; some you must put together yourself. The idea is to have the jacket and skirt in different fabrics. The jacket may be a nice, soft tweed and the skirt a solid that picks up a color from the jacket tweed. The jacket might also be a fine pin stripe and the skirt solid. Look around for unmatched suits and for parts and pieces you can put together yourself.

DON'T DRESS TO "LOOK YOUR AGE"

Somehow as soon as a woman passes thirty, she seems to feel that many kinds of clothes—and attitudes—are off limits. She feels, in other words, as though she must look her age. It's part of deciding that it's time to be mature and settle down. There's nothing wrong with feeling a need to push yourself to maturity, but somehow this attitude has often been reflected in a look that can only be defined as matronly. The tendency to fall into this trap is dropping away, thanks to the growing number of women in the work force and the women's movement. Still, a great many women feel that if they are to call themselves mature, they must assume a certain severity of style. Often we go through a period when we feel we look great. The clothes we wear, the hair style, the makeup, all seem to combine to create a perfect image. Then styles change, fashion moves on, but we don't. Out of fear or laziness, we cling to a look that once worked, but no longer does. We're stuck in a terrible rut and haven't the courage or confidence to climb out. To get out of such a rut requires time, patience, and courage—the courage to see yourself in new ways. If you're the least bit suspicious that you may have fallen into such a rut, here's how you can get out.

Start by really studying yourself: your clothes, your hair, your makeup. How do they compare to what you see worn by women you consider attractive and contemporary? Look at magazines. Not the fashion fantasy magazines, but those that show believable, real-looking women and clothes and see how you compare to what you see there. If you're honest with yourself and if you discover that you are not contemporary in your look, start forcing yourself to change. Go on a shopping trip and avoid the stores and departments you usually shop in. You'll just fall back into the same old trap if you go to favorite haunts. Instead go to shops you know have a fresh contemporary image. Look at what is being sold. Try on things, look at yourself with a fresh eye. Then—and this is the hard part—force yourself to buy something new, something you would never have bought before. Don't make it the most far-out thing you see. You'll never wear that, but do make it something that has a slightly younger, fresher look. Make yourself wear it. Get used to how you look in it. Get comfortable in it. Then, little by little, make more changes. You can start with small things: some different, more contemporary accessories, a single skirt, a blouse. Slowly, you'll begin to feel comfortable in new looks and you'll be able to create a new image for yourself.

If you're prepared to spend a little money, a personal shopper can be an enormous help here. Go to a shop that offers this service—and more and more do—and tell the shopper that you feel your image is out of date. Say that you'd like to change, to look more contemporary, but you'd like to move into the change step by step. A good personal shopper will suggest individual pieces that will spruce up what you already own, and keep in touch with you as new merchandise arrives. This service is usually free, but in all fairness, if you don't intend to buy a few new clothes, it's not fair to take up the shopper's time. You don't have to spend a fortune, however. You can make it clear that you do intend to buy, but over a period of time.

LEARN WHAT MAKES YOU FEEL GREAT

You can read a dozen rules for dressing young and they can, of course, be helpful, but one of the best ways to find *your* best look is to be aware of what makes you feel good when you wear it. We all have days when we get ourselves together and go out the door feeling absolutely wonderful. You sail through the day feeling good about the way you look—and because of that, generating lots of compliments—and you go home feeling that you've had an absolutely wonderful day, in spite of all the things that may have gone wrong. Why did you feel so good? Chances are you wore something that looked especially good on you. For some subtle reason, it flattered you as nothing else seems to, made you feel feminine, competent, just great. The next time you have this feeling, be aware of what you're wearing. Try to figure out what it is about the clothes that make you feel good. Is it the color, the cut, the fit, the style? If you keep focusing on it, you'll be able to discover exactly the elements that make this look exceptional for you. Now, try to duplicate some of these elements in something else. If you decided it is the color, then buy something else in that color. If it's the style, try to find something else in a similar style. Obviously, you don't want an entire wardrobe of look-alike clothes. Chances are, however, there are enough different things that make you feel good to give you variety in your wardrobe.

PLAYING IT SMART WITH COLOR

Every season, colors come and go. This year, neutrals may be hot; next season, it may be the brights. Most of us are interested enough in fashion that we want to reflect some of these trends, but I advise caution. Earlier in this book, I suggested a basic plan of picking two or three colors you like and sticking with them for most of your basics. This will make dressing easier because you'll have more things that go together and, ideally, the colors you pick will be flattering. I recommend you stick with this philosophy. It really works. If a color is flattering to you, it makes you look young and fresh. If you want to reflect the current "new" color, buy one piece in this color—a blouse, a belt, a pair of shoes. This way you can feel "with it" but you won't fall victim to the ever-changing whims of fashion or end up with a closet full of clothes that don't coordinate.

MAKE ACCESSORIES WORK FOR YOU

Accessories can often turn something fairly run-of-the-mill into something sensational. The secret is to pick just one focus piece—a belt, a wonderful necklace, a scarf. If you really like the accessory and it works well with what you're wearing, it can make a big improvement in your look. No one can give you rules for picking accessories. You need to experiment with what you own and you also need to be aware of what's fashionable. New-looking accessories can help update less-than-new clothes. Look in the stores; look at fashion magazines. Do a little research.

A WORD ABOUT SHOES

Shoes are something you should become really savvy about. They make an enormous difference in the way an outfit looks. Heavy, clunky shoes are never going to make you look feminine. They won't do a thing for anyone's legs, either. As a rule, a medium heel that is slender, not chunky, is most flattering and is also comfortable to wear. Even when you're buying flats, avoid the most clunky, heavy styles unless you're buying something for serious outdoor wear. Look for styles with low-cut throats. They are extremely flattering to legs; they can even help slim thick ankles. Stay away from ankle straps and high-cut throats unless you have sensational legs. Stay away from ultra–high-heeled shoes. They are uncomfortable and make almost any woman assume an unsightly posture.

LINGERIE, YOUR HIDDEN SECRET

Your attitude can make an enormous difference in the way you look. If you feel good about yourself, it shows in your face, in the way you carry yourself, in the way you relate to others. Pretty lingerie is a magic little secret that can make you feel terrific about yourself. Stretched-out, dryer-destroyed elastic, gray nylon bras and panties won't do a thing for your morale. Treat yourself to some really pretty and sexy underwear. Try matching bra and panties. Buy a gorgeous half slip or a sexy teddy. Even though you may be forced to wear fairly conservative clothes because of the work you do, you can feel feminine and good in pretty lingerie. Your mother had the right idea when she told you to wear good underwear. Her reasoning may have been wrong—no one will care what you are wearing in the hospital after an accident—but your morale will be lifted and that's important.

TO THE RESCUE

- Roll the sleeves of a jacket or dress. Just roll them a turn or two. Instant style! Any but the most severely tailored jackets will get a style boost from this treatment, especially jackets or dresses with wide, loose sleeves.
- Add shoulder pads to shirts, dresses, sweaters, and jackets for a style lift. Don't buy the biggest ones—a medium-size style is best. Investigate the ones that simply snap on a bra strap, allowing you to wear them with many outfits.
- Add a belt. Stiff, "matronly" looking clothes can often be softened by the addition of the right belt. Experiment with what you have. Don't be afraid to try things you feel are off-beat. That might be just the touch you need.
- When you're bored, add a scarf. Accumulate a collection of wonderful-looking scarves to tie at the neck of a sweater or plain blouse, over the shoulders of a jacket, at the hip of a slim skirt, or over the shoulders of a coat.

The Sexy Sarong

The sarong wrap skirt here is a more contemporary version of the classic wrap. Some fake the sarong wrapping with hooks and eyes or snaps, others actually have a loose end that you tuck inside the waist to create the sarong look. Either one looks terrific and is ageless. The skirts with some kind of fastening at the waist are easier to wear than those that just tuck in.

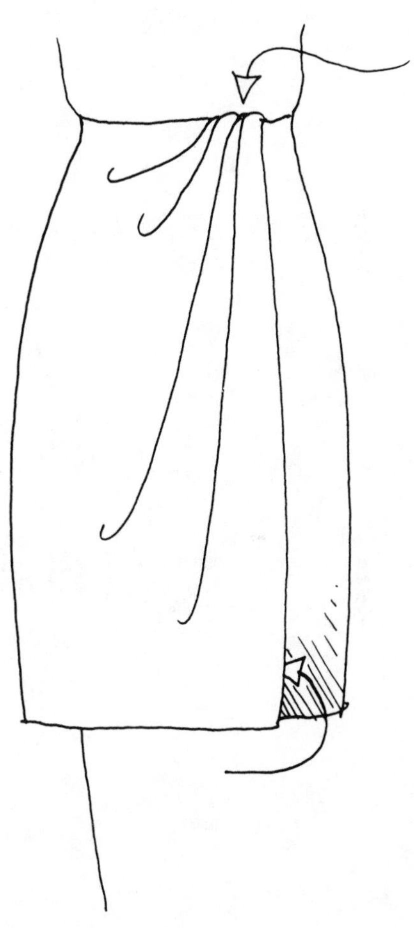

Tailored but Chic

The jewel-neck blouse here is tailored, but soft enough to look feminine. It is a style that will endure for seasons and a woman of twenty looks as attractive in it as a woman of fifty. The tight push-up sleeves give this version some added dash.

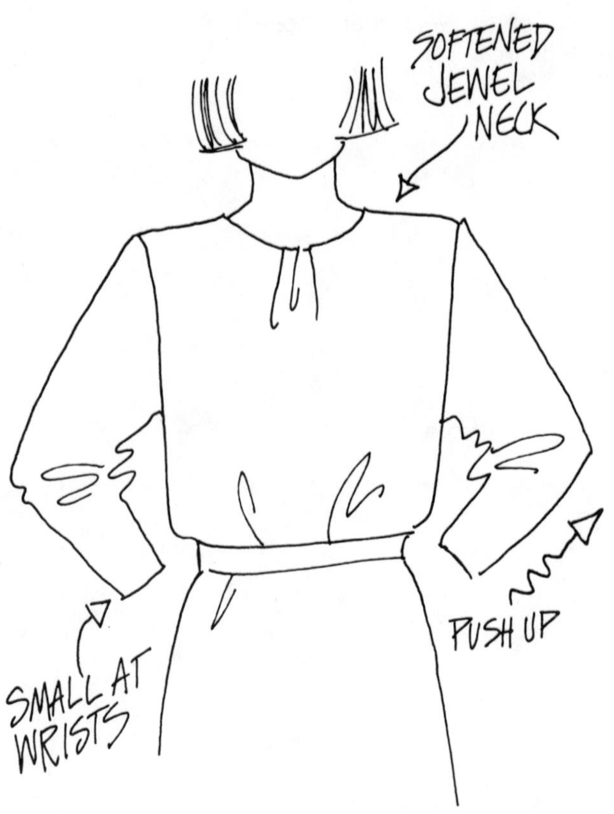

Soft and Feminine

A blouse that is feminine is ageless. This one has a soft cowl neck and loose rolled sleeves. It's not excessively frilly, yet it delivers the kind of soft sexiness that's appropriate at any age.

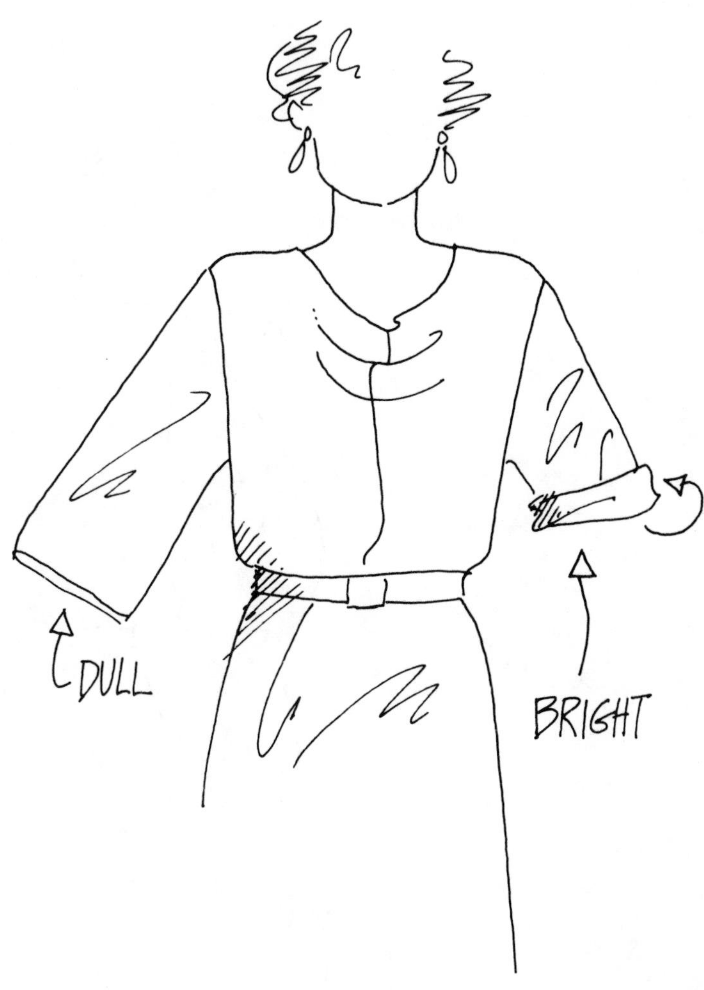

A Classic

You can't have too many classic notched-collar shirts. At least one in white belongs in every wardrobe and from there you can add variations of color and nuances of style. Wear them with pants, skirts, or suits—wonderful!

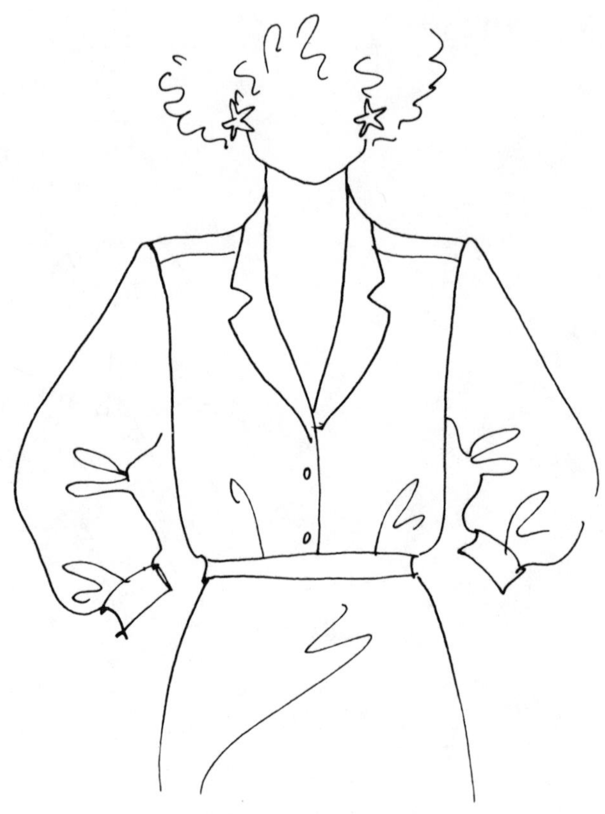

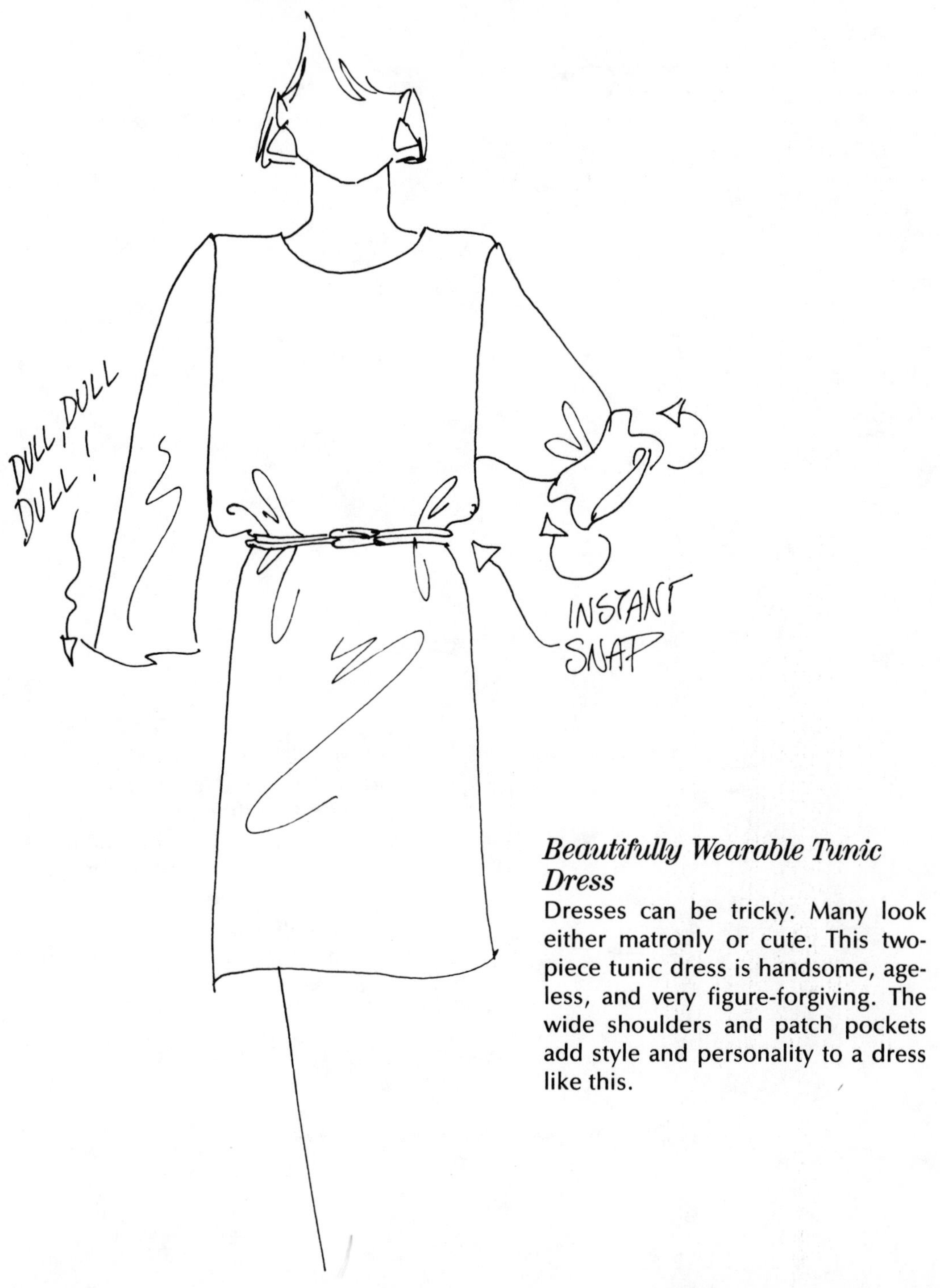

Beautifully Wearable Tunic Dress

Dresses can be tricky. Many look either matronly or cute. This two-piece tunic dress is handsome, ageless, and very figure-forgiving. The wide shoulders and patch pockets add style and personality to a dress like this.

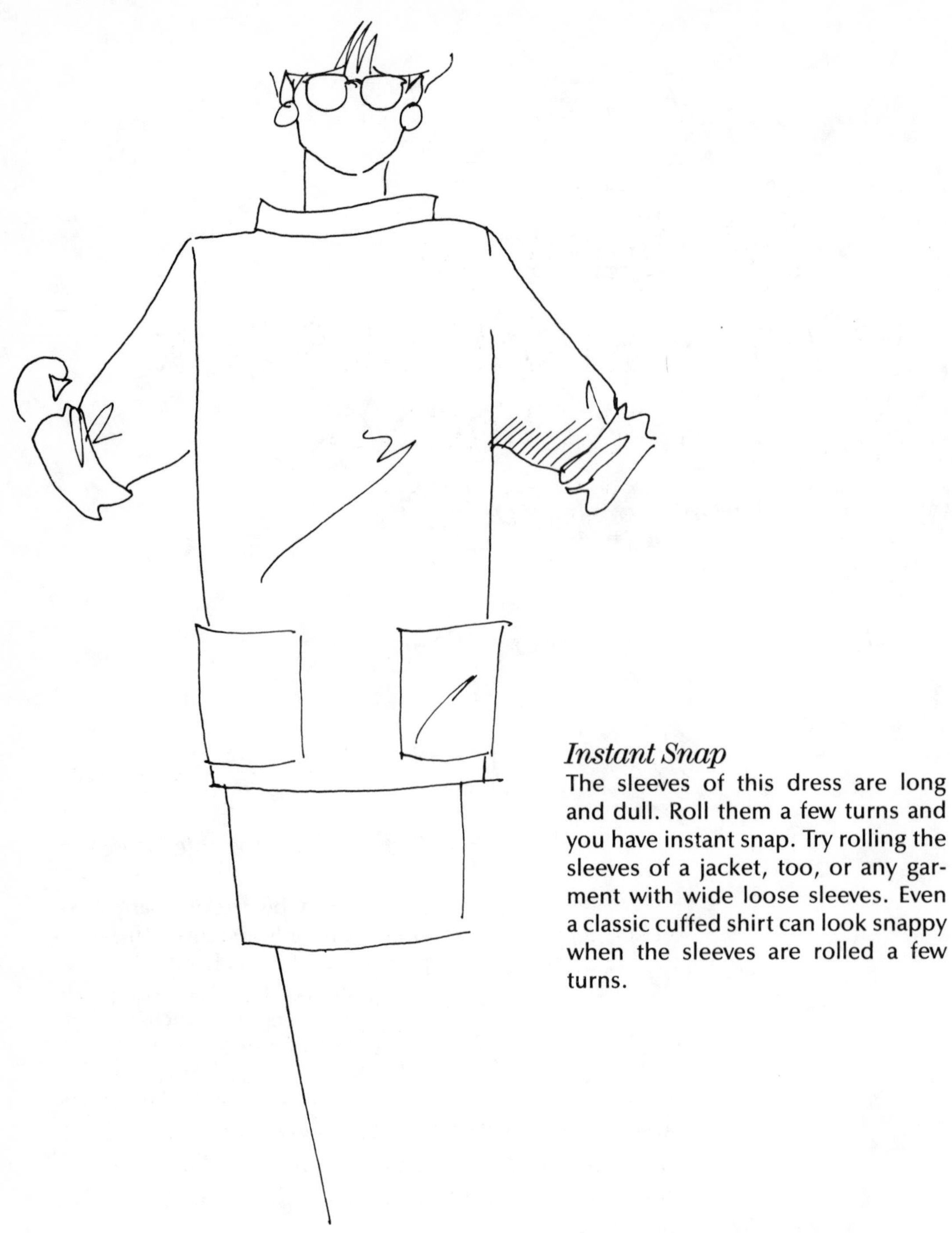

Instant Snap

The sleeves of this dress are long and dull. Roll them a few turns and you have instant snap. Try rolling the sleeves of a jacket, too, or any garment with wide loose sleeves. Even a classic cuffed shirt can look snappy when the sleeves are rolled a few turns.

9 SPECIAL STRATEGIES FOR WORKING WOMEN

All of the dress-thinner-and-younger strategies outlined in this book work beautifully for working women—they work for all women. There are, however, many women who work in very conservative workplaces, such as large corporations, insurance firms, law offices, and brokerage houses. For these women, some kind of dress-for-success suit is almost obligatory.

The dress-for-success suit has become a working woman's cliché. Back in the seventies, when so many women entered the workforce determined to have a man's career, women were made to feel that they had to look like a man to be taken seriously. Fortunately, much of that has changed. A suit is still a wise choice in many instances, but the suit of choice is now a far cry from the strictly tailored one of the seventies.

In the seventies, a suit meant a strictly tailored jacket and matching tailored skirt teamed with conservative shoes and very little jewelry. For most working women, even those in very conservative workplaces, a suit can now have many looks.

THE NEW DRESS-FOR-SUCCESS SUIT

A suit looks newest, freshest, and most flattering when the jacket and skirt clearly look as though they go together, but don't actually match. A tweedy jacket and a skirt in one of the tweed's colors is one way this look works. Another might be a houndstooth-check jacket and a skirt in one of the check's colors. A dress and jacket can also function as a suit. The jacket should be tailored; the dress can be soft and feminine and should look good under the jacket. Although I don't really think shirtwaist dresses do much for most women, they do work well under a tailored jacket, and if they are in a soft, silky fabric, it's a good look for work. A sweater-jacket also looks wonderful over a silky shirt and tailored skirt for work.

WHEN A SUIT IS A MUST, AND WHEN IT'S NOT

A suit can be a wonderful, very pulled-together look, but the idea of wearing a very tailored one to work day after day is not very appealing to most women. We feel somewhat stifled and constrained. Most of us long for something more feminine. Happily, working women from all kinds of conservative work areas are reporting a loosening up of the dress code. This is because a woman's place in an upwardly mobile working world is much more accepted. Women feel more sure of their competence and less need to hide the fact that they are feminine. Many women say they would always wear a tailored suit for a job interview. Most would opt for a suit in any situation where they would be working with business clients and for meetings with superiors. For all other ordinary work days, they feel that a well-cut, rather conservatively styled dress is appropriate. Many women feel that well-cut tailored separates are acceptable in their firms on most days. A dress and jacket is increasingly acceptable, even when clients are involved.

One of the surest ways to figure out the dress code in your company is to be very aware of what women who are already successful are wearing for various kinds of business days. If you follow their lead, you won't go wrong. If you've already moved up the ladder yourself, be a trendsetter. Be a bit more adventuresome and try wearing the most conservative clothes on the most important work days and wearing something a little looser the rest of the time.

LOOKING YOUNGER, SLIMMER IN TAILORED CLOTHES

Very tailored clothes have a hard-edged image that must be overcome in subtle ways if you are to look good in them. More important, they need some softening up if you are to feel womanly in them. But let's start with the basics of what is flattering and what is not.

Any jacket, whether it's a suit jacket or one you wear over a dress or separates, must be flattering. Usually that means hip length. Most women carry their excess weight below the waist and a short jacket only exposes that weight. Always be certain that your jacket is long enough to cover any tummy or hip bulge. A loosely cut blazer-type jacket is usually the best idea here. Although some of the trendiest suits now have shorter jackets, they are not very flattering for the majority of women. Don't buy one unless you're sure it's flattering from all angles. A three-way mirror is a must when trying on such a jacket.

Skirts for tailored suits tend to be straight and very conservative. You've learned that a slim skirt can make you look trim if it's beautifully cut and fits you perfectly. Make sure it doesn't bind or cut over the buttocks. Watch that it doesn't accent a tummy bulge in front. Usually a skirt with pleats, tucks, or some gathering will look softer and be more slimming.

Be very careful about the length of your skirt. Since hemlines in general are creeping up, you can be a bit more adventuresome, but no matter what the current trend, the proportion of the suit and the proportion of your body are what's important. A loose, boxy blazer jacket looks young and slimming over a slim skirt that hits about midknee. If your knees don't bear inspection, don't expose them. Let your skirt hit just below the kneecap. If the jacket looks best over a longer skirt—shorter, closer-to-the-body jackets do—make sure the skirt hits your calf at a flattering spot, usually about midcalf. The idea is to allow the curve that begins here to show. A straight skirt is going to look dowdy worn this long. A full, bias-cut skirt won't.

SOFT IDEAS

One of the easiest ways to soften the hard edges of a tailored look is to pick a wonderful color. For the most part, you can forget the old rules about dark clothes only for on-the-job wear. Most working women, even lawyers and brokers, say they can wear bright colors and they feel much more feminine when they do. A red jacket and black skirt looks sensational. Most any bright jewel-colored jacket will look good with a black skirt. Pick the color that flatters you. A soft, pastel tweed jacket with a pale, solid-colored skirt is another flattering option. If you feel you must wear the traditional dark colors or you already own suits in these colors, don't despair. Wear a bright blouse in the softest style and fabric you can find. A cowl-necked silky blouse can do wonders to soften a strict, navy blue suit, for example. Avoid high necks and round necks, which look very uptight. A classic notched-collar shirt in a soft, silky fabric can also look wonderful. Soften it some more with pretty pearls or gold chains.

If you wear crisply tailored clothes, especially in traditional colors, be certain your hair and makeup are soft. The beauty chapters in this book will be of special help to you because this is an area you can't afford to overlook.

YOUR SEXY SECRET

Working women by the dozens have told me they have a special secret way of making themselves feel more feminine in very tailored clothes. They wear sexy underwear! In spite of splashy ads for man-tailored cotton underwear, the big boom in lingerie in the past five years has been in pretty, feminine underwear: sexy, lace-trimmed teddies, pretty camisoles, bikini panties, lacy slips. When you have something soft and sensuous next to your skin, it makes you feel good. You communicate this feminine feeling in your attitude and demeanor. It will go a long way toward softening your entire look.

DRESSING UP YOUR SUIT

One of the biggest problems working women have with tailored clothes is how to make them look feminine for after-work occasions—those times when you are going out

TO THE RESCUE

- Keep extras of all makeup items in your office for quick touch-ups or unexpected dates.
- A gentle, light fragrance will make you feel feminine in hard-edged clothes.
- Try a big, bright silk scarf tied attractively at the neck of any classic dark-colored suit.
- One—but only one—wonderful piece of jewelry can enliven even the dreariest suit.

to dinner, or to a concert or the theater. You can work wonders very easily. You might consider carrying a change of jewelry and shoes to work when you're going out later, or better yet, keep an extra pair or two in a desk drawer for unexpected dates. A pair of dramatic earrings can help, too. Try wearing your suit jacket without the blouse. Many jackets look wonderfully sexy this way. You can fill in the neckline with strands of pearls or other jewelry. Sometimes a big, showy pin on the lapel will do the trick. Some jackets also belt well. A blazer won't but a long slim jacket often looks fabulous with no blouse and a belt. Experiment at home in front of your mirror to see what works.

10 HOPE IN TUBES, BOTTLES, AND JARS?

If women are preoccupied with being slim, we are no less preoccupied with being beautiful—in this day and age this means looking young. Why are we all so terribly eager to look good? A certain amount of pride in appearance is, of course, part of good self-esteem and mental health, but many would argue that women have taken the desire for beauty far beyond the bounds of healthy self-esteem. The most basic reason for our preoccupation is a society that clearly does not believe beauty is only skin deep. Those who are beautiful are also considered good, and smart, and are treated better. It starts at birth. Cute babies are cuddled more than homely ones; good-looking toddlers are forgiven for misbehaving more easily than ordinary-looking ones. Attractive students are assumed to be smarter and are often given the benefit of the doubt when it comes to a passing grade. Attractive job applicants have it all over homely ones, providing they are not blatantly sexual in their approach to job-finding. The truth is, we simply grow up being pressured to be beautiful. Women are described positively as beautiful, soft, pretty, delicate. Men are described as strong, smart, successful. An overwhelming amount of research shows that throughout childhood and adolescence, girls receive more attention for their looks than boys do. Beauty is so closely and inescapably tied to our self-esteem that we cannot help but search endlessly for ways to improve our lot in this area. Although times are changing and women are being recognized for brains as well as beauty and men are becoming more and more aware of their appearance, women are still in search of a fountain of youth, a jar of good looks. And, for most of us, the old adage "hope springs eternal" is still true. Belief in this adage keeps millions of dollars flowing into the cash registers of cosmetic companies all over the world. The hottest selling cosmetic products today are not the lipstick and blusher of years ago. What sell most today are the "hope" products, high-tech concoctions that are supposed to do many things, but promise above all to make you look younger.

I am certainly not saying that it is wrong to want to look younger and better. Whether we like it or not, those who look best get more of the good things in this world. So long as we do not become preoccupied with our looks and spend endless time lamenting things we cannot change, the desire to look young and attractive is healthy. That brings us back to the jars and bottles of hope. Do they work?

This is a question that can't be answered by a categorical yes or no. Advertising claims are no longer always pie-in-the-sky words. The advertising industry is heavily regulated and if a claim is made, a company had better be able to substantiate it. This sometimes makes for some very interesting and hedgy copy. To understand what the array of claims is all about, it is necessary to know a little about what makes skin look young and fresh. The skin is a living, growing structure. The top layer, the one we see, is composed of cells that have made their way up from deeper layers where new cells are generated. When we are young, new cells are generated rapidly and these have a great capacity to hold moisture, giving skin a fresh, dewy, young look. As we age, the rate at which new cells are produced slows down, and each individual cell lives longer. These older cells are less able to hold moisture than young cells. As a result, skin looks dry and tiny lines form. Since new cells are not constantly pushing through the many layers of our skin, a collection of old, dead cells accumulates on the skin's surface, giving it a dull, dry appearance. This is a vast simplification of the skin's complexities, but it gives you a general idea of what happens as we age. Knowing this, you can understand the importance of a good moisturizer to help replace the moisture that skin loses as cells age. You can also see the importance of getting rid of the dead outer layer of cells that dulls skin's appearance. With this understanding of the problem, look at the advertisements for many skin treatment products. The promises they make are all focused on moisturizing, sloughing off the dull outer layer, and increasing cell turnover.

Since these are the days of high-tech testing, we are bombarded by all sorts of interesting ways to measure a product's effectiveness. Skin softness can now be measured by the "Twistometer"; the "Magiscan" can magnify the surface of a skin sample and count the peaks and valleys to measure smoothness; the "Evaporimeter" can measure how much moisture a skin sample holds. These sophisticated testing instruments do work with a high degree of accuracy, but there is a catch. Just because a sophisticated testing instrument shows that a product causes some peaks and valleys in a skin sample to be smoothed out or another test shows skin holding "measurably" more moisture, are these measurements translatable into improved skin appearance? Not necessarily. Many of the measurements are too fine to be perceived by human touch or sight, though this doesn't mean the measurement isn't accurate. It may only be meaningless in terms of what we consider visible skin improvement.

So what is a consumer to do? It seems almost every month a new product emerges surrounded by convincing test results. We plunk down our $50 or $75 or even more and hurry home to try the miracle substance. Sometimes we convince ourselves that something wonderful is happening. Sometimes it is. All too often, however, the product is relegated to the back of the medicine chest and we tell ourselves that we will never fall prey to another hype.

Actually, science is making gains in finding new products that moisturize more successfully and, therefore, make the skin feel and look better. What you must remember as a wise consumer is that price doesn't guarantee superior results. Some of the inexpensive products have good moisturizing properties and an ordinary washcloth or abrasive face puff will remove the dead outer layer of skin cells. As for speeding up cell turnover, there is evidence that some products do speed up the process somewhat, but whether they speed it up enough to make a visible difference in the appearance of skin is another matter. The best advice I can give you is to experiment with a variety of products, and they needn't be the most expensive ones. Since most of the moisturizing products on the market now work well, it gets down to a matter of taste and esthetics. What you like, what makes you feel good, should be what you use. For women forty and over, I do believe in sloughing the skin, that is, using a product, either chemical or mechanical, to remove dead surface cells and polish the outer layer of the skin. These sloughing products exist in abundance and most are not expensive. Experiment with them to find those you like best.

WHAT TO LOOK FOR

Faced with such a vast selection of products and ingredients, a woman is tempted to run from the cosmetic counter screaming. Don't. The choice can be quite simple. At this moment, any product that visibly improves your skin will do so only temporarily. As soon as you stop using the product, you will stop getting the results. No product can offer you permanency. Almost all products work pretty much as they say they do, but the results are subtle, not dramatic as you may be led to believe. Knowing this, you can get down to the business of choosing a product you like. Many moisturizers and skin creams contain collagen and elastin. Both are found in our skin naturally and their purpose, among other things, is to give skin support and resiliency. As we age, we lose collagen and elastin, and sagging and wrinkles result. Reading between the lines of many cosmetic claims, a woman is lead to believe that the collagen and elastin in a product will counteract the effects of the natural loss of these substances. This is not true, unfortunately. Collagen is an excellent moisturizer and temporarily helps skin to retain larger amounts of moisture. It is a tricky substance to work with chemically, however, and so far, science has not been able to put it into a form that is absorbed deeply enough in the skin to replace collagen lost through aging. Because of its complex chemical nature, collagen tends to turn into an insoluble gel when heated and most companies get around this problem by adding the collagen to the product last, after it has already been heated. Still, it's a good idea to buy a middle-of-the-line product in terms of cost to be certain the collagen has been handled properly and you get all the benefits you should. Elastin in a cosmetic preparation does help smooth out tiny lines, but once again, it is not a miracle worker. Its effects are subtle, but visible.

There are dozens of new ingredients in treatment products today in addition to elastin and collagen. Some are pure hype, claims just waiting to be challenged by the Federal Food and Drug Administration (FDA) and by a determination made by the courts with laboratory substantiation. Other products offer some benefits. All, however, offer only temporary benefits and none works wonders. Expect subtle results. Save your expectations of dramatic changes for cosmetic surgery. This is the only procedure that offers dramatic, "permanent" results, although here, too, permanence is doubtful. As soon as a cosmetic operation is finished, skin begins to age again.

HOW SHOULD YOU CARE FOR YOUR SKIN?

A good, basic skin-care routine is fairly simple. It involves gentle, but thorough cleansing. If your skin is normal to oily, use a mild-complexion soap. If you have dry skin, use a cream or cleansing lotion. Most women over thirty have skin that is dry enough to require some moisturizing. If you have or have had very oily skin, moisturize only in the dry areas, usually around eyes, across chin and at perimeters of the face. If your skin is dry or normal, moisturize all over. You can use a cream or lotion. The choice is really only a matter of esthetics. Experiment to find one that suits your needs and your taste.

Finally, a third step is the one I consider most important because so many women skip it. Any woman over thirty and especially women over forty should use some sort of sloughing product. You can use a lotion—ask at your favorite cosmetic counter for recommendations—or buy a facial puff with a slightly abrasive surface in any drug store. If you use a puff, use it only once a day; if you use a lotion, use it according to directions. This step helps remove the dry outer layer of skin, leaving you with a better surface for makeup. Think of it as the polishing step, because this is truly what it is. It polishes your skin, refining the surface texture.

If you have dry skin, a thorough cleansing, moisturizing, and sloughing at night should be sufficient. In the morning, simply splash your face with water and remoisturize. If your skin is normal or oily, cleanse again in the morning and moisturize. Slough only once a day, unless the product you choose calls for more frequent use. Even so, some skins are irritated by too much sloughing. You have to experiment a bit to see which routine works best for you.

TO THE RESCUE

- When your skin is especially dry, either in winter or in summer after too much sun exposure, apply a heavy moisturizing cream or lotion and sit in a hot tub for ten minutes. The steam will help the moisturizer penetrate.
- If you awaken with puffy eyes in the morning, take an extra five minutes to apply icy cold compresses to your closed eyes. Consciously try to blink more frequently for the first twenty minutes you're up. It will help the body naturally carry away the water that is retained in delicate under-eye skin. It is this water retention that causes puffiness.
- Change your moisturizer seasonally. Use a heavier one in cold weather, a lighter one in warm weather.

11 HOW TO FIGHT YOUTH'S WORST ENEMY

Although you've probably heard it many times, this book wouldn't be doing its job if it didn't tell you one more time: Sun exposure is skin's worst eneny. Sun will age your skin much faster than passing years. In fact, there is a lot of evidence that shows that our skins would look younger, even in old age, if we didn't expose ourselves to the sun.

An instant test on your body: Look at the skin on your breasts and buttocks and notice how much smoother it looks and feels than the skin elsewhere on your body. Notice that the skin on the backs of your hands and upper chest probably looks and feels the roughest and shows age the most. This is because these parts of the body usually get the most sun exposure while breasts and buttocks get the least.

It is not realistic to expect that we will never enjoy the sun and the wonderful sense of well-being that basking in it produces. But you can enjoy the sun more safely than you probably do. Anyone who lies in the sun for the sole purpose of getting a tan is deliberately aging her skin. A tan is visible proof of sun damage. A sunburn is visible—and painful—proof of lunacy. Not only do you age your skin unnecessarily; excessive sun exposure contributes to the development of skin cancer. Since 1930, for example, the incidence of malignant melanoma, a serious and often fatal form of skin cancer, has risen from 1 in every 1,500 people to the current rate of 1 in every 150 people! Doctors are also seeing melanomas in younger and younger women, and the conclusion can only be that our enduring love affair with the sun is one that must end.

In the last chapter, you learned that as you age, your skin loses elastin and collagen, causing it to sag and wrinkle. Sun exposure causes damage to both collagen and elastin in your skin in the deepest layers, thus undermining the skin's support system and causing wrinkles, bags, and crinkles. Actually, this wrinkled look has more to do with sun exposure than it does with aging.

The fairer you are, the more prone you are to sun damage of all kinds. The trickiest aspect of this is eye color. Many women with dark hair and medium skin or even dark hair and skin feel they are safe from sun damage. Not so. If you have pale eyes—blue, hazel, or green—regardless of your skin color, take care. Your skin is very susceptible to sun damage. In truth, everyone's skin is susceptible to sun damage and there is no such thing as safe exposure. We used to believe that if we took sun exposure gradually and slowly worked up a tan, we were protecting our skin. Scientists have since learned that both the ultraviolet B-rays (those that burn) and ultraviolet A-rays (those that combine with B-rays and do damage to the skin's structure) are damaging to the skin. We used to think that only the B-rays caused damage and the use of a sunscreen protected against these rays. A tan, we thought, further protected our skin from damage. Unfortunately, a tan is actually evidence that the sun's burning rays have penetrated skin deeply enough to cause damage.

Since you clearly will spend time out of doors, the only solution is not to venture forth without the protection of a good sunscreen. Pick one of the newest ones that offers protection from both ultraviolet B- and A-rays. Use a high SPF (sun protection factor) number. A number 15 is essentially a sun block and should always be used on your face. If you are dark-skinned and dark-eyed, you can probably use an 8 or 10 on your body. Fair-eyed and fair-skinned women should use a 15 all over. If you want a slight tan, you can reduce the SPF number to a 10 or an 8 later in the sun season. This will allow you to get a tan. You must, however, weigh the pleaures of a tan with the reality of sun damage to your skin. Any burn or tan means that you are damaging your skin to some extent. If you're willing to endure the damage because you must have the tan, so be it. A tan and moderate sun damage is one thing, but skin cancer, especially melanoma, is another. Taking the sun for long periods of time without protecting your skin is foolish. Some scientists have actually hypothesized that one severe sunburn as a child can increase the risk of developing melanoma significantly. You must be the judge of how much risk you're willing to take.

MAKE YOUR SUNSCREEN A CONSTANT PARTNER

Because cosmetic companies realize the importance of sunscreens, many are making products that include a sunscreen. Many moisturizers and foundations now include a sunscreen as do some lipsticks and many lip balms. It is wise to pick such a product. If you consider how much your face is exposed to the sun in normal activity—going to and from work, shopping, walking outdoors—you will see that you are exposed to a considerable amount of sun simply because you're alive. Why not take advantage of the help you can get? If your favorite moisturizer or foundation is not available with a sunscreen, you can always apply one on a daily basis. Pick a lightweight one that won't compete with makeup or moisturizer.

TANNING SALONS: STAY AWAY

Recently, many health clubs have opened tanning salons. Tanning salons with no health club facilities are also appearing in many cities. You tan with the aid of sun lamps and reflectors. These are perhaps more dangerous than ordinary sun exposure. The reflectors intensify the ultraviolet exposure, and in a tanning salon you don't even have the advantage of being outdoors enjoying some activity. Don't make the mistake of thinking these places are offering you anything healthy. On the contrary, they are offering a fast route to sun-damaged skin.

TO THE RESCUE

- Make applying a sunscreen or a beauty product that contains one as much a part of your daily routine as brushing your teeth.
- Confine your sports sun exposure to the hours of 9–11 A.M. and after 4 P.M. Never stay outdoors between 12 and 3 P.M. if you can help it. The sun's rays are most damaging during these hours.
- Don't forget the old-fashioned pleasure of a sun hat. There's nothing like one to shade your face. A big straw brim is wildly flattering. If you're playing sports, choose a visor style that will stay on if it gets windy or when you are very active.

12 MAKEUP THAT TAKES OFF YEARS

When it comes to makeup, the trouble with most adults is that we still think like adolescents. As adolescents, making up meant covering up. We covered pimples, large pores, all sorts of real or imagined blemishes. As we matured, we never lost the idea of makeup as cover-up. The only difference is that now we are trying to cover up little lines and wrinkles instead of pimples. Actually, we should be thinking "less is more." The less makeup you use, the better your skin will look. That doesn't mean you shouldn't wear the works: foundation, blush, eye shadow, and lip color. It does mean you should apply it with a light hand.

WHAT YOU NEED TO DO THE JOB

- Good quality cosmetic sponges
- Good quality sponge-tipped eye shadow applicator with a brush on one end
- Foundation
- Translucent powder
- Good quality blush and powder brushes
- Powder blush
- Powder eye shadow
- Dark brown or black mascara
- Lip-lining pencil
- Lipstick

PREPARING YOUR FACE FOR COLOR

What makes eyes sparkle, cheeks glow, lips look inviting? Color. The colors you wear can make or break a great look. But before you get to the color, you need a background for it. This is where the right foundation comes in. Foundation of some kind or a tinted moisturizer will even out skin tone and make your complexion look better. Pick a lightweight foundation, oil-based if you have dry skin, water-based if you have oily skin. When you're buying foundation, test the color on your face. It's the only place you can really test color. Your hand or your neck is not the same color as your face. Apply foundation with a light hand. One sure way to get a light, even application is to apply it with a slightly dampened cosmetic sponge. After you have applied foundation all over your face, use the sponge to blend it. This gives you the sheerest mist of coverage. When you have blended the foundation well, press a clean facial tissue over your face, especially across forehead and nose to absorb any excess foundation. Now, dust on a translucent powder with a brush. Translucent powder is always best because it doesn't add any additional color and its texture is light. If you dust powder on with a good quality brush, you will get a soft glow, not a matte look. Dust off any excess powder with a clean brush.

GOOD COLORS/ BAD COLORS

No matter how skillful you are at applying makeup, if you apply the wrong colors, the effect isn't going to work. Just as many women grow up believing that they can cover up with makeup, many also grow up with a poor color sense. Somehow eyeshadow colors such as turquoise, bright blue, and bright green, symbolize glamour to many women. The same is true for deep brown or bright pink and red blushes and very dark or very pale lip colors, especially the frosted shades. Nothing could be less glamorous than these overly frosted bright colors that end up looking artificial on almost any woman. Good makeup should make you look as though you were born looking terrific. It looks natural. Most of that naturalness comes from the right colors. For eye shadows, always stick to smokey shades of gray, brown and possibly deep green or deepest blue-gray. If you have green or hazel eyes, smokey browns, rusts, and deep green look wonderful. (Think of rust as a lighter member of the brown family and you won't err by picking too light or bright a shade of rust.) If your eyes are blue, smokey grays or deep smokey blues are good choices. If your eyes are brown, you can wear any of the smokey browns or rusts. It's best not to venture from these colors unless you have an unerring eye for color and for what looks natural. Stay away from frosted colors, especially pastels. Subtly frosted, smokey eye shadow colors can be pretty if the frosting is very subtle.

Strong red, bright pink, or deep brown blushers are to be avoided at all costs. Instead, think tawny, earthy, or sandy tones. Almost any woman looks good in soft, subtle colors. There are tawny pinks, peaches, and rusts to choose from in both lip and cheek colors. The chart here will help you

Hair/Eye Color	Eye Shadow	Blush	Lip Color
Blond/blue eyes	Smokey gray/blue	Tawny peach/pink	Tawny pink/peach
Blond/green eyes	Smokey brown/ rust/green	Tawny peach	Tawny peach/ russet
Blond/brown eyes	Smokey brown/ rust	Tawny peach/ russet	Tawny peach/ russet
Brown/hazel eyes	Smokey brown/ rust/green	Tawny peach/ russet	Tawny peach/ russet
Brown/brown eyes	Smokey brown/ rust	Tawny peach/ russet	Tawny peach/ russet
Dark brown/ brown eyes	Smokey brown	Tawny peach/ russet/clear, soft red	Russet/red
Dark brown/blue eyes	Smokey gray/blue	Soft red/tawny pink	Tawny pink/soft red
Red	Smokey brown/ rust	Tawny peach	Tawny peach/ russet

pick the most becoming shades of tawny colors for your skin and hair.

Lip color is just as crucial as any other color you're applying to your face. I think almost any woman, regardless of her age, looks best in realistic lip colors. Gloss usually looks messy, and unsophisticated pale colors look as artificial as darks. Peach, pink, and reddish browns look best. Think of apricots, shrimp, the color of autumn leaves, all of which are in the tawny family. True brunettes can wear a bright red lip color well, but almost no one else can. Most frosted lip colors simply don't work; they look too artificial. Occasionally, a frosted color can work for evening, if the effect is very subtle, but most frosted lip colors are anything but subtle. If the color looks emphatically frosted on your lips, don't wear it.

PERFECT EYES

Your eyes should be the focus of your face. They are the primary conveyors of expression and emotion and you should not overlook making them as appealing as possible. Unfortunately, your eyes are surrounded by your face's most fragile skin. It is supplied with fewer oil glands than skin elsewhere on your face. What this means is that the skin around the eyes of even a relatively young woman can look less than good all too soon. What happens is largely a matter of heredity, so all the expensive eye creams in the world aren't going to be of much use. Keep the skin here well moisturized with your regular moisturizer and treat skin gently when applying and removing makeup. This is the best advice anyone can give you. If you develop hereditary bags or puffiness around your eyes, or if the skin on your upper eyelid becomes droopy, you can use makeup to help compensate, but the problem will not go away. Cosmetic surgery is the only real solution here, but this is a book about instant results, so let's stick to makeup. If you are a youngish woman and the skin around your eyes is in good shape, you can take advantage of a good makeup job to bring out your eyes. Many techniques have been advanced for round eyes, deep-set eyes, wide-set eyes, and the like. True, you can create a scheme for each of these conditions, but it's really not necessary and most women simply aren't going to apply six different colors to a dozen different areas of the eyes. Who has that kind of time and patience? What I'm about to give you is a basic technique with a few variations that will always work and won't take an undue amount of time.

If your eyes are relatively smooth, this is the application technique to use. It will give you gorgeous eyes in a jiffy. Start with the appropriate color, using a powder shadow. Most creams do not give a long-lasting effect. For the most part, you can toss out the applicators that come with shadow. They are either too small, too large, or don't have enough body in the applicator tip. Using a good quality sponge-tipped applicator, apply shadow to the applicator. If you're using a shadow compact with several shades, don't be afraid to mix them on the applicator for a better effect than any single color would give you. Tap the applicator against the case to remove excess shadow. Now, using the edge of the applicator, run it under your lower lid from the center of your eye to just beyond the outer corner, finishing with an upward stroke. Use a cotton-tipped swab to remove any excess shadow. Then, using the flat part of the applicator, apply shadow evenly across the upper lid, extending it to meet the shadow you've applied to lower lid. You can make this application slightly deeper in color if you like. Apply color up to but not above the crease in your lid, allowing the color to fade in intensity as you reach the crease. Now use the brush end of your applicator to even the color and remove just a bit so you end up with a very subtle effect. Finally, using the other flat side of your sponge applicator, apply a very light misting of shadow up to your brow. If you have a compact that has several tones of the same color, use the lightest to do this. If you don't have this kind of shadow, buy a second compact with a very pale shade of the color you've used on the lids. The idea is for the intensity of color to be concentrated just below and above your eye. Color should fade away to nothing at your brow. Do *not* use a pale irridescent shadow under your brow as so many women tend to do. It gives an artificial, old-fashioned look. Using all one tone in varying intensities on your upper lid will give you a much prettier, subtler effect. Always finish with several coats of good quality dark brown or black mascara and apply to both your top and bottom lashes.

If the skin around your eyes is lined or droopy, there is another application technique that will work very well. The idea is to use less shadow and confine it to the area just above and below your lashes. You can use a powder shadow, but a powdery pencil—*not* a creamy one—will work very well for you. Draw the crayon or edge of the sponge applicator under lower lashes, starting at the center of your eye and extending it to the corner of the eye, finishing with an upward stroke. Limit the color to a narrow band. Now do the same thing on the upper lid, starting at the inner corner of the eye. Do not extend color up to the crease, just form a subtle band of color next to the lashes. Using the brush end of your applicator, smooth out the color and remove any excess. Now draw the brush across the shadow, using the lightest tone you have of the color you've just used and very, very lightly dust color over the rest of your lid. If even this amount of color draws attention to the crepey-ness of your eyelid skin, forget this step and stop when you've applied color to top and bottom lids. Finish with several coats of dark brown or black mascara.

If your brows are pale or sparse, don't fill them in with pencil; instead use a powder brow makeup. If you can't find one made for brows—though there are plenty available—use a pale brown shadow. The effect is much subtler than a pencil.

PERFECT BLUSH

You can put blush on the "apples" of your cheeks, in the cheek hollows, in triangles, circles—in a dozen different places and shapes. The most important thing to remember is that blush should look like the flattering flush cold air gives you or the glow a compliment brings to your cheeks. It shouldn't be used to contour or create cheekbones. This simply doesn't work, except occasionally for photographic purposes. It always looks artificial in real life. The prettiest way to apply blush is to put it where you normally blush. If you don't know where your cheeks blush naturally, try to find out by checking yourself in a mirror at an appropriate time. Basically it should go in a sort of kidney shape that starts just under the outer corner of your eye and ends at the center of your eye and extends down to the tip of your nose. This is the area where a natural blush shows up on most people and it's the placement that looks most natural and flattering. I believe that a powder blush is always easier to work with. You can blend it better, it lasts longer, and it is easier on your skin because it doesn't clog pores as a cream blush can.

PAINT A PERFECT MOUTH

Mouths come in all shapes and sizes and we are pretty much stuck with what we've got no matter whether the current vogue may be for big pouty lips or little cupid's bows. Nature gave you the mouth that works for your face and you may as well accept it. If your lips are very full or very thin, you can help nature along just a bit, but you should never try a big change on a mouth. It just doesn't work. Here is a basic technique that works for everyone. I recommend using a lip-lining pencil because it gives a clean sharp line and it also helps stop lipstick from bleeding, especially if you use a good quality hard pencil that won't smear. *Always* use a tawny lip pencil. Red, pinks, and other colors look artificial. If you use a soft, lip-toned shade it will never look fake. To outline your lips, first find the two highest points of your upper lip and make a small dot at each point. Then do the same for the lowest points on the lower lip. Now put a dot just inside each of the four corners of your mouth. Connect these dots and you have a perfectly drawn mouth to fill in with lip color. If your lips are very thin, you can put these dots just slightly outside your natural lip line to give a fuller illusion, and if your lips are very full, put the dots just slightly inside. Never do any more than this to adjust the size and shape of your mouth. Fill in with a pretty lip color. If you want the most staying power, blot your lips once, powder lightly, and reapply lip color.

What I've just given you is a basic, natural-looking contemporary makeup technique. If you follow it, you will look fresh and contemporary. So many women go wrong by continuing to use makeup colors and routines that no longer look contemporary or flattering. If you follow the advice given here, you'll avoid this pitfall. However, in addition to a fresh up-to-date look, there are certain basics that you need to know about what will make you look younger and what won't.

TO THE RESCUE

- Always carry a little loose translucent powder and a small brush with which to apply it.
- Always carry a small blush brush and a small blush powder compact with you.
- Always wear lip color and mascara, even when you're too busy to do a real makeup job.
- Learn how to use under-eye concealer carefully, that is, with a light hand. Use a shade that *matches* your skin color, not a darker or lighter color. Apply it only in the area directly under eyes to help conceal dark shadows. It won't do a thing for bags.

WHAT AGES/ WHAT DOESN'T

- Matte makeup looks masklike and ages even the youngest, prettiest woman.
- Lip color that is harsh and bright ages.
- Too much eye makeup ages.
- Soft, glowing makeup that reflects light—look for translucent formulas—look dewy and young on all women.
- Tawny pinks, peaches, and russets look soft and young on almost any skin.
- A little blush stroked down the center of the nose and across the chin gives a sunny, youthful look.
- Lip color with a sheen looks more flattering than very matte color. This doesn't mean you should use frosted colors, unless the frosting is very subtle. It also doesn't mean that gooey lip gloss is a solution.

Perfect Blush Placement
The kidney-shaped area shaded in the sketch here shows you the perfect blush application. This is the area where a natural blush shows up in most women, and using it as a guide for replacement of either powder or cream blush will help give you pretty, natural-looking results. Don't be afraid to let blush color fade into your hairline. An abrupt edge looks artificial.

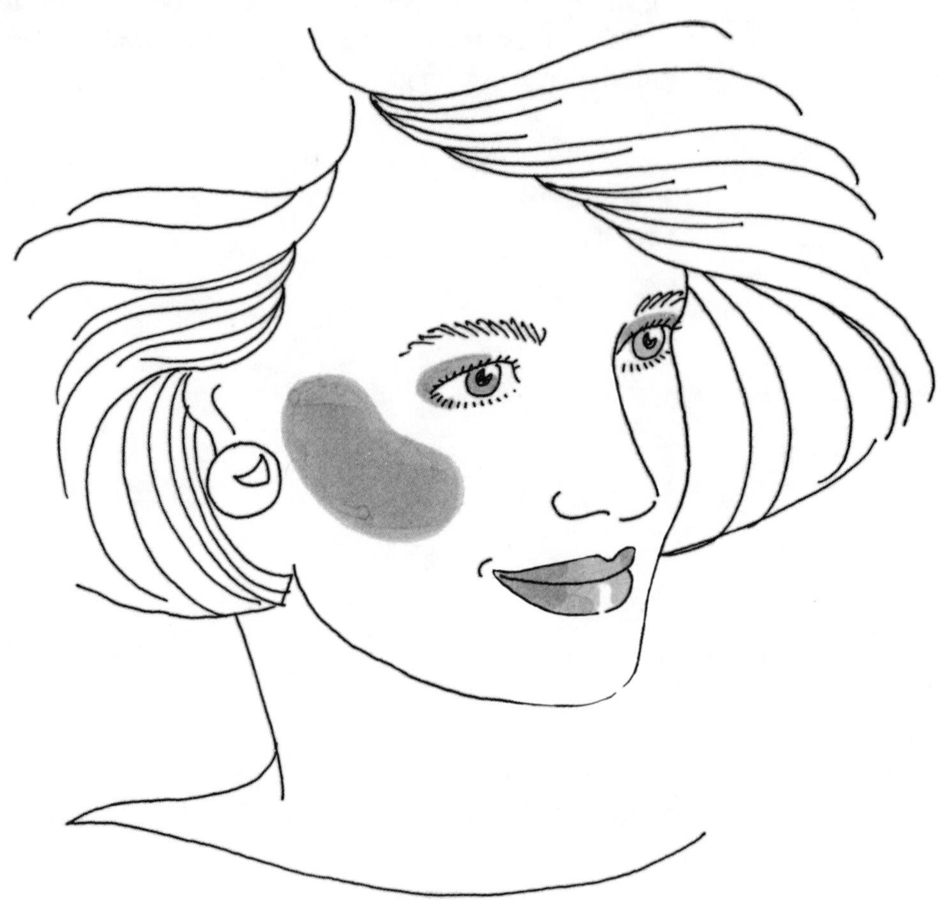

Shadowing Pretty Eyes

If your eyelids are smooth, rather than saggy or crepelike, use the sketch here as a guide for shadow placement. With a top quality sponge-tipped or sable-brush applicator, shadow the lower lid as shown, being sure to keep the shadow color confined mostly to the outer half of the lid. Extend color just slightly beyond the eye corner. Now apply shadow on the top lid as shown in sketch. Blend color to smooth it. A cotton-tipped swab is a good tool for this.

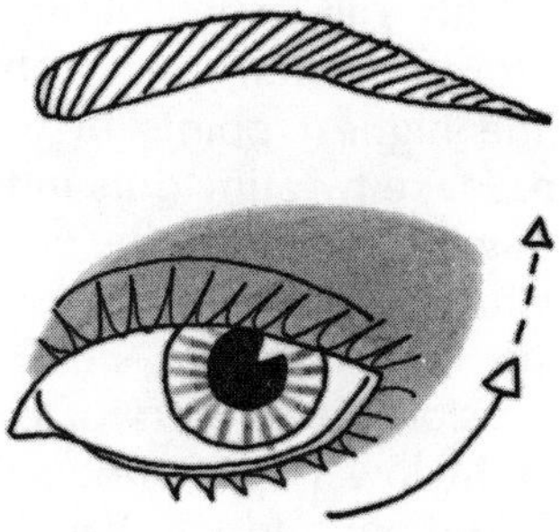

Shadowing Difficult Eyes

If your eyelids are slightly droopy or crepelike, try this method of shadow application. Using a good quality shadow applicator, apply a thin line of shadow under the lower lid, confining color primarily to the outer corner of the eye and extending it slightly beyond the corner. Now shadow the top lid as shown in the sketch. Blend color well.

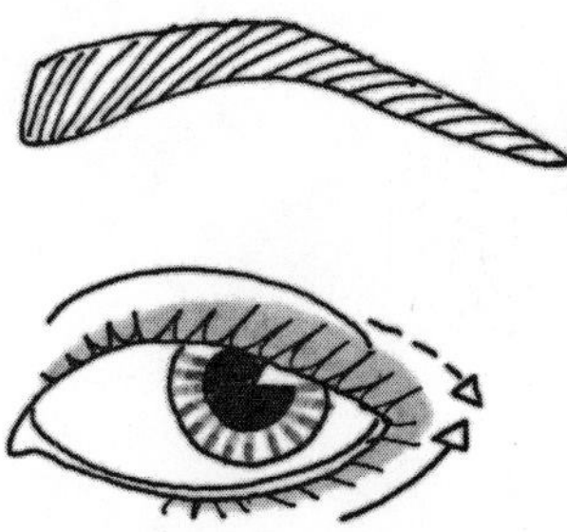

Draw the Perfect Mouth

Lips always look better when they are lined with a lip pencil. Using a tawny-colored pencil, make two dots at the highest points of your upper lip. Make two tiny dots in the corners of your mouth, on the upper lip. Now put two dots on your lower lip, at the lowest points. Put two dots just inside the corners of your mouth on the lower lip. Connect the dots with lip liner and you have the perfect outline to fill in with color. Make your dots small so they won't show in the finished outline.

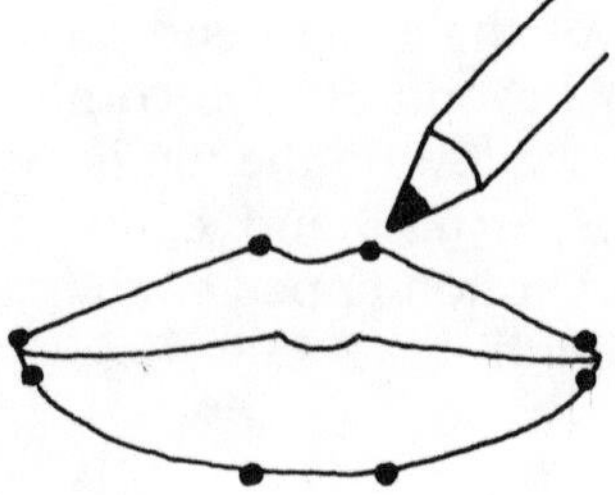

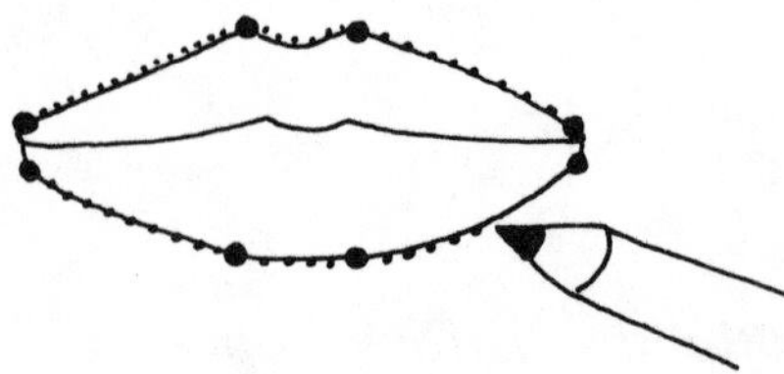

13 10-YEARS-YOUNGER HAIR

This is one of the most important chapters in this book. Unless your hair style looks up to date, anything else you do with yourself suffers. You may scoff and say I'm exaggerating when I say that if your hair is wrong, your entire look is off, but there are some classic examples of this. If you have ever seen "Golden Girls," one of TV's popular comedy shows, you'll know what I mean. Betty White, one of the stars, is trim and incredibly pretty. She has been a beauty all her life. But her hair! It is a teased froth of blond that looks like 1960. It makes this beautiful woman look very out of date. On the same show, Rue McClanahan, approximately the same age, looks much better simply because her hair is contemporary. She has a short up-to-date hair cut, and though she's actually not as trim as Betty White, she looks younger and fresher. Young women can look just as "off" with the wrong hair style.

Remember the two Nixon daughters who were young and pretty in their White House days, yet both looked twenty going on forty, mostly because of their too "done," too uptight hair styles. Even the legendary looks of Jackie Kennedy are beginning to suffer because she hasn't changed her hair style in decades. But you don't have to look to celebrities of any era to find examples of hair spoiling a look. Watch the women you see on the street. What makes some so much more attractive than others? Chances are, those who look appealing look that way in part because they have an up-to-date hair style that flatters their features.

HOW UP TO DATE IS YOUR HAIR STYLE? AN INSTANT TEST

Take just a minute to ask yourself a few questions that will immediately pinpoint how up to the minute your hair style is.

1. Have you changed your hair style in the past five years?
2. Do you see young, attractive women with hair styles similar to yours?
3. Do you keep reverting to one basic look no matter how often you attempt to change your style?
4. Does your hair style represent a certain era—the fifties or the sixties, for example?

If you haven't changed your hair style in five years, it's bound to look somewhat behind the times. This doesn't mean you have to make a major change, but you should make some adjustment, some concession to what's in style at least every five years. Perhaps you can change the length or the part; you can curl your hair more or less. These aren't drastic changes, but they do represent a change in your look.

If you don't see anyone young and attractive with a hair style similar to yours, you'd better ask yourself why. Chances are your style is out of date.

If you keep reverting to one basic style—say a shoulder-length pageboy or a side-parted-ends-turned-up style—it's probably because you are stuck in an era. You found yourself happy with the look of a certain time and you can't get your looks or your mind into the current era. Young women who had very long hair in college often drift into a similar trap. Long straight hair can look wonderful on a college sophomore. It doesn't do much for a twenty-eight-year-old woman.

Let us assume you'd like a change of hair style. How do you go about finding something that's appropriate for you? The first thing to ask yourself is what kind of hair you have. The most important rule for great looking hair is: *Don't fight its texture or tendency to curl or not.* If you have fine, straight hair, it's foolhardy to try to achieve a complicated curly hair style. On the other hand, if you have very curly, coarse hair, it's just as foolish to try to achieve a sleek, straight hair style. In both cases, you're fighting your hair. The look you get will be less than satisfactory *and* you'll also end up spending a great deal of time trying to get your hair to behave. In many ways, the quality and texture of your hair will dictate its style. Here are some clues about what your hair may be telling you.

IF YOUR HAIR IS FINE AND STRAIGHT

Pick a relatively uncomplicated style. Something sleek and straight works well. This kind of hair absolutely must be cut well. The cut is what gives it its look. A blunt cut, one in which the ends are cut straight across rather than tapered, will give your hair the illusion of more body and volume. Though a very layered cut is not the best idea for this kind of hair, you can benefit by a few wispy layers cut around your face to vary the look of straight and sleek. Another caveat for this kind of hair: Don't wear it more than chin to midneck length. Longer than this will give you a stringy look and the ends will not stay together. A soft bodywave is an option for this kind of hair. Be careful though, since your hair will become frizzy if the permanent is not left on exactly the correct amount of time. What you want is body, not curl. Setting lotions, setting gels, and mousses will help give body to fine, straight hair, but don't overdo them. They can make your hair look dirty after only a day. Use just a little and avoid the tendency to pour them on in the hope of giving your hair extra body.

IF YOUR HAIR IS FINE AND CURLY

Fine hair is often curly, but usually not supercurly. What nature frequently hands out are waves rather than curls. These waves gives you the option of picking a slightly curlier hair style than the woman with fine, straight hair, but you should still stick to a simple, uncomplicated style. Use a brush and blow-dryer or a curling iron to make the most of your curl. Trying to increase the amount of curl in your hair with a permanent is usually not a good idea. You are too likely to end up with frizz instead of soft curl. Setting lotions and gels, used sparingly, will increase the curliness of your hair when you blow it dry or set it.

IF YOUR HAIR IS MEDIUM TEXTURED AND STRAIGHT

Lucky woman. This is probably the ideal kind of hair to have because it offers the most options. You can wear it short or long, curly or sleek. Your hair will take a good permanent if you want a curly look. You can have it cut blunt for volume or layered and wispy for softness. Enjoy. Nature was good to you.

IF YOUR HAIR IS MEDIUM TEXTURED AND CURLY

Once again, you are lucky. You have many options. Your hair will look wonderful if you just allow the curl to guide the style. A soft cloud of curls around your face is a wonderful look, and if you have enough style to carry it off, you can go to a shoulder-length style that just curls away as your hair dictates.

IF YOUR HAIR IS COARSE AND STRAIGHT

The main problem with this type of hair is its tendency to become unruly. If it's cut too short, it tends to stick out instead of lying flat. If it's worn too long, it tends to look bushy. The best options are medium-length styles with some softness layered into the hair around the face. A good cut is essential for this kind of hair, too. It will tame the tendency to unruliness. Styling aids such as softening conditioners are a good idea for your kind of hair. They help tame bushiness. Although your hair can take a successful permanent, you must be careful. Two disasters might occur: The permanent won't take at all or it will add to the bushiness. A soft curl is what you want and you should discuss your needs carefully with your hair stylist. Make sure you feel he or she understands the final look you want and that the limitations of your hair are taken into consideration. Five minutes of conversation should tell you whether or not you are in good hands.

IF YOUR HAIR IS CURLY AND COARSE

This is difficult hair. If you let the curl have its way totally, you are going to end up with a bushy look. Actually if you have the face, figure, and style for it, this can be a hallmark of your style, but not too many women can carry it off. This hair type benefits by a chemical straightening. Here, as in the case of permanenting coarse hair, you must be careful to get the very best job. Don't attempt to end up with straight hair. Instead, your goal should be to relax the curl just a bit so that you can make your hair more manageable. Softening conditioners will also help tame the curl. This kind of hair should not be worn too long. A very short cut that allows the hair to curl all around your head can be good, so can anything down to about chin length or just a bit longer. A blow-dryer and brush are your best styling tools.

FINDING THE RIGHT STYLE

Now that you know the limitations of your particular hair type, how do you decide on exactly what style will work for you? Much has been written about hair style and face shape. I feel the same way about this as I do about using makeup to create or change features. Most face shapes can wear some variation of most any hair style. It is the texture of your hair that really determines style limitations. The best way to decide which direction to go is to have a look around you. Go into the really good department stores or boutiques in your town. Notice what kind of hair styles attractive women are wearing. Buy a supply of the latest fashion magazines and look at the styles pictured here. Read what they have to say about hair styles. This will give you a good overview of what's current. Tear out pictures of the styles you really like. Watch especially for those on women who have your kind of look. Now that you have an idea of what you like and want, start eliminating. Eliminate those that are impossible for your hair. Those that are too curly or too straight, too short or too long should be pulled out of your pile. What's left? These are the real options. They are looks you like and looks that will work for your hair. Try to eliminate the options so that you have three or four really good choices. Most important, see if it's possible to find any common element in the styles you like. Are all of them wispy and soft, sleek and sophisticated? If you can find a theme that runs throughout, you know that you are responding to a particular element, and the style that's right for you should incorporate that element. Perhaps it's bangs or a kind of soft, face-framing quality. Whatever it is, this is something you should point out to your hair stylist.

MAKING THE CHANGE

Whether you're looking for a major change or just a variation on what you already have, you should make an appointment for a consultation with your hair stylist before scissors are put to your hair. Don't be afraid to take up the stylist's time. If necessary, you can pay a consultation fee, but most stylists will gladly talk to you for five minutes a few days before you actually have your hair cut. It's best to have your consultation before the day of the cut. This gives you time to think over what was said and to be sure you know exactly how you want to proceed. Be sure that you and the stylist both agree on what's wanted and that you both feel the new style will work for your life style and your hair type. Discuss how much time maintaining your new style will take, and be certain that you're willing to spend whatever amount of time is needed.

If you're planning on a major change, you might want to consider making it in two steps. If you're going much shorter, for example, you might want to start with a cut that's slightly longer than the shortest length to see how you like the look, how it works for your hair and face. It all goes well, you can cut it shorter next time.

SOME DO'S AND DON'TS

Although I don't believe in tailoring a hair style to a face shape, there are a few caveats that you'd do well to consider:

DON'T pick an off-the-face style if you have a long, narrow face.

DON'T wear bangs straight across your forehead if you have a round face.

DON'T wear your hair exactly at chin length if you have a round face.

DO wear bangs to soften a broad forehead or an uneven hairline.

DO wear some kind of bangs if you have large eyes. The bangs will act as a frame for your eyes and make them look even bigger and more appealing.

DO pick a style that shows off high cheekbones if you have them. Hair brushed back at the sides will do it. Wispy pieces sliding onto the cheek will also accent good cheekbones.

WHAT ABOUT COLOR?

Like facial features, hair color is something nature is fairly wise about. The color you have is what blends with your skin tone and your eye color. This doesn't mean you can't help nature along. It simply means you shouldn't double-cross nature by changing your color completely. This usually ends up looking very unnatural and costs a fortune because such a drastic change requires so much upkeep.

In general, it's best not to go more than two shades lighter or darker than your natural color. The older you are, the better you'll look going a bit lighter rather than darker. Darker colors can look harsh. The hair that benefits most from color is what I call "mouse brown." This hair color is usually pretty drab and a little color lift can do wonders for it. You might opt for an all-over color that is just slightly lighter or you could try highlights, perhaps just around your face. Upkeep on the highlights is simpler and less expensive. Whatever you do, don't end up with old-fashioned-looking ultrapale "frosting." This harks back to the sixties and wasn't pretty even then. Unfortunately, many salons, especially those outside major cities, are still giving women these unattractive streaks. Highlighting or color streaking on any shade of brown hair should be gold or amber. Amber is pretty on darker shades of brown hair. Dark brown hair can look smashing with reddish highlights, but these must be done by a good colorist. Too many highlights or too red a color can look artificial. Highlights "painted" on with henna can look very pretty on deep brown hair. Real carrot-top redheads can soften the effects of their hair color by adding a few golden blond highlights around the face.

Any color, even highlighting, will add body and volume to your hair, so if lack of body is a problem for you, hair color can be a plus.

WHAT ABOUT GRAY?

Depending on their hair, many women begin to get gray hair in their twenties. On very dark, thick hair, silver strands look marvelous and I wouldn't change them. However, if in your thirties you begin to get quite gray, you might want to consider coloring your hair to get rid of the gray. Gray hair can be very beautiful esthetically, but, unfortunately, most of us equate gray with "old" and since I have advocated being pragmatic in this book, it does seem to make sense to color gray hair if you feel it's making you look older than you are. If you have enough gray hair to reach the point of deciding whether to color it or not, I feel the decision, if you opt for coloring, should be for a permanent color, not one of the temporary ones made just for covering gray. The trouble with these products is that they fade in about six weeks, and the last ten days before you recolor can find you with hair that looks "off." Depending on your natural color, you may find there is occasionally a slight greenish or bluish cast to your hair just prior to recoloring it. This

TO THE RESCUE

- Wash your hair frequently. This may sound like stating the obvious, but most hair doesn't really look great for more than two or three days after a shampoo. If you really want marvelous-looking hair, wash it at least every three days. It's worth the time and trouble.
- If your hair is straight, and especially if it's fine and tends to lose its curl quickly, carry one of the portable butane-fueled curling irons with you. You can tuck one in a bag or briefcase and touch up instantly on damp days.
- If you color your hair, try one of the colored setting mousses just before you're ready to recolor. It keeps roots from looking unsightly. It can get you gracefully through the week before touch-up.
- Just for fun, for a big event, try spray-on highlights. Blond or red is pretty sprayed on medium to dark brown hair. Just "paint" on a few streaks around your face. The color dries quickly, washes out with the next shampoo. You can even brush it out without shampooing if you want.

cast is most noticeable in bright sunlight and you don't often check your hair color when you're outdoors in this kind of light. If you're uncertain about whether you want to color your hair, these temporary colors are a good test. If you don't like the color, it will eventually wash out. If you start with permanent color and don't like it, you must wait for the color to grow out and this can be very unattractive.

Fine Straight Hair

If your hair is straight and fine, you're best off with a short cut. Too much length and this kind of hair loses its line. Here, two ways to wear a short cut. The hair here is left to fall straight, its beautiful shape coming from a superb cut.

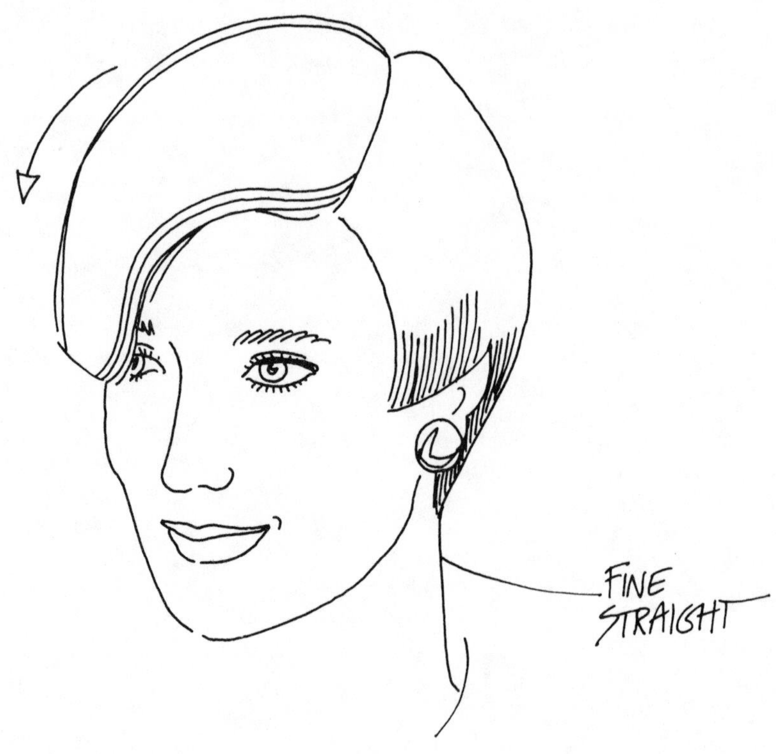

This is basically the same cut as the straight look, but here it's curled softly. Since the hair is short, it should hold the curl easily. The shortness also helps keep maintenance down. Curl with a curling iron when hair is almost dry; this style takes only a few minutes to dry.

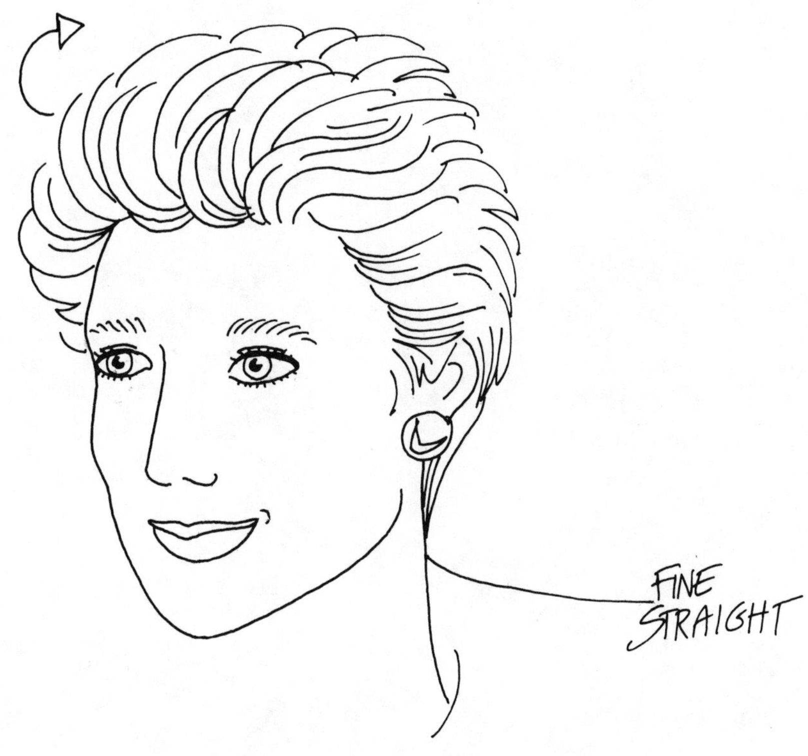

Fine Curly Hair

If your hair is fine and has some curl, you might try a very short cut like the one here. The hair is left to dry naturally so that it curls softly all around the face.

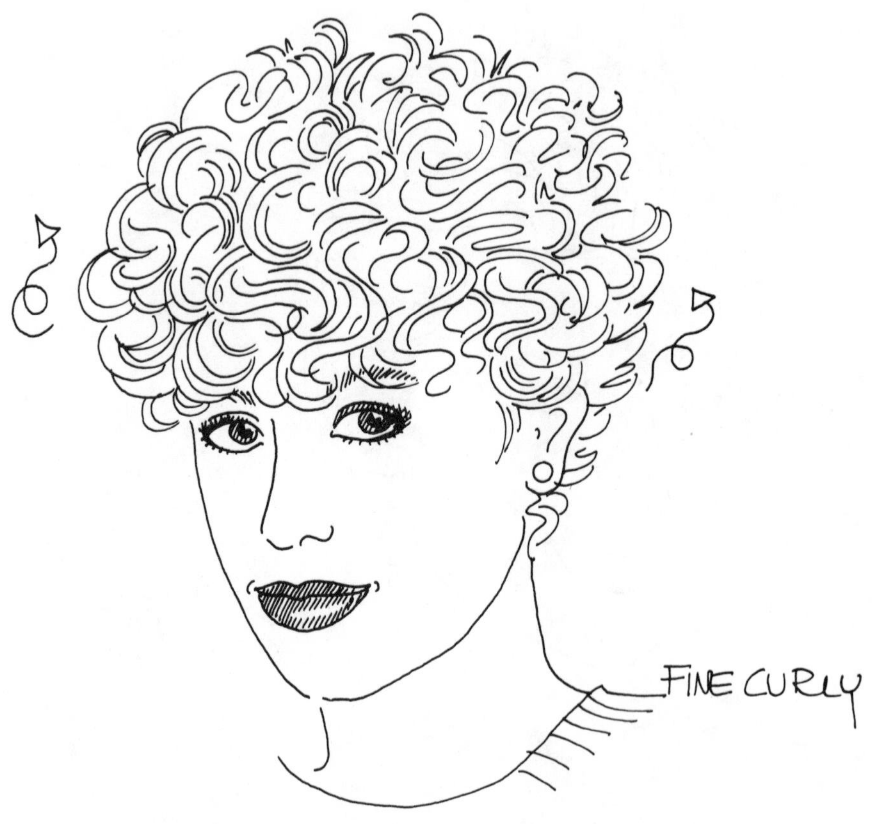

Here, a slightly longer style for fine, curly hair. Fine hair, even when it's curly, shouldn't be any longer than this if you want a polished look. When hair is longer, the length pulls out the curl and your style loses its shape.

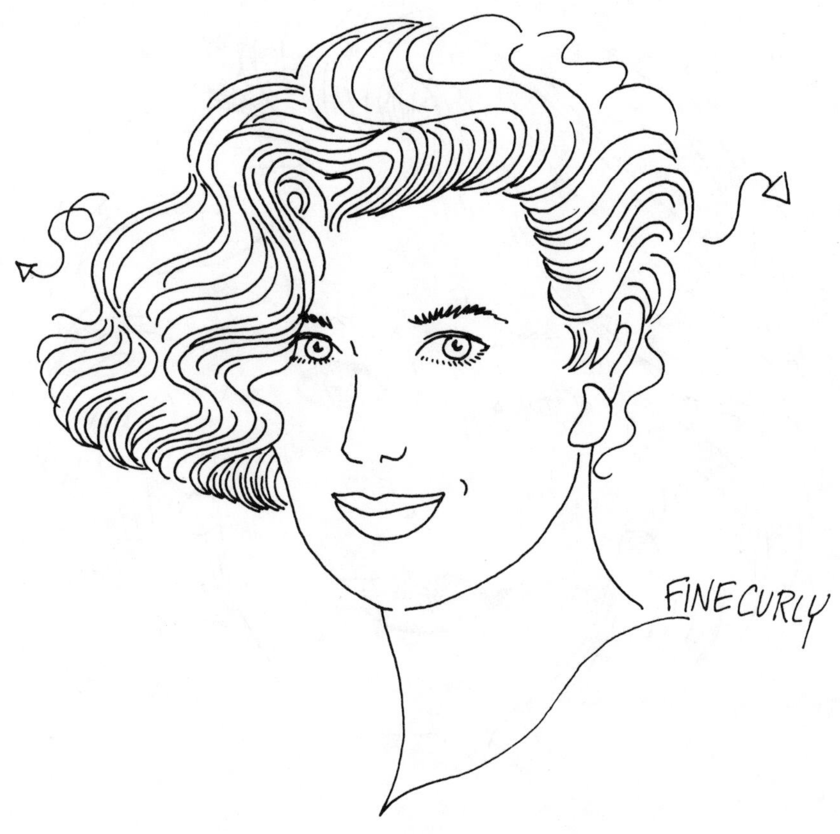

Medium-Textured Straight Hair

Hair that is medium textured is easy to work with and can be styled many ways. This cut is particularly versatile. More hair can be combed down on the forehead, the part can be switched to the center, sides can be pulled back. Any of these variations change the look of this good basic cut for straight hair.

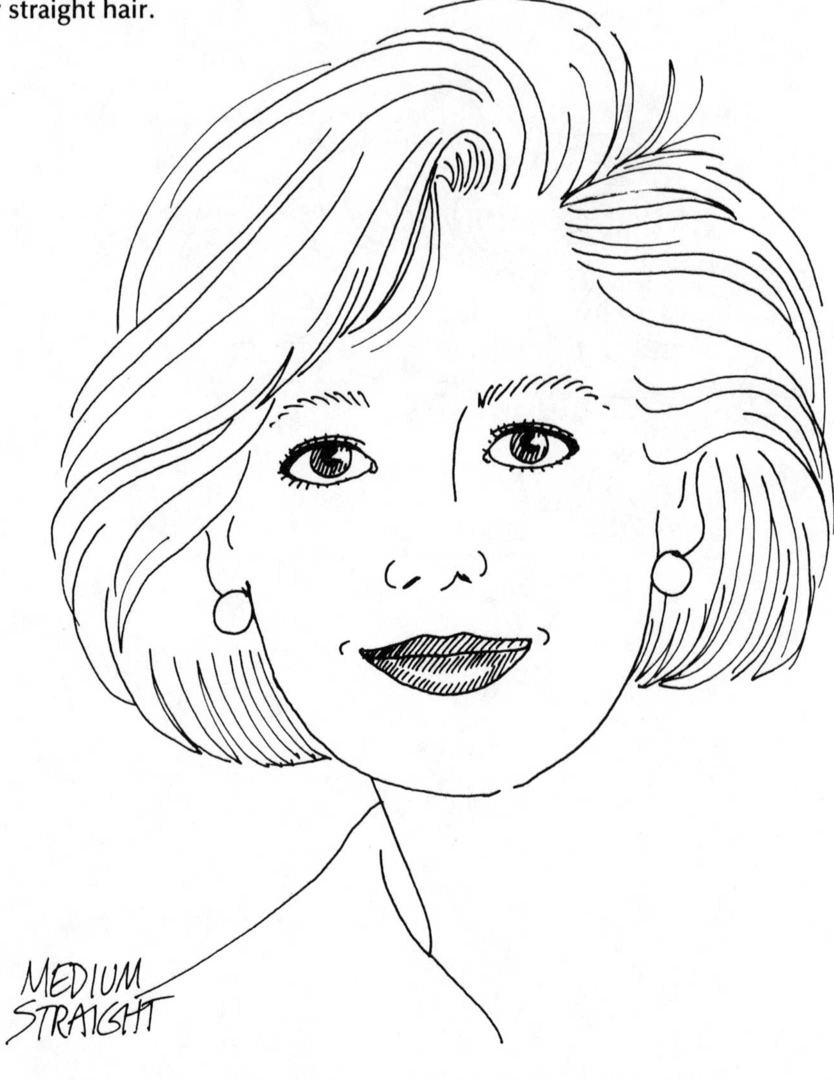

Medium-Textured Curly Hair

Once again, medium-textured hair with curl is very versatile. Since a curly "halo" like this one is very fashionable now, it's a good style to try. The hair can be allowed to dry naturally for this look. "Scrunch" the curls between your fingers as hair dries to encourage more curl.

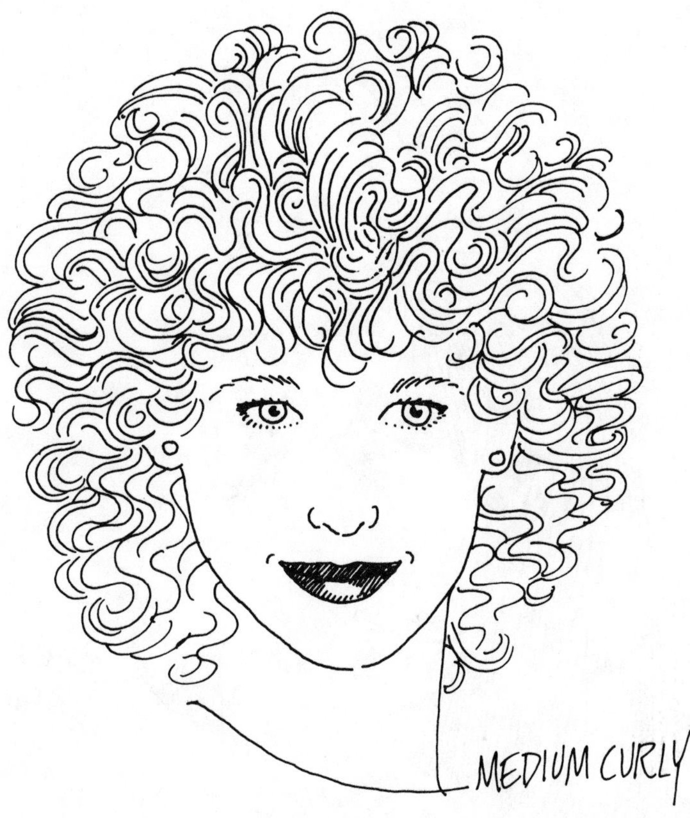

Coarse Straight Hair

Coarse hair, whether straight or curly, can be tricky to handle. The cut should be first-rate and kept simple. This is an excellent length for this kind of hair. When your cut is too short, you're apt to get a bristly look. When it's too long, you get a bushy look. This then is a good in-between length, and the shortness around the face adds softness, something this kind of hair needs.

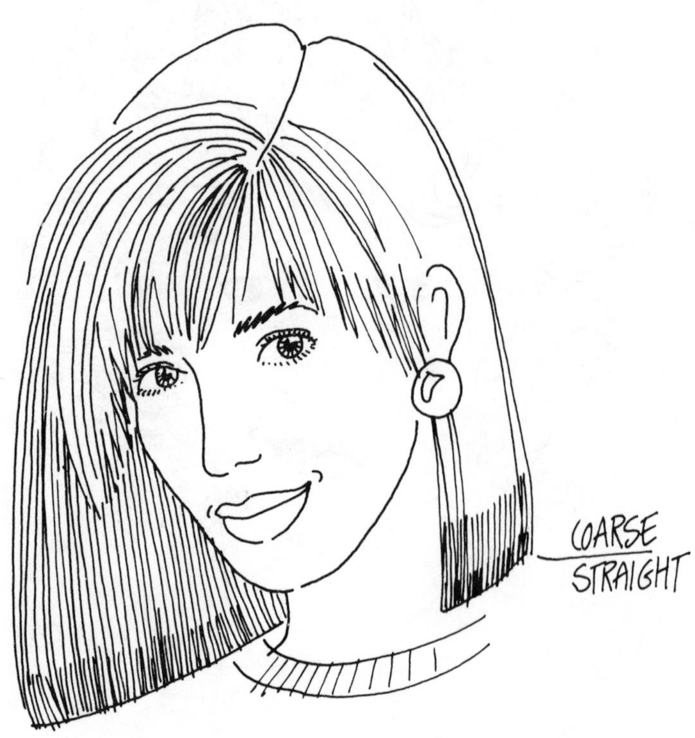

Coarse Curly Hair

This "halo" of curls can be a wonderful look for a woman who can carry it off. It looks fresh and contemporary and takes full advantage of the curl. If your hair is coarse and curly, it's fruitless to try a straight style. You'll be fighting your hair's natural tendency to curl. If you feel you can't carry this much length, opt for a short curly style. It will be just as successful. Just let hair dry naturally, scrunching curl with your fingers as hair dries.

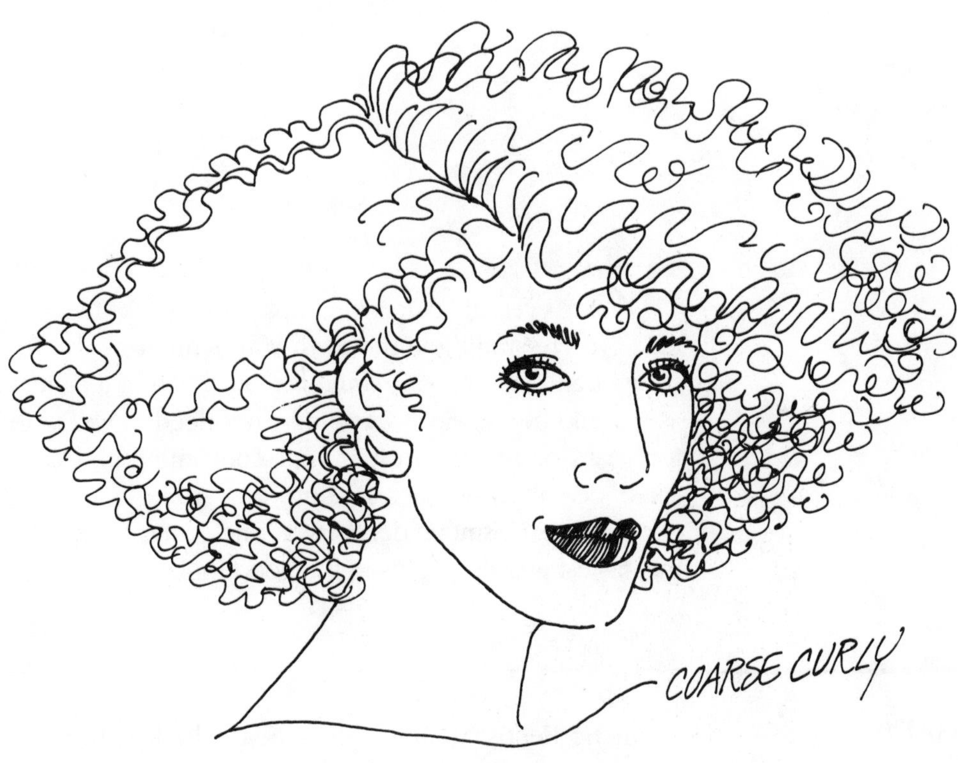

14 TURN YOUR SMILE INTO AN INSTANT BEAUTY LIFT

Your eyes light up, your lips curve back invitingly—you're smiling. If the teeth your smile reveals are not straight and bright, your smile isn't as much of a beauty lift as it could be. Nowadays, you may not need to wear braces for years or resort to other time-consuming and complicated dental techniques to put your smile instantly into good shape. Cosmetic dentistry is one of the fastest changing, fastest growing fields in the good looks business today.

WHAT IS COSMETIC DENTISTRY?

Cosmetic dentistry aims to make you look better almost instantly. It achieves this goal without sacrificing anything to dental health, and, in many cases, the cosmetic work actually makes teeth stronger and healthier in the bargain.

Not many years ago, it you wanted to have a broken or damaged tooth fixed, you had to have it capped. To get a cap, you had to spend hours in the dentist's chair and weeks waiting for the finished product to arrive. In addition, you probably had to have the broken or damaged tooth filed down to almost nothing so that the cap could be fitted around the tooth. Today, you could visit a good dentist and leave the office a few hours later with a bonded tooth, a tooth that did not have to be filed down, does not have to be treated with kid gloves and one that looks just like the surrounding teeth. This is all thanks to the new cosmetic dentistry.

Bonding is not the only option cosmetic dentistry has to offer. Porcelain veneers are the other primary option. A veneer is a porcelainlike shield that is bonded to the front of your tooth or teeth to repair damage, to "straighten" crooked teeth, or to fill in spaces between teeth. Bonding involves sculpting a tooth with a composite-resin bonding material. This material is soft when it is applied to allow the dentist to sculpt the repair. When the dentist achieves the desired effect, the resin is hardened with a beam of ultraviolet light.

WHO NEEDS WHAT AND WHY

Bonding and porcelain veneers are the mainstays of cosmetic dentistry. With these two tools, a good dentist can correct many cosmetic defects. Crooked teeth can be "straightened," stained or discolored teeth can be instantly brightened, broken teeth can be fixed, gaps between teeth can be reduced or eliminated.

Your dentist is actually the best judge of which technique is best for you. In general, major cover-up jobs are usually done best with a veneer. A veneer must be applied to a tooth with good enamel. If your tooth enamel is badly worn, your tooth may first have to be bonded to smooth the enamel. Also, if a tooth is badly broken, there is not enough tooth surface for a veneer to adhere, so bonding is a better option. Bonding is best used to "straighten" crooked teeth and to fill in spaces between teeth. Bonding is somewhat more "instant" than using a veneer because the bonding can be applied on the first visit to the dentist. A mold of the tooth must first be taken before a veneer can be made. Veneering takes much less time than capping. Per tooth, bonding and veneering usually cost about half of what a cap costs.

PROS AND CONS

There are very few cons to having cosmetic dental procedures performed, though there are a few things to keep in mind. Bonding materials do tend to be stained by dark liquids, especially tea, coffee, and red wines. Smoking also stains bonded teeth. New bonding materials are considerably more stain resistant that those originally used, but you must still exercise caution. Careful brushing with a good toothpaste is required; this is also a prerequisite for good dental health. There is at least one toothpaste on the market now (called SuperSmile) made especially for bonded teeth, which virtually eliminates the staining problem; it is also a good all-round toothpaste because it is a real plaque fighter. Stains can also be periodically buffed away. Although porcelain veneers are more stain resistant, they are more fragile because there is sometimes a problem making the veneer adhere properly. Also, if the veneer is not carefully fitted at the gum line, you may get a narrow ridge of staining at the gum line, which is difficult to remove.

Neither bonding nor veneering is totally permanent. Nor, for that matter, is a cap. Bonding will last for many years if it's well taken care of, if you do not use your teeth as tools, and if you have stains professionally buffed every so often. Since bonding is a new process, it's hard to predict precisely how long it will last in any given case.

WHY GOOD TEETH SUBTRACT YEARS

A beautiful smile is an asset at any age, but as we age, that smile is bound to age, too. Many of the changes are very subtle, but our eyes have learned to associate these changes with aging. For example, at twenty, most of us have nice white teeth, but over thirty, our teeth begin to show the effects of coffee, tea, wine, and tobacco. They can look yellow and stained. A more important and much less subtle effect of age is the gradual wear of the teeth at the cutting edge, producing teeth that are slightly shorter than those we started out with. We have learned to associate this look with age. A good cosmetic dentist can add just a bit of length to front teeth, which instantly makes a major difference in looks.

FINDING THE RIGHT DENTIST

Not every good dentist is a good cosmetic dentist. A good cosmetic dentist must be an artist as well as a technician. If you are having your teeth bonded, the dentist must literally sculpt the bonding material to form a new tooth, and not every dentist is skilled in this. If you are having a veneer made, a mold of your tooth is taken, but some artistic judgment is still involved in the appearance of the finished product. The best way to find a dentist with an artistic hand is through word of mouth. Try to find someone who has had work done and is satisfied. Look at this person's teeth and make your own judgment about how good the work is. If you cannot find a dentist this way, ask your own dentist if he or she does cosmetic dentistry. Ask how much of this kind of work he or she has done and if there are any "before" and "after" pictures you can look at. If your dentist doesn't do much cosmetic work, ask for the names of dentists who do. You might also call your local dental society or the dentistry school of a large nearby university to ask for recommendations.

Cosmetic dentistry comes about as close to being an instant cure-all for unsightly teeth as anything can. It cannot, however, correct gum and jawline problems. Teeth that protrude greatly or those that curve inward dramatically cannot be helped by cosmetic dentistry. Teeth that curve in only slightly can be helped. If you're in doubt about whether this new field can help you, consult your dentist.

15 FAST FAT FIGHTING

If you wanted to be on a diet, you'd be on one. Most of us have been on and off diets for much of our adult lives, trying to lose those miserable five or ten extra pounds that always seem to creep on. We lose them. We gain them back. We lose them. We gain them back. There is another way! You can change your eating habits—and I don't mean turn yourself into a carrot cruncher. No one is really going to do that for any length of time. There is another alternative, one that is quick, efficient, lasting, and healthy to boot.

What I am talking about is getting rid of excess fat. "But," you say, "that's what I've been trying to do!" When I say getting rid of fat, I don't mean the fat on your body. There is no doubt that you will lose some of the fat on your body, but the way to do this most effectively is to lose some of the fat in your diet. Americans are a fat-eating group. We consume mounds of fast food and we eat in conventional restaurants a great deal. Restaurant food is notoriously high in fat, and in fast-food restaurants, much of the food is fried.

NOT ALL CALORIES ARE EQUAL

Why, you might ask should you be so concerned about fat, other than the fact that too much is unhealthy? What you may not know is that a gram of fat contains nine calories compared to only four calories for a gram of carbohydrates or protein. That means that for every gram of fat you consume, you're getting more than twice the calories you get eating carbohydrates or proteins. Doesn't it make sense, then, to cut back on fats? As you cut back, you cut way back on calories, too. Eating a diet high in fat packs a double wallop. Dietary fats are more readily stored by your body as fat than either carbohydrates or proteins. Carbohydrates must first be changed into fats by your body before they can be stored as fat. This process requires body energy, which translates into calorie usage. You can now begin to see what a bargain carbohydrates are. They provide you with energy first and foremost and are only stored as fat when your body fails to use all their energy; they also have fewer calories than fat, are healthy, and taste wonderful. The good healthy carbohydrates are the complex ones found in whole grains and, of course, in fruits and vegetables. As researchers have been looking more and more at the body's use of fats because of the role they play in many diseases, they have also learned other things about fats and weight control. That's what this chapter is all about.

CUTTING DOWN

Cutting down on fats is not as simple as it might seem. We are all used to the idea that it's wise to trim our steak of excess fat—in fact, we know it's wise not to eat steak too often. What you may not know is where all the fat in your diet comes from, aside from the obvious places. Here are some ways to help you find the fat and fight back.

In Restaurants

The rules for cutting back on fats in restaurants are fairly simple and straightforward. They are, however, extremely valuable if you want to cut back both on fat and calories.

- Order chicken or fish. Both have less fat than other meats.
- Order your meat, fish, or chicken grilled whenever possible.
- If an entrée comes with a sauce, ask to have the sauce on the side, so you can add it sparingly.
- Ask to have salad dressings (loaded with fat) on the side, so you can control the amount you consume.
- Skip anything fried.
- Avoid fast-food restaurants whenever you can. Their food is a calorie nightmare. For example, there are a whopping 340 calories in an Egg McMuffin from McDonald's, and 42 percent of those calories come from fat. At Burger King, a Croissan'wich with sausage yields 496 calories, 69 percent of these come from fat.
- When you do eat in a fast-food restaurant, pick one that offers some grilled foods—maybe a grilled rather than a fried hamburger. Don't eat the fried coating on breaded entrées. Most of the calories come from the fat in the coating.
- Skip dessert unless you can have fresh fruit. Most cakes, pies, and pastries are loaded with shortening—read that as fat. It's not only the sugar in them that makes them so caloric.

At Home

You may think it's simple to cut back on fats at home because you are in control of what comes into your kitchen, what you cook, and how you cook it. That's true, but chances are you're missing the hidden fats in innocent looking foods that sit on your pantry shelf or in your refrigerator. For instance, did you know that many of those crisp, tasty, innocent-looking crackers in your pantry are loaded with fat? Many have almost as much fat as potato chips. Most snack foods are loaded with fat. Cheese-flavored crackers, chips, or other cheesy snacks are fat laden. The only way to be certain how much fat a commercial food contains is to read the package label. Foods are carefully labeled in this country, thanks to government regulations. Look for the ingredients list and notice how close to the top fat is listed. The closer to the top, the more fat there is. You must remember that "fat" comes in many forms, so look for oils or shortening of any kind. A label may say, for example, that the food contains hydrogenated vegetable oil, shortening, corn oil, palm oil, butter, or lard. All are fat, and if any of them are listed near the top of the ingredients list, the food is high in fat, and you should either avoid it altogether or eat it sparingly. If you become an avid label reader, you'll educate yourself so that you can automatically eliminate high-fat foods from your kitchen—and your diet.

Foods to Be Suspicious Of

Certain kinds of foods are more likely to fool you with high-fat content than others. Here are some food categories that pack hidden surprises:

- *Salad dressings.* Most of their calories come from oils.
- *Breads.* Most breads are low-fat foods, but watch out for muffins, croissants, and similar innocent-sounding goodies. They are full of fats.
- *Processed meats.* These are much higher in fat than regular cuts of meat. Avoid salami, bologna, and sausages, which are very fatty.

- *Crackers.* They are usually high in fat. Read the ingredients list to see how close to the top oil or shortening is listed.
- *Granolas.* These are often high in nuts and coconut, both of which are fatty.
- *Salty snacks.* Chips are obvious, but many of their "relatives" are just as fatty, even more so. You should avoid these foods altogether. Their high calorie content is not worth the little nutrition they provide.
- *Hard cheeses.* Most of us know that soft creamy cheeses such as Triple Creme, cream cheese, or Brie are high in fat. We are usually less aware of the fat in such hard cheeses as cheddar. To convince yourself that these cheeses are just as fatty as soft ones, melt some. Notice the pool of oil the surrounds the melted cheese. Convinced?

In addition to becoming an avid label reader and an alert consumer, there are other ways you can cut down on fats and still enjoy many of the things you like.

- Buy skim milk rather than homogenized or low-fat milk.
- Buy low-fat ice cream rather than regular. Be suspicious of some "healthy" sweets in this area. Tofutti, for example, contains almost twice the fat of ice cream; ice milk contains less than half and low-fat yogurt one-tenth as much fat as ice cream.
- Buy "light" salad dressings. The calorie reduction here comes from virtually eliminating the oils.
- Buy "light" mayonnaise. Much of the fat is eliminated.
- Spray-on pan coatings provide adequate fat to cook with, but greatly reduce the amount you would normally use.
- Buy "light" sour cream instead of regular. You can even buy "light" cream cheese.
- Buy "light" cheese slices. They contain half the fat and calories of regular cheese.

THE BENEFITS OF FIGHTING DIETARY FAT

I won't focus on the health benefits here because this is a book about instant good looks. Still, it would be unfair not to point out that by lowering the amount of fat you consume, you are giving yourself an enormous health boost. A diet too high in fats contributes to most of the circulatory and heart disease in this country. A high-fat diet has also been associated with a higher incidence of breast and colon cancer. Need I say more?

The American Heart Association Guidelines recommend restricting your fat intake to 30 percent of your total caloric intake (50 to 55 percent should come from carbohydrates, with an emphasis on complex carbohydrates, and 15 percent from proteins). Most Americans actually consume almost 40 to 50 percent of their calories from fat. By following the guidelines just given, you should easily be able to cut your fat calories to around 30 percent of your diet. By cutting back as outlined, you can automatically cut your calories by 10 to 20 percent—without going on any kind of diet! You get the point? If you cut back your calories by this much, you simply *must* lose weight. What's more, you'll keep it off if you continue to eat this way. This kind of eating is not deprivational. You can happily eat many good things, including pasta for example, and still cut calories. Sound like magic? Well it is, and it's healthy magic, too.

THE EXERCISE BOOST

Most of us hear the word *exercise* and we groan. We think of down-on-the-floor calisthenics or heart-racing aerobics. I'm not knocking either of these: The former will help you firm your body and the latter will do wonders for your cardiovascular health. But I promised you instant results in this book, so although I recommend both calisthenics and aerobic exercise, I realize that many women simply are not motivated to do either. So what can you do? You might try doing a bit more walking, which is, hands down, about the best kind of exercise there is, and it's fun, easy, and addictive, too. You probably don't give much thought to how you might get more exercise. It's a lot easier than you think—try the following:

- Walk to work if you can. It saves bus fare, too. If the walk is too long, ride or drive part way and walk the rest.
- Walk in your office. Don't pick up the phone every time you want to talk to someone. Walk to an office instead, and deliver a memo instead of putting it in interoffice mail. All this may not amount to many miles, but it *will* give you more exercise than sitting at your desk.
- Walk at home. Make it a point to get up and walk around your house or apartment regularly. Do it during commercials while you watch TV. Do it every half hour while you read.
- Walk up stairs. This is fabulous exercise and burns up lots of calories. Get off the elevator a couple of floors below yours at work or in your apartment and take the stairs a few floors. If you live in a two-story house, make it a point to walk up and down the stairs at least ten times every day.
- Take a walk. It's fun, stimulating, allows you to see new things, and it's wonderful exercise. Make it a point to take a brisk walk every weekend.

All this obviously can't replace good regular exercise, but it can get you moving more and help work off calories. This, combined with cutting back on your daily fat intake, can make a substantial difference in your weight very quickly. Try it.

TO THE RESCUE

- If you're a snacker, make it a point to cultivate some tasty low-fat snacks, such as frozen yogurt, real-fruit popsicles, low-fat crackers, or fruit.
- Try eating red meat only twice a week. Eat chicken, fish, and pasta the rest of the time. Stick to low-fat sauces, such as tomato-based sauces rather than creamy ones for pasta.
- Make the dietary changes suggested in this chapter with a friend who also wants to lose a little weight.

16 ANSWERS TO YOUR QUESTIONS

Most of this book has been devoted to the general rules of looking slimmer and more attractive. Since there are literally hundreds of specific questions that relate to this topic, I can't attempt to answer them all, but here are the answers to some that I've heard asked most often. Maybe yours is here.

FASHION

Bra Bulge

I have large breasts and though I'm not more than five pounds overweight, I always seem to get a roll at the top and bottom of my bra. This limits what I can wear—what can I do?

You need a good, support bra if you have large breasts, but that doesn't mean you need one that will produce a roll.

The fleshiest parts of the back on even normal-weight women are just above the bra line, under the armpit, and in the center of the back. If a bra hits you here, it is going to produce a roll. Look for an underwire bra—it will give you the support you need—with a lowish cut under the arm and a wide band in back. The wider the band, the more support it offers and the lower on your back the bottom edge will come. This lower area is not as fleshy as the area just above it and won't produce a roll as readily.

Bikini Tummy

I love bikini panties, but even at my good weight, I get a bulge above the elastic at the top. Do I have to give them up?

No. Your bikinis may be shrinking as a result of washing them in very hot water. Try washing them by hand in lukewarm water and see if this helps. Also, look for a very low-cut bikini. One that hits just above the pubic hairline will not cause a bulge because most women are not fleshy here.

Panty Line

I can't stand wearing pantyhose without underwear. How can I avoid the "panty line" I always get when I wear pants?

Many women don't like the feel of pantyhose with no underwear. Yet, pantyhose are the only solution to a smooth pants line. One idea you might try is wearing a sanitary panty shield in your pantyhose. This will give you the feeling of something between you and the hose, but won't spoil your look in pants.

Love Handles

I have a good collection of cashmere and lambswool sweaters in conventional shapes. I love wearing them with pants and skirts, but my thick middle seems so obvious when I wear them, and belting them only makes the problem worse. How should I wear them?

There is no real solution for these sweaters. It is the nature of their fit that they cling. You might try tucking in your sweaters and wearing a pretty silk shirt open over them. This is a nice look and will hide your problem. As you add new sweaters, consider buying some of the wonderful looking oversize styles around now. They look fashionable and won't emphasize a thick middle.

Pants for Hippy Women

I am "hippy" and I thought the very full-hipped pants that are in style now would look terrific on me because the fullness would hide my problem. Not so—they just make me look hippier. What kind of pants should I wear?

Your best bet is a pair of pleat-front trousers that fit you *perfectly.* Don't try for too much fullness, just enough to keep everything smooth. If you're careful what kind of top you wear with them, this style will work well. A loose, boxy sweater is one good choice. A soft silk blouse is another. You might also try tucking in a thin sweater and wearing a silk shirt open over the sweater.

Help for Thick Ankles

I am not really overweight, but I have thick ankles that make my legs look fat. How can I disguise them?

The length of your skirt is very important. If you're going to wear a short skirt, it should barely graze your knees so that there is a long expanse of leg and you get the benefit of the taper of the calf muscles. If you wear a long skirt, it should be worn quite long, almost ankle length, and the style should be intended for that length. Another trick: Keep your stockings, skirt, and shoes in the same color family. Boots, in winter, are always a good and fashionable solution. Also, watch shoe styles. A high-cut throat or tie oxford will emphasize thick ankles. A low-cut throat will help your ankles look slim.

Swimsuit for a Tummy Bulge

I am not at all overweight; in fact, I'm quite slender. Nevertheless, in a swimsuit, I have a tummy bulge. It looks especially unattractive because I'm so thin everywhere else. What should I do?

If you are truly slim everywhere else, your tummy bulge is definitely caused by habitual poor posture. You can't solve this problem unless you're willing to pay attention to your posture, at least when you're wearing a bathing suit. Pull in your tummy and tighten your buttock muscles. Try to remember to do this as often as you can. In the long run, it would be better if you tackled this problem once and for all. Habitual bad posture tends to weaken back muscles over time and leads to back problems. You might get a book of back exercises to help strengthen your back and then do twenty-five sit-ups daily in addition to the back exercises.

What Length Skirt

Skirts seem to have gotten short again and I don't want to look old and dowdy. Should I shorten my skirts, or not?

Skirt lengths are always changing, but since the big change with the mini back in the sixties, fashion designers have learned that women want a choice of lengths, and you will always find that there is a choice in stores and there is a choice among your own clothes. The best advice I can give you is not to worry too much about the fashion of it, instead think about the proportion of it. In general, slim skirts look best worn shorter. They are dowdy when worn too long. The bottom of the kneecap or a little above or below, depending on the fashion and your legs, is best. Full-cut bias skirts should be worn long and graceful. Midcalf is a good length for this kind of skirt. If you are wearing an evening skirt, just above the ankle is a good length. Always be sure the hem allows some of the curve of the ankle to show. It's more graceful. The exception would be a floor-length formal dress.

Professional Looking Cover-ups

I live in the South and work in a very conservative law office. Some of the other women wear tailored short-sleeve dresses, but I feel my arms don't look attractive enough for this kind of dress. What can I wear without feeling so hot in the warmest weather?

Air circulation is crucial to staying cool in hot weather. Find some long, open-weave, full-sleeve dresses or shirts that will cover your arms, but won't cling. That way air can circulate. Voile is a good fabric for both its femininity and its coolness. Avoid synthetics, which will be hot. You might also find that a well-cut and well-tailored lightweight cotton jacket will work. Pick one with wide, straight sleeves and roll the sleeves back a few turns. This is a snappy look and is also cooler than it sounds. The loose sleeves let air circulate.

Bare Legs for Work?

It gets very hot in my city in the summer and many women come to the office wearing no stockings. I think this is in poor taste. What are the rules here?

Wearing no stockings to anything but the most informal office with no air conditioning is not going to do a thing to move you ahead in your career. It looks unprofessional, and unless you have great legs with no visible veins, it is aging to go without stockings. Think of stockings as a beauty aid, because that's what they are. A few manufacturers make "summer-weight" pantyhose, and though they are still uncomfortable on very sticky days, they are an improvement over many other, heavier kinds.

Exposing Heavy Thighs

I have fairly good calves, but my thighs are heavy, starting just above the knee. I like wearing skirts knee length, but when I sit, they ride up and expose my fat thighs. Can you help?

Slim skirts will ride up, especially if they are worn quite short. Look for those that have a pleat either in front or in back at the hem. A back slit will help, too. Front slits "sit" very poorly. Avoid them. The best solution if you like the look of a slim skirt worn short is a wrap skirt. You will have to be sure the wrap is closed as you sit, but once that's done, this kind of skirt looks graceful and shouldn't expose your thighs.

Wrinkled Skin at the Neck

I look good for my forty-two years, but I hate the way the skin on my neck looks. It's much more wrinkled than my face. I have trouble finding enough high-necked blouses and sweaters to cover the problem. What else can I do?

Skin on the neck often becomes wrinkled before the rest of your skin. Your neck twists and turns hundreds of times a day. The skin here is also thinner than that on the face, especially in fair, thin-skinned women. Wearing high-necked clothes is not really a good solution. With the exception of a soft turtleneck sweater, most high-necked clothes look uptight and constricting. Try bearing a little more rather than covering up and you'll find you will look better. Surprisingly enough, clothes with a lower neck look better because they create a soft, feminine line and expose a bit of smooth chest skin. A V-necked, notched-collar shirt gives a pretty line and is appropriate for almost any kind of wear. A soft cowl neck also give a pretty line.

Don't focus on your neck. It is just one part of the overall package. If you are well put together overall, no one is going to focus on your neck.

Slipping Shoulder Pads

I have very narrow shoulders and broad hips, so I find tops with shoulder pads help to even out my proportions. The trouble is, the pads slip around, especially in lightweight clothes such as silk shirts. This looks terrible and feels worse. What can I do?

First of all, don't buy clothes with super-large shoulder pads. If you love something, but it has "football shoulders," replace the pads with something smaller. You will probably find it is worth investing in a pair of shoulder pads with snaps attached. The snap goes around your bra strap and holds the pads in place. Most notions departments in department stores carry them.

Sun Spots

As a result of sun exposure over the years, I have several brownish pigment spots on my cheeks and one under my eye. They are not terribly dark, but they show through normal makeup. Heavy cover-sticks look like a mask—is there anything better?

These spots are easily and quickly removed by a good dermatologist and will not return, though you may develop new ones in other spots. If you want a simpler solution, look for a cover-up that comes in a wand, very much like a mascara wand. These products are only slightly heavier than regular makeup and they cover very well. Several cosmetic companies make them, so you should have no trouble finding one.

Body for Fine Hair

My hair is so fine that no hair style really seems to hold, and I feel my whole look is spoiled. Is there any style that will work?

Fine hair can indeed be very troublesome, but there are more ways to help now than ever. I presume you've tried the obvious solutions—a body wave or body-building setting lotions. If you haven't found these work for you, you might investigate some of the "thickening" products on the market. There are a couple of thickening mousses available that add a great deal of body to fine hair and help it hold a line. There are also many thickening shampoos around that also add a lot of body. The one drawback to all these products is that they tend to make hair look dirty very quickly. You will probably need to shampoo your hair every other day. This actually shouldn't be much of a drawback because fine hair should be shampooed frequently to give it the volume it needs. After a day or two, fine hair usually looks lank no matter what products you use on it. The best solution for your problem is one of these thickening products and a very good short haircut. Short hair cuts down on maintenance time and is usually a good solution to lack of body, because fine, clean, short hair holds a set longer than fine, clean, longer hair. The added length weighs hair down and pulls out curl.

Solution for Eye Shadow Problem

I use a cream eye shadow and it always cakes in the crease of my eyelid. What should I use instead?

Cream shadows have a tendency to crease on the lid. This happens partly because of the constant movement of the eyelid combined with the texture of the shadow. Since you continue to wear a cream shadow in spite of the problem, you probably do not like powder shadows. Powders will crease less, especially the very fine-textured ones. If you insist on a cream, try one of the creamy eye crayons. The consistency is creamy, but not overly so. This may solve your problem.

Lipstick Bleed

My lipstick always "bleeds" into the fine lines above my upper lip. How can I prevent this?

This is an annoying problem that is intensified when you eat. First of all, try a lip pencil to line your lips before you apply color. Pick one in a neutral, tawny color—this applies for all lipsticks—and a hard texture. Soft pencils will bleed as much as your lipstick. Carefully line your lips, blot pencil outline, and then apply lip color. This should help, even if it won't totally prevent the problem.

Spotty Blush

When I apply my cream blush, how can I prevent the color from sinking into my pores and giving my cheeks a blotchy appearance?

This is not an unusual problem for both cream and liquid blushes, especially in deeper shades. The only real solution is to switch to a powder blush. Applied with a large, soft brush, the powder should give you a smooth, glowing blush. If you still prefer a cream blush, you might try switching to a slightly lighter color. The paler the blush, the less likely you are to encounter this problem.

Smudgy Mascara

My mascara always smudges onto my skin, just under the lower lid. What can I do about this?

This is undoubtedly caused by the oils in your skin mixing with the mascara. Every time you blink, your upper lashes press on the lower ones, causing some lashes to touch the skin and deposit a film of mascara. This is most likely to happen with an oil-based mascara. Switch to a water-based product. You can tell the difference by looking at the label on your mascara. If the first ingredient is some kind of petroleum oil, look for one with water listed first. This will surely help.

Disappearing Makeup

I use all the appropriate makeup—foundation, powder, blush, eye makeup, and lipstick—but an hour after I apply it, it has "disappeared" into my skin. Why does this happen and what can I do about it?

Redheads and blondes, especially those with dry skin, seem to suffer most often from this problem. This kind of skin seems almost to absorb the makeup. To solve this, don't overapply makeup. That will just give you a masklike look. Instead, look for makeup colors with more intensity. Concentrate on blush and lipstick color, because if you can keep color on cheeks and lips, you'll retain a more finished look. A powder blush in a tawny color is good. Look for a tawny color with some intensity, not a pastel hue. Dust on blush liberally, then use a clean blush brush to even out the color. Then, apply just a bit more blush. Experiment with lipstick formulations. You should be looking for the least greasy formula you can find. Stay away from shiny formulas or glosses. They will not work for your kind of skin. Pick a tawny coral shade with intensity; this will allow you to get the most from the color without looking overdone.

If your skin is especially fair, which is often the case for women who experience this problem, don't overlook the possibility of going just a shade deeper in foundation. This will give you a base of natural color to work with. Be careful here, however. Don't go more than one shade darker than your natural skin tone and don't do even this unless you are quite fair to begin with.

Thinning Hair

My hair seems to be thinning out noticeably, though I'm only forty-five. What could be causing this and what can I do?

As we age, we do tend to lose more hair, but at forty-five this should not be a real problem. For some as-yet-not-understood reason, many women seem to lose more hair in the fall than at any other time of year, but this is not a significant enough loss to cause your hair to look thinned out. You should first check with a good dermatologist to determine whether there is any medical problem that is causing hair loss. If there is not, you may be overreacting to normal hair loss, either seasonal or just normal daily loss.

There are several cosmetic solutions you might also try. Having your hair colored will give it more body, thus making it look fuller. If you don't want to try this, a permanent will give straight hair more body and make it look fuller. Most important of all, get a good haircut. A shorter style that is soft and full will make the most of hair that tends to be thin. It would probably be worth your while to go to a first-rate hair stylist for a consultation. He or she can suggest styles and might also reassure you if you are overreacting to normal hair loss.

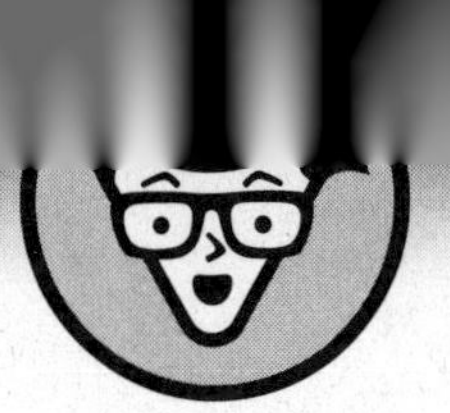

Java®

7th Edition

by Barry Burd, PhD

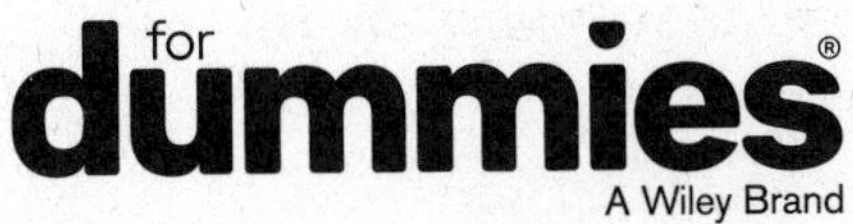

Java® For Dummies®, 7th Edition

Published by: **John Wiley & Sons, Inc.,** 111 River Street, Hoboken, NJ 07030-5774, www.wiley.com

For general information on our other products and services, please contact our Customer Care Department within the U.S. at 877-762-2974, outside the U.S. at 317-572-3993, or fax 317-572-4002. For technical support, please visit https://hub.wiley.com/community/support/dummies.

Wiley publishes in a variety of print and electronic formats and by print-on-demand. Some material included with standard print versions of this book may not be included in e-books or in print-on-demand. If this book refers to media such as a CD or DVD that is not included in the version you purchased, you may download this material at http://booksupport.wiley.com. For more information about Wiley products, visit www.wiley.com.

Library of Congress Control Number: 2017932837

ISBN: 978-1-119-23555-2; 978-1-119-23558-3 (ebk); 978-1-119-23557-6 (ebk)

Manufactured in the United States of America

10 9 8 7 6 5 4 3 2

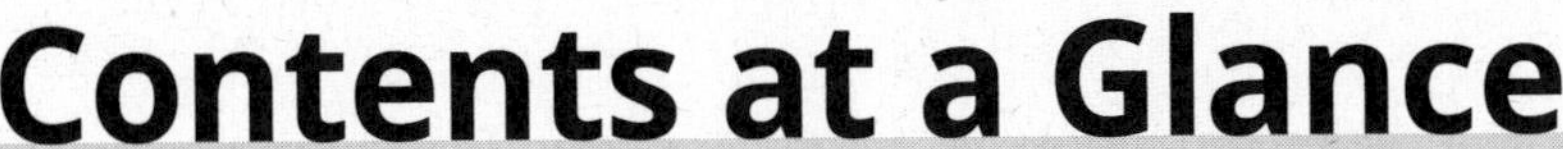

Contents at a Glance

Table of Contents

Introduction

Java is good stuff. I've been using it for years. I like Java because it's orderly. Almost everything follows simple rules. The rules can seem intimidating at times, but this book is here to help you figure them out. So, if you want to use Java and you want an alternative to the traditional techie, soft-cover book, sit down, relax, and start reading *Java For Dummies*, 7th Edition.

How to Use This Book

I wish I could say, "Open to a random page of this book and start writing Java code. Just fill in the blanks and don't look back." In a sense, this is true. You can't break anything by writing Java code, so you're always free to experiment.

But let me be honest. If you don't understand the bigger picture, writing a program is difficult. That's true with any computer programming language — not just Java. If you're typing code without knowing what it's about and the code doesn't do exactly what you want it to do, you're just plain stuck.

In this book, I divide Java programming into manageable chunks. Each chunk is (more or less) a chapter. You can jump in anywhere you want — Chapter 5, Chapter 10, or wherever. You can even start by poking around in the middle of a chapter. I've tried to make the examples interesting without making one chapter depend on another. When I use an important idea from another chapter, I include a note to help you find your way around.

In general, my advice is as follows:

- If you already know something, don't bother reading about it.
- If you're curious, don't be afraid to skip ahead. You can always sneak a peek at an earlier chapter, if you really need to do so.

Conventions Used in This Book

Almost every technical book starts with a little typeface legend, and *Java For Dummies*, 7th Edition, is no exception. What follows is a brief explanation of the typefaces used in this book:

- New terms are set in *italics.*
- If you need to type something that's mixed in with the regular text, the characters you type appear in bold. For example: "Type **MyNewProject** in the text field."
- You also see this `computerese` font. I use computerese for Java code, filenames, web page addresses (URLs), onscreen messages, and other such things. Also, if something you need to type is really long, it appears in computerese font on its own line (or lines).
- You need to change certain things when you type them on your own computer keyboard. For instance, I may ask you to type

  ```
  public class Anyname
  ```

  which means that you type **public class** and then some name that you make up on your own. Words that you need to replace with your own words are set in *`italicized computerese`*.

What You Don't Have to Read

Pick the first chapter or section that has material you don't already know and start reading there. Of course, you may hate making decisions as much as I do. If so, here are some guidelines that you can follow:

- If you already know what kind of an animal Java is and know that you want to use Java, skip Chapter 1 and go straight to Chapter 2. Believe me, I won't mind.
- If you already know how to get a Java program running, and you don't care what happens behind the scenes when a Java program runs, skip Chapter 2 and start with Chapter 3.
- If you write programs for a living but use any language other than C or C++, start with Chapter 2 or 3. When you reach Chapters 5 and 6, you'll probably find them to be easy reading. When you get to Chapter 7, it'll be time to dive in.

- If you write C (not C++) programs for a living, start with Chapters 2, 3, and 4 and just skim Chapters 5 and 6.
- If you write C++ programs for a living, glance at Chapters 2 and 3, skim Chapters 4 through 6, and start reading seriously in Chapter 7. (Java is a bit different from C++ in the way it handles classes and objects.)
- If you write Java programs for a living, come to my house and help me write *Java For Dummies,* 8th Edition.

If you want to skip the sidebars and the Technical Stuff icons, please do. In fact, if you want to skip anything at all, feel free.

Foolish Assumptions

In this book, I make a few assumptions about you, the reader. If one of these assumptions is incorrect, you're probably okay. If all these assumptions are incorrect . . . well, buy the book anyway:

- **I assume that you have access to a computer.** Here's the good news: You can run most of the code in this book on almost any computer. The only computers that you can't use to run this code are ancient things that are more than ten years old (give or take a few years).
- **I assume that you can navigate through your computer's common menus and dialog boxes.** You don't have to be a Windows, Linux, or Macintosh power user, but you should be able to start a program, find a file, put a file into a certain directory . . . that sort of thing. Most of the time, when you practice the stuff in this book, you're typing code on the keyboard, not pointing and clicking the mouse.

  On those rare occasions when you need to drag and drop, cut and paste, or plug and play, I guide you carefully through the steps. But your computer may be configured in any of several billion ways, and my instructions may not quite fit your special situation. When you reach one of these platform-specific tasks, try following the steps in this book. If the steps don't quite fit, consult a book with instructions tailored to your system.
- **I assume that you can think logically.** That's all there is to programming in Java — thinking logically. If you can think logically, you've got it made. If you don't believe that you can think logically, read on. You may be pleasantly surprised.

» **I make few assumptions about your computer programming experience (or your lack of such experience).** In writing this book, I've tried to do the impossible: I've tried to make the book interesting for experienced programmers yet accessible to people with little or no programming experience. This means that I don't assume any particular programming background on your part. If you've never created a loop or indexed an array, that's okay.

  On the other hand, if you've done these things (maybe in Visual Basic, Python, or C++), you'll discover some interesting plot twists in Java. The developers of Java took the best ideas in object-oriented programming, streamlined them, reworked them, and reorganized them into a sleek, powerful way of thinking about problems. You'll find many new, thought-provoking features in Java. As you find out about these features, many of them will seem quite natural to you. One way or another, you'll feel good about using Java.

How This Book Is Organized

This book is divided into subsections, which are grouped into sections, which come together to make chapters, which are lumped finally into five parts. (When you write a book, you get to know your book's structure pretty well. After months of writing, you find yourself dreaming in sections and chapters when you go to bed at night.) The parts of the book are listed here.

Part 1: Getting Started with Java

This part is your complete, executive briefing on Java. It includes some "What is Java?" material and a jump-start chapter — Chapter 3. In Chapter 3, you visit the major technical ideas and dissect a simple program.

Part 2: Writing Your Own Java Program

Chapters 4 through 6 cover the fundamentals. These chapters describe the things that you need to know so that you can get your computer humming along.

If you've written programs in Visual Basic, C++, or any another language, some of the material in Part 2 may be familiar to you. If so, you can skip some sections or read this stuff quickly. But don't read too quickly. Java is a little different from some other programming languages, especially in the things that I describe in Chapter 4.

Part 3: Working with the Big Picture: Object-Oriented Programming

Part 3 has some of my favorite chapters. This part covers the all-important topic of object-oriented programming. In these chapters, you find out how to map solutions to big problems. (Sure, the examples in these chapters aren't big, but the examples involve big ideas.) In bite-worthy increments, you discover how to design classes, reuse existing classes, and construct objects.

Have you read any of those books that explain object-oriented programming in vague, general terms? I'm proud to say that *Java For Dummies*, 7th Edition, isn't like that. In this book, I illustrate each concept with a simple-yet-concrete program example.

Part 4: Smart Java Techniques

If you've tasted some Java and you want more, you can find what you need in this part of the book. This part's chapters are devoted to details — the things that you don't see when you first glance at the material. After you read the earlier parts and write some programs on your own, you can dive in a little deeper by reading Part 4.

Part 5: The Part of Tens

The Part of Tens is a little Java candy store. In the Part of Tens, you can find lists — lists of tips for avoiding mistakes, for finding resources, and for all kinds of interesting goodies.

Icons Used in This Book

If you could watch me write this book, you'd see me sitting at my computer, talking to myself. I say each sentence in my head. Most of the sentences, I mutter several times. When I have an extra thought, a side comment, or something that doesn't belong in the regular stream, I twist my head a little bit. That way, whoever's listening to me (usually nobody) knows that I'm off on a momentary tangent.

Of course, in print, you can't see me twisting my head. I need some other way of setting a side thought in a corner by itself. I do it with icons. When you see a Tip icon or a Remember icon, you know that I'm taking a quick detour.

Here's a list of icons that I use in this book:

TIP

A tip is an extra piece of information — something helpful that the other books may forget to tell you.

WARNING

Everyone makes mistakes. Heaven knows that I've made a few in my time. Anyway, when I think people are especially prone to make a mistake, I mark it with a Warning icon.

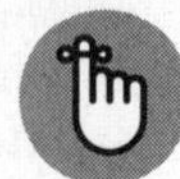
REMEMBER

Question: What's stronger than a Tip, but not as strong as a Warning?

Answer: A Remember icon.

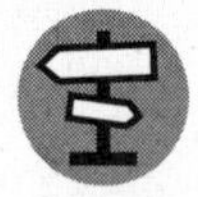
CROSS REFERENCE

"If you don't remember what such-and-such means, see blah-blah-blah," or "For more information, read blahbity-blah-blah."

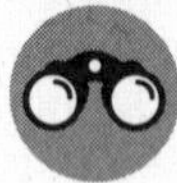
TRY IT OUT

Writing computer code is an activity, and the best way to learn an activity is to practice it. That's why I've created things for you to try in order to reinforce your knowledge. Many of these are confidence-builders, but some are a bit more challenging. When you first start putting things into practice, you'll discover all kinds of issues, quandaries, and roadblocks that didn't occur to you when you started reading about the material. But that's a good thing. Keep at it! Don't become frustrated. Or, if you do become frustrated, visit this book's website (`www.allmycode.com/JavaForDummies`) for hints and solutions.

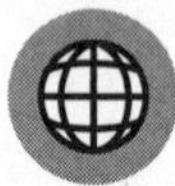

This icon calls attention to useful material that you can find online. Check it out!

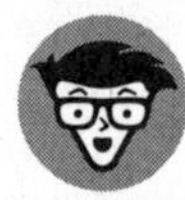
TECHNICAL STUFF

Occasionally, I run across a technical tidbit. The tidbit may help you understand what the people behind the scenes (the people who developed Java) were thinking. You don't have to read it, but you may find it useful. You may also find the tidbit helpful if you plan to read other (more geeky) books about Java.

Beyond the Book

In addition to what you're reading right now, this book comes with a free access-anywhere Cheat Sheet containing code that you can copy and paste into your own Android program. To get this Cheat Sheet, simply go to `www.dummies.com` and type **Java For Dummies Cheat Sheet** in the Search box.

Where to Go from Here

If you've gotten this far, you're ready to start reading about Java application development. Think of me (the author) as your guide, your host, your personal assistant. I do everything I can to keep things interesting and, most importantly, to help you understand.

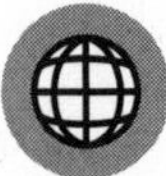

If you like what you read, send me a note. My email address, which I created just for comments and questions about this book, is JavaForDummies@allmycode.com. If email and chat aren't your favorites, you can reach me instead on Twitter (@allmycode) and on Facebook (www.facebook.com/allmycode). And don't forget — for the latest updates, visit this book's website. The site's address is www.allmycode.com/JavaForDummies.

1 Getting Started with Java

IN THIS PART . . .

Find out about the tools you need for developing Java programs.

Find out how Java fits into today's technology scene.

See your first complete Java program.

» **Where Java came from**

» **Why Java is so cool**

» **How to orient yourself to object-oriented programming**

Chapter 1
All about Java

Say what you want about computers. As far as I'm concerned, computers are good for just two simple reasons:

» **When computers do work, they feel no resistance, no stress, no boredom, and no fatigue.** Computers are our electronic slaves. I have my computer working 24/7 doing calculations for `Cosmology@Home` — a distributed computing project to investigate models describing the universe. Do I feel sorry for my computer because it's working so hard? Does the computer complain? Will the computer report me to the National Labor Relations Board? No.

  I can make demands, give the computer its orders, and crack the whip. Do I (or should I) feel the least bit guilty? Not at all.

» **Computers move ideas, not paper.** Not long ago, when you wanted to send a message to someone, you hired a messenger. The messenger got on his or her horse and delivered your message personally. The message was on paper, parchment, a clay tablet, or whatever physical medium was available at the time.

  This whole process seems wasteful now, but that's only because you and I are sitting comfortably in the electronic age. Messages are ideas, and physical things like ink, paper, and horses have little or nothing to do with real ideas; they're just temporary carriers for ideas (even though people used them to carry ideas for several centuries). Nevertheless, the ideas themselves are paperless, horseless, and messengerless.

The neat thing about computers is that they carry ideas efficiently. They carry nothing but the ideas, a couple of photons, and a little electrical power. They do this with no muss, no fuss, and no extra physical baggage.

When you start dealing efficiently with ideas, something very nice happens. Suddenly, all the overhead is gone. Instead of pushing paper and trees, you're pushing numbers and concepts. Without the overhead, you can do things much faster and do things that are far more complex than ever before.

What You Can Do with Java

It would be so nice if all this complexity were free, but unfortunately, it isn't. Someone has to think hard and decide exactly what to ask the computer to do. After that thinking takes place, someone has to write a set of instructions for the computer to follow.

Given the current state of affairs, you can't write these instructions in English or any other language that people speak. Science fiction is filled with stories about people who say simple things to robots and get back disastrous, unexpected results. English and other such languages are unsuitable for communication with computers, for several reasons:

- **An English sentence can be misinterpreted.** "Chew one tablet three times a day until finished."
- **It's difficult to weave a very complicated command in English.** "Join flange A to protuberance B, making sure to connect only the outermost lip of flange A to the larger end of the protuberance B, while joining the middle and inner lips of flange A to grommet C."
- **An English sentence has lots of extra baggage.** "Sentence has unneeded words."
- **English is difficult to interpret.** "As part of this Publishing Agreement between John Wiley & Sons, Inc. ('Wiley') and the Author ('Barry Burd'), Wiley shall pay the sum of one-thousand-two-hundred-fifty-seven dollars and sixty-three cents ($1,257.63) to the Author for partial submittal of *Java For Dummies,* 7th Edition ('the Work')."

To tell a computer what to do, you have to use a special language to write terse, unambiguous instructions. A special language of this kind is called a *computer programming language.* A set of instructions written in such a language is called a *program.* When looked at as a big blob, these instructions are called *software* or *code.* Here's what code looks like when it's written in Java:

```
public class PayBarry {

    public static void main(String args[]) {
        double checkAmount = 1257.63;
        System.out.print("Pay to the order of ");
        System.out.print("Dr. Barry Burd ");
        System.out.print("$");
        System.out.println(checkAmount);
    }
}
```

Why You Should Use Java

It's time to celebrate! You've just picked up a copy of *Java For Dummies*, 7th Edition, and you're reading Chapter 1. At this rate, you'll be an expert Java programmer* in no time at all, so rejoice in your eventual success by throwing a big party.

To prepare for the party, I'll bake a cake. I'm lazy, so I'll use a ready-to-bake cake mix. Let me see . . . add water to the mix and then add butter and eggs — hey, wait! I just looked at the list of ingredients. What's MSG? And what about propylene glycol? That's used in antifreeze, isn't it?

I'll change plans and make the cake from scratch. Sure, it's a little harder, but that way I get exactly what I want.

Computer programs work the same way. You can use somebody else's program or write your own. If you use somebody else's program, you use whatever you get. When you write your own program, you can tailor the program especially for your needs.

Writing computer code is a big, worldwide industry. Companies do it, freelance professionals do it, hobbyists do it — all kinds of people do it. A typical big company has teams, departments, and divisions that write programs for the company. But you can write programs for yourself or someone else, for a living or for fun. In a recent estimate, the number of lines of code written each day by programmers in the United States alone exceeds the number of methane molecules on the planet Jupiter.** Take almost anything that can be done with a computer. With the right amount of time, you can write your own program to do it. (Of course, the "right amount of time" may be very long, but that's not the point. Many interesting and useful programs can be written in hours or even minutes.)

---

*In professional circles, a developer's responsibilities are usually broader than those of a programmer. But, in this book, I use the terms programmer and developer almost interchangeably.

**I made up this fact all by myself.

Getting Perspective: Where Java Fits In

Here's a brief history of modern computer programming:

- **1954–1957: FORTRAN is developed.**

  FORTRAN was the first modern computer programming language. For scientific programming, FORTRAN is a real racehorse. Year after year, FORTRAN is a leading language among computer programmers throughout the world.

- **1959: Grace Hopper at Remington Rand develops the COBOL programming language.**

  The letter *B* in COBOL stands for *Business,* and business is just what COBOL is all about. The language's primary feature is the processing of one record after another, one customer after another, or one employee after another.

  Within a few years after its initial development, COBOL became the most widely used language for business data processing.

- **1972: Dennis Ritchie at AT&T Bell Labs develops the C programming language.**

  The "look and feel" that you see in this book's examples comes from the C programming language. Code written in C uses curly braces, `if` statements, `for` statements, and so on.

  In terms of power, you can use C to solve the same problems that you can solve by using FORTRAN, Java, or any other modern programming language. (You can write a scientific calculator program in COBOL, but doing that sort of thing would feel really strange.) The difference between one programming language and another isn't power. The difference is ease and appropriateness of use. That's where the Java language excels.

- **1986: Bjarne Stroustrup (again at AT&T Bell Labs) develops C++.**

  Unlike its C language ancestor, the language C++ supports object-oriented programming. This support represents a huge step forward. (See the next section in this chapter.)

- **May 23, 1995: Sun Microsystems releases its first official version of the Java programming language.**

  Java improves upon the concepts in C++. Java's "Write Once, Run Anywhere" philosophy makes the language ideal for distributing code across the Internet.

  Additionally, Java is a great general-purpose programming language. With Java, you can write windowed applications, build and explore databases, control handheld devices, and more. Within five short years, the Java programming language had 2.5 million developers worldwide. (I know. I have a commemorative T-shirt to prove it.)

- **November 2000: The College Board announces that, starting in the year 2003, the Computer Science Advanced Placement exams will be based on Java.**

  Wanna know what that snot-nosed kid living down the street is learning in high school? You guessed it — Java.

- **2002: Microsoft introduces a new language, named C#.**

  Many of the C# language features come directly from features in Java.

- **June 2004: Sys-Con Media reports that the demand for Java programmers tops the demand for C++ programmers by 50 percent (**`http://java.sys-con.com/node/48507`**).**

  And there's more! The demand for Java programmers beats the combined demand for C++ and C# programmers by 8 percent. Java programmers are more employable than Visual Basic (VB) programmers by a whopping 190 percent.

- **2007: Google adopts Java as the primary language for creating apps on Android mobile devices.**

- **January 2010: Oracle Corporation purchases Sun Microsystems, bringing Java technology into the Oracle family of products.**

- **June 2010: *eWeek* ranks Java first among its "Top 10 Programming Languages to Keep You Employed" (**`www.eweek.com/c/a/Application-Development/Top-10-Programming-Languages-to-Keep-You-Employed-719257`**).**

- **2016: Java runs on 15 billion devices (**`http://java.com/en/about`**), with Android Java running on 87.6 percent of all mobile phones worldwide (**`www.idc.com/prodserv/smartphone-os-market-share.jsp`**).**

  Additionally, Java technology provides interactive capabilities to all Blu-ray devices and is the most popular programming language in the TIOBE Programming Community Index (`www.tiobe.com/index.php/content/paperinfo/tpci`), on PYPL: the PopularitY of Programming Language Index (`http://sites.google.com/site/pydatalog/pypl/PyPL-PopularitY-of-Programming-Language`), and on other indexes.

  Well, I'm impressed.

Object-Oriented Programming (OOP)

It's three in the morning. I'm dreaming about the history course that I failed in high school. The teacher is yelling at me, "You have two days to study for the final exam, but you won't remember to study. You'll forget and feel guilty, guilty, guilty."

Suddenly, the phone rings. I'm awakened abruptly from my deep sleep. (Sure, I disliked dreaming about the history course, but I like being awakened even less.) At first, I drop the telephone on the floor. After fumbling to pick it up, I issue a grumpy, "Hello, who's this?" A voice answers, "I'm a reporter from the *New York Times*. I'm writing an article about Java, and I need to know all about the programming language in five words or less. Can you explain it?"

My mind is too hazy. I can't think. So I say the first thing that comes to my mind and then go back to sleep.

Come morning, I hardly remember the conversation with the reporter. In fact, I don't remember how I answered the question. Did I tell the reporter where he could put his article about Java?

I put on my robe and rush out to my driveway. As I pick up the morning paper, I glance at the front page and see this 2-inch headline:

Burd Calls Java "A Great Object-Oriented Language"

Object-oriented languages

Java is object-oriented. What does that mean? Unlike languages, such as FORTRAN, that focus on giving the computer imperative "Do this/Do that" commands, object-oriented languages focus on data. Of course, object-oriented programs still tell the computer what to do. They start, however, by organizing the data, and the commands come later.

Object-oriented languages are better than "Do this/Do that" languages because they organize data in a way that helps people do all kinds of things with it. To modify the data, you can build on what you already have rather than scrap everything you've done and start over each time you need to do something new. Although computer programmers are generally smart people, they took a while to figure this out. For the full history lesson, see the sidebar "The winding road from FORTRAN to Java" (but I won't make you feel guilty if you don't read it).

THE WINDING ROAD FROM FORTRAN TO JAVA

In the mid-1950s, a team of people created a programming language named FORTRAN. It was a good language, but it was based on the idea that you should issue direct, imperative commands to the computer. "Do this, computer. Then do that, computer." (Of course, the commands in a real FORTRAN program were much more precise than "Do this" or "Do that.")

In the years that followed, teams developed many new computer languages, and many of the languages copied the FORTRAN "Do this/Do that" model. One of the more popular "Do this/Do that" languages went by the 1-letter name *C*. Of course, the "Do this/Do that" camp had some renegades. In languages named SIMULA and Smalltalk, programmers moved the imperative "Do this" commands into the background and concentrated on descriptions of data. In these languages, you didn't come right out and say, "Print a list of delinquent accounts." Instead, you began by saying, "This is what it means to be an account. An account has a name and a balance." Then you said, "This is how you ask an account whether it's delinquent." Suddenly, the data became king. An account was a thing that had a name, a balance, and a way of telling you whether it was delinquent.

Languages that focus first on the data are called *object-oriented* programming languages. These object-oriented languages make excellent programming tools. Here's why:

- Thinking first about the data makes you a good computer programmer.
- You can extend and reuse the descriptions of data over and over again. When you try to teach old FORTRAN programs new tricks, however, the old programs show how brittle they are. They break.

In the 1970s, object-oriented languages, such as SIMULA and Smalltalk, were buried in the computer hobbyist magazine articles. In the meantime, languages based on the old FORTRAN model were multiplying like rabbits.

So in 1986, a fellow named Bjarne Stroustrup created a language named C++. The C++ language became very popular because it mixed the old C language terminology with the improved object-oriented structure. Many companies turned their backs on the old FORTRAN/C programming style and adopted C++ as their standard.

(continued)

(continued)

But C++ had a flaw. Using C++, you could bypass all the object-oriented features and write a program by using the old FORTRAN/C programming style. When you started writing a C++ accounting program, you could take either fork in the road:

- Start by issuing direct "Do this" commands to the computer, saying the mathematical equivalent of "Print a list of delinquent accounts, and make it snappy."
- Choose the object-oriented approach and begin by describing what it means to be an account.

Some people said that C++ offered the best of both worlds, but others argued that the first world (the world of FORTRAN and C) shouldn't be part of modern programming. If you gave a programmer an opportunity to write code either way, the programmer would too often choose to write code the wrong way.

So in 1995, James Gosling of Sun Microsystems created the language named *Java.* In creating Java, Gosling borrowed the look and feel of C++. But Gosling took most of the old "Do this/Do that" features of C++ and threw them in the trash. Then he added features that made the development of objects smoother and easier. All in all, Gosling created a language whose object-oriented philosophy is pure and clean. When you program in Java, you have no choice but to work with objects. That's the way it should be.

Objects and their classes

In an object-oriented language, you use objects *and* classes to organize your data.

Imagine that you're writing a computer program to keep track of the houses in a new condominium development (still under construction). The houses differ only slightly from one another. Each house has a distinctive siding color, an indoor paint color, a kitchen cabinet style, and so on. In your object-oriented computer program, each house is an object.

But objects aren't the whole story. Although the houses differ slightly from one another, all the houses share the same list of characteristics. For instance, each house has a characteristic known as *siding color.* Each house has another characteristic known as *kitchen cabinet style.* In your object-oriented program, you need a master list containing all the characteristics that a house object can possess. This master list of characteristics is called a *class.*

So there you have it. Object-oriented programming is misnamed. It should be called "programming with classes and objects."

Now notice that I put the word *classes* first. How dare I do this! Well, maybe I'm not so crazy. Think again about a housing development that's under construction. Somewhere on the lot, in a rickety trailer parked on bare dirt, is a master list of characteristics known as a blueprint. An architect's blueprint is like an object-oriented programmer's class. A blueprint is a list of characteristics that each house will have. The blueprint says, "siding." The actual house object has gray siding. The blueprint says, "kitchen cabinet." The actual house object has Louis XIV kitchen cabinets.

The analogy doesn't end with lists of characteristics. Another important parallel exists between blueprints and classes. A year after you create the blueprint, you use it to build ten houses. It's the same with classes and objects. First, the programmer writes code to describe a class. Then when the program runs, the computer creates objects from the (blueprint) class.

So that's the real relationship between classes and objects. The programmer defines a class, and from the class definition, the computer makes individual objects.

What's so good about an object-oriented language?

Based on the preceding section's story about home building, imagine that you've already written a computer program to keep track of the building instructions for houses in a new development. Then, the big boss decides on a modified plan — a plan in which half the houses have three bedrooms and the other half have four.

If you use the old FORTRAN/C style of computer programming, your instructions look like this:

```
Dig a ditch for the basement.
Lay concrete around the sides of the ditch.
Put two-by-fours along the sides for the basement's frame.
...
```

This would be like an architect creating a long list of instructions instead of a blueprint. To modify the plan, you have to sort through the list to find the instructions for building bedrooms. To make things worse, the instructions could be scattered among pages 234, 394–410, 739, 10, and 2. If the builder had to decipher other peoples' complicated instructions, the task would be ten times harder.

Starting with a class, however, is like starting with a blueprint. If you decide to have both three- and four-bedroom houses, you can start with a blueprint called the house blueprint that has a ground floor and a second floor, but has no indoor walls drawn on the second floor. Then you make two more second-floor blueprints — one for the three-bedroom house and another for the four-bedroom house. (You name these new blueprints the *three-bedroom house* blueprint and the *four-bedroom house* blueprint.)

Your builder colleagues are amazed with your sense of logic and organization, but they have concerns. They pose a question. "You called one of the blueprints the 'three-bedroom house' blueprint. How can you do this if it's a blueprint for a second floor and not for a whole house?"

You smile knowingly and answer, "The three-bedroom house blueprint can say, 'For info about the lower floors, see the original house blueprint.' That way, the three-bedroom house blueprint describes a whole house. The four-bedroom house blueprint can say the same thing. With this setup, we can take advantage of all the work we already did to create the original house blueprint and save lots of money."

In the language of object-oriented programming, the three- and four-bedroom house classes are *inheriting* the features of the original house class. You can also say that the three- and four-bedroom house classes are *extending* the original house class. (See Figure 1-1.)

The original house class is called the *superclass* of the three- and four-bedroom house classes. In that vein, the three- and four-bedroom house classes are *subclasses* of the original house class. Put another way, the original house class is called the *parent class* of three- and four-bedroom house classes. The three- and four-bedroom house classes are *child classes* of the original house class. (Refer to Figure 1-1.)

Needless to say, your homebuilder colleagues are jealous. A crowd of homebuilders is mobbing around you to hear about your great ideas. So, at that moment, you drop one more bombshell: "By creating a class with subclasses, we can reuse the blueprint in the future. If someone comes along and wants a five-bedroom house, we can extend our original house blueprint by making a five-bedroom house blueprint. We'll never have to spend money for an original house blueprint again."

"But," says a colleague in the back row, "what happens if someone wants a different first-floor design? Do we trash the original house blueprint or start scribbling all over the original blueprint? That'll cost big bucks, won't it?"

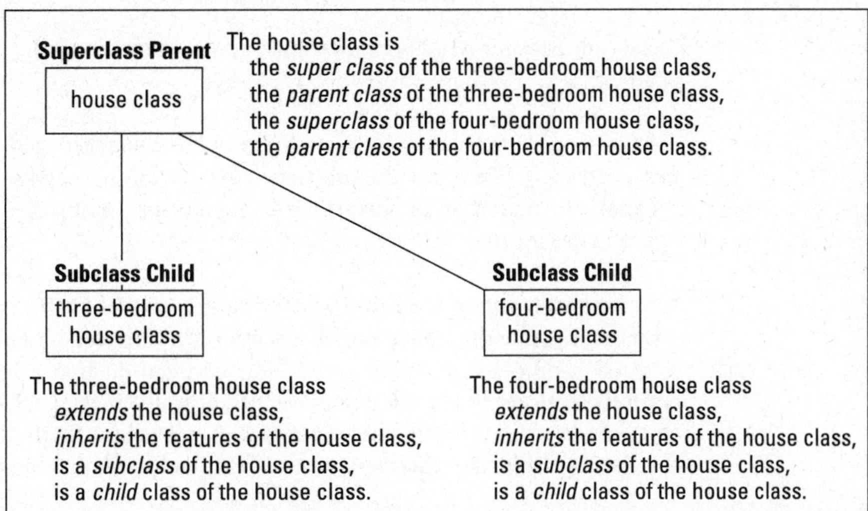

Superclass Parent
house class
The house class is
the super class of the three-bedroom house class,
the parent class of the three-bedroom house class,
the superclass of the four-bedroom house class,
the parent class of the four-bedroom house class.
Subclass Child
three-bedroom house class
Subclass Child
four-bedroom house class
The three-bedroom house class
extends the house class,
inherits the features of the house class,
is a subclass of the house class,
is a child class of the house class.
The four-bedroom house class
extends the house class,
inherits the features of the house class,
is a subclass of the house class,
is a child class of the house class.

FIGURE 1-1: Terminology in object-oriented programming.

In a confident tone, you reply, "We don't have to mess with the original house blueprint. If someone wants a Jacuzzi in his living room, we can make a new, small blueprint describing only the new living room and call this the *Jacuzzi-in-living-room house* blueprint. Then, this new blueprint can refer to the original house blueprint for info on the rest of the house (the part that's not in the living room)." In the language of object-oriented programming, the Jacuzzi-in-living-room house blueprint still *extends* the original house blueprint. The Jacuzzi blueprint is still a subclass of the original house blueprint. In fact, all the terminology about superclass, parent class, and child class still applies. The only thing that's new is that the Jacuzzi blueprint *overrides* the living room features in the original house blueprint.

In the days before object-oriented languages, the programming world experienced a crisis in software development. Programmers wrote code, and then discovered new needs, and then had to trash their code and start from scratch. This problem happened over and over again because the code that the programmers were writing couldn't be reused. Object-oriented programming changed all this for the better (and, as Burd said, Java is "A Great Object-Oriented Language").

Refining your understanding of classes and objects

When you program in Java, you work constantly with classes and objects. These two ideas are really important. That's why, in this chapter, I hit you over the head with one analogy after another about classes and objects.

Close your eyes for a minute and think about what it means for something to be a chair . . . .

A chair has a seat, a back, and legs. Each seat has a shape, a color, a degree of softness, and so on. These are the properties that a chair possesses. What I describe is *chairness* — the notion of something being a chair. In object-oriented terminology, I'm describing the `Chair` class.

Now peek over the edge of this book's margin and take a minute to look around your room. (If you're not sitting in a room right now, fake it.)

Several chairs are in the room, and each chair is an object. Each of these objects is an example of that ethereal thing called the `Chair` class. So that's how it works — the class is the idea of *chairness*, and each individual chair is an object.

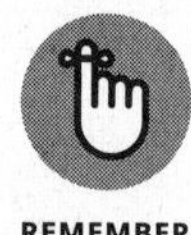

REMEMBER

A class isn't quite a collection of things. Instead, a class is the idea behind a certain kind of thing. When I talk about the class of chairs in your room, I'm talking about the fact that each chair has legs, a seat, a color, and so on. The colors may be different for different chairs in the room, but that doesn't matter. When you talk about a class of things, you're focusing on the properties that each of the things possesses.

It makes sense to think of an object as being a concrete instance of a class. In fact, the official terminology is consistent with this thinking. If you write a Java program in which you define a `Chair` class, each actual chair (the chair that you're sitting on, the empty chair right next to you, and so on) is called an *instance* of the `Chair` class.

Here's another way to think about a class. Imagine a table displaying all three of your bank accounts. (See Table 1-1.)

TABLE 1-1 **A Table of Accounts**

Account Number	Type	Balance
16-13154-22864-7	Checking	174.87
1011 1234 2122 0000	Credit	–471.03
16-17238-13344-7	Savings	247.38

Think of the table's column headings as a class, and think of each row of the table as an object. The table's column headings describe the `Account` class.

According to the table's column headings, each account has an account number, a type, and a balance. Rephrased in the terminology of object-oriented programming, each object in the `Account` class (that is, each instance of the `Account` class) has an account number, a type, and a balance. So, the bottom row of the table is an object with account number *16-17238-13344-7*. This same object has type *Savings* and a balance of *247.38*. If you opened a new account, you would have another object, and the table would grow an additional row. The new object would be an instance of the same `Account` class.

What's Next?

This chapter is filled with general descriptions of things. A general description is good when you're just getting started, but you don't really understand things until you get to know some specifics. That's why the next several chapters deal with specifics.

So please, turn the page. The next chapter can't wait for you to read it.

» **Selecting the version of Java that's right for you**

» **Preparing to write and run Java programs**

Chapter 2
All about Software

The best way to get to know Java is to do Java. When you're doing Java, you're writing, testing, and running your own Java programs. This chapter gets you ready to do Java by describing the *general* software setup — the software that you must have on your computer whether you run Windows, Mac, Linux, or Joe's Private Operating System. This chapter *doesn't* describe the specific setup instructions for Windows, for a Mac, or for any other system.

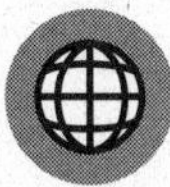

For setup instructions that are specific to your system, visit this book's website (`www.allmycode.com/JavaForDummies`).

Quick-Start Instructions

If you're a seasoned veteran of computers and computing (whatever that means), and if you're too jumpy to get detailed instructions from this book's website, you can try installing the required software by following this section's general instructions. The instructions work for many computers, but not all. And this section provides no detailed steps, no if-this-then-do-that alternatives, and no this-works-but-you're-better-off-doing-something-else tips.

To prepare your computer for writing Java programs, follow these steps:

1. **Install the Java Development Kit.**

   To do so, visit `www.oracle.com/technetwork/java/javase/downloads`.

   Follow the instructions at that website to download and install the newest Java SE JDK.

   REMEMBER

   Look for the Standard Edition (SE). Don't bother with the Enterprise Edition (EE) or any other such edition. Also, go for the JDK, not the JRE. If you see a code number, such as 9u3, this stands for "the 3rd update of Java 9." Generally, anything marked Java 9 or later is good for running the examples in this book.

2. **Install an integrated development environment.**

   An *integrated development environment* (IDE) is a program to help you compose and test new software. For this book's examples, you can use almost any IDE that supports Java.

   Here's a list of the most popular Java IDEs:

   - *Eclipse*

     According to `www.baeldung.com/java-ides-2016`, 48.2 percent of the world's Java programmers used the Eclipse IDE in mid-2016.

     To download and use Eclipse, follow the instructions at `http://eclipse.org/downloads`. Eclipse's download page may offer you several different packages, including Eclipse for Java EE, Eclipse for JavaScript, Eclipse for Java and DSL, and others. To run this book's examples, you need a relatively small Eclipse package — the Eclipse IDE for Java Developers.

     Eclipse is free for commercial and noncommercial use.

   - *IntelliJ IDEA*

     In Baeldung's survey of Java IDEs (`http://www.baeldung.com/java-ides-2016`), IntelliJ IDEA comes in a close second, with 43.6 percent of all programmers onboard.

     When you visit `www.jetbrains.com/idea`, you can download the Community Edition (which is free) or the Ultimate Edition (which isn't free). To run this book's examples, you can use the Community Edition. You can even use the Community Edition to create commercial software!

- *NetBeans*

  Baeldung's survey of Java IDEs (`http://www.baeldung.com/java-ides-2016`) gives NetBeans a mere 5.9 percent. But NetBeans is Oracle's official Java IDE. If the site offers you a choice of download bundles, choose the Java SE bundle.

  To get your own copy of NetBeans, visit `https://netbeans.org/downloads`.

  NetBeans is free for commercial and noncommercial use.

3. **Test your installed software.**

   What you do in this step depends on which IDE you choose in Step 2. Anyway, here are some general instructions:

   a. Launch your IDE (Eclipse, IntelliJ IDEA, NetBeans, or whatever).

   b. In the IDE, create a new Java project.

   c. Within the Java project, create a new Java class named `Displayer`. (Selecting File ⇨ New ⇨ Class works in most IDEs.)

   d. Edit the new `Displayer.java` file by typing the code from Listing 3-1 (the first code listing in Chapter 3).

   For most IDEs, you add the code into a big (mostly blank) editor pane. Try to type the code exactly as you see it in Listing 3-1. If you see an uppercase letter, type an uppercase letter. Do the same with all lowercase letters.

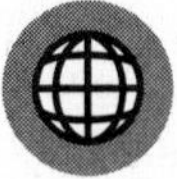

   What? You say you don't want to type a bunch of code from the book? Well, all right then! Visit this book's website (`www.allmycode.com/JavaForDummies`) to find out how to download all the code examples and load them into the IDE of your choice.

   e. Run `Displayer.java` and check to make sure that the run's output reads `You'll love Java!`.

That's it! But remember: Not everyone (computer geek or not) can follow these skeletal instructions flawlessly. So you have several alternatives:

» **Visit this book's website.**

Do not pass Go. Do not try this section's quick-start instructions. Follow the more detailed instructions that you find at `www.allmycode.com/JavaForDummies`.

» **Try this section's quick-start instructions.**

You can't hurt anything by trying. If you accidentally install the wrong software, you can probably leave the wrong software on your computer. (You don't have to uninstall it.) If you're not sure whether you've installed the software correctly, you can always fall back on my website's detailed instructions.

» **E-mail your questions to me at** `JavaForDummies@allmycode.com`**.**

» **Tweet me at** `@allmycode`**.**

» **Visit my** `/allmycode` **Facebook page.**

I like hearing from readers.

What You Install on Your Computer

I once met a tool-and-die maker. He used tools to make tools (and dies). I was happy to meet him because I knew that, one day, I'd make an analogy between computer programmers and tool-and-die makers.

A computer programmer uses existing programs as tools to create new programs. The existing programs and new programs might perform very different kinds of tasks. For example, a Java program (a program that you create) might keep track of a business's customers. To create that customer-tracking program, you might use an existing program that looks for errors in your Java code. This general-purpose error-finding program can find errors in any kind of Java code — customer-tracking code, weather-predicting code, gaming code, or the code for an app on your mobile phone.

So how many tools do you need for creating Java programs? As a novice, you need three tools:

» **You need a compiler.**

A *compiler* takes the Java code that you write and turns that code into a bunch of instructions called *bytecode*.

Humans can't readily compose or decipher bytecode instructions. But certain software that you run on your computer can interpret and carry out bytecode instructions.

» **You need a Java Virtual Machine (JVM).**

A *Java Virtual Machine* is a piece of software. A Java Virtual Machine interprets and carries out bytecode instructions.

» **You need an integrated development environment (IDE).**

An *integrated development environment* helps you manage your Java code and provides convenient ways for you to write, compile, and run your code.

To be honest, you don't actually *need* an integrated development environment. In fact, some programmers take pride in using plain, old text editors such as Windows Notepad, Macintosh TextEdit, or the vim editor in Linux. But, as a novice programmer, a full-featured IDE makes your life much, much easier.

The World Wide Web has free, downloadable versions of each of these tools:

» When you download the Java SE JDK from Oracle's website (`www.oracle.com/technetwork/java/javase/downloads/index.html`), you get the compiler and the JVM.

» When you visit the Eclipse (`www.eclipse.org/downloads`), IntelliJ IDEA (`www.jetbrains.com/idea`, or NetBeans (`https://netbeans.org/downloads`) site, you get an IDE.

You may find variations on the picture that I paint in the preceding two bullets. Many IDEs come with their own JVMs, and Oracle's website may offer a combined JDK+NetBeans bundle. Nevertheless, the picture that I paint with these bullets is useful and reliable. When you follow my instructions, you might end up with two copies of the JVM, or two IDEs, but that's okay. You never know when you'll need a spare.

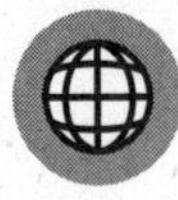

This chapter provides background information about software you need on your computer. But the chapter contains absolutely no detailed instructions to help you install the software. For detailed instructions, visit this book's website (`www.allmycode.com/JavaForDummies`).

The rest of this chapter describes compilers, JVMs, and IDEs.

What is a compiler?

A compiler takes the Java code that you write and turns that code into a bunch of instructions called bytecode.

—*BARRY BURD*, JAVA FOR DUMMIES, *7TH EDITION*

You're a human being. (Sure, every rule has exceptions. But if you're reading this book, you're probably human.) Anyway, humans can write and comprehend the code in Listing 2-1.

LISTING 2-1: Looking for a Vacant Room

```
// This is part of a Java program.
// It's not a complete Java program.
roomNum = 1;
while (roomNum < 100) {
    if (guests[roomNum] == 0) {
        out.println("Room " + roomNum + " is available.");
        exit(0);
    } else {
        roomNum++;
    }
}
out.println("No vacancy");
```

The Java code in Listing 2-1 checks for vacancies in a small hotel (a hotel with room numbers 1 to 99). You can't run the code in Listing 2-1 without adding several additional lines. But here in Chapter 2, those additional lines aren't important. What's important is that, by staring at the code, squinting a bit, and looking past all the code's strange punctuation, you can see what the code is trying to do:

```
Set the room number to 1.
As long as the room number is less than 100,
    Check the number of guests in the room.
    If the number of guests in the room is 0, then
        report that the room is available,
        and stop.
    Otherwise,
        prepare to check the next room by
        adding 1 to the room number.
If you get to the nonexistent room number 100, then
    report that there are no vacancies.
```

If you don't see the similarities between Listing 2-1 and its English equivalent, don't worry. You're reading *Java For Dummies,* 7th Edition, and like most human beings, you can learn to read and write the code in Listing 2-1. The code in Listing 2-1 is called *Java source code.*

So here's the catch: Computers aren't human beings. Computers don't normally follow instructions like the instructions in Listing 2-1. That is, computers don't follow Java source code instructions. Instead, computers follow cryptic instructions like the ones in Listing 2-2.

LISTING 2-2: **Listing 2-1 Translated into Java Bytecode**

```
aload_0
iconst_1
putfield Hotel/roomNum I
goto 32
aload_0
getfield Hotel/guests [I
aload_0
getfield Hotel/roomNum I
iaload
ifne 26
getstatic java/lang/System/out Ljava/io/PrintStream;
new java/lang/StringBuilder
dup
ldc "Room "
invokespecial java/lang/StringBuilder/<init>(Ljava/lang/String;)V
aload_0
getfield Hotel/roomNum I
invokevirtual java/lang/StringBuilder/append(I)Ljava/lang/StringBuilder;
ldc " is available."
invokevirtual
  java/lang/StringBuilder/append(Ljava/lang/String;)Ljava/lang/StringBuilder;
invokevirtual java/lang/StringBuilder/toString()Ljava/lang/String;
invokevirtual java/io/PrintStream/println(Ljava/lang/String;)V
iconst_0
invokestatic java/lang/System/exit(I)V
goto 32
aload_0
dup
getfield Hotel/roomNum I
iconst_1
iadd
putfield Hotel/roomNum I
aload_0
getfield Hotel/roomNum I
```

(continued)

LISTING 2-2: *(continued)*

```
bipush 100
if_icmplt 5
getstatic java/lang/System/out Ljava/io/PrintStream;
ldc "No vacancy"
invokevirtual java/io/PrintStream/println(Ljava/lang/String;)V
return
```

The instructions in Listing 2-2 aren't Java source code instructions. They're *Java bytecode* instructions. When you write a Java program, you write source code instructions (like the instructions in Listing 2-1). After writing the source code, you run a program (that is, you apply a tool) to your source code. The program is a *compiler.* The compiler translates your source code instructions into Java bytecode instructions. In other words, the compiler takes code that you can write and understand (like the code in Listing 2-1) and translates it into code that a computer has a fighting chance of carrying out (like the code in Listing 2-2).

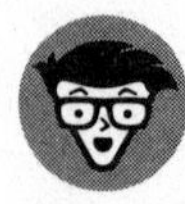
TECHNICAL STUFF

You might put your source code in a file named `Hotel.java`. If so, the compiler probably puts the Java bytecode in another file named `Hotel.class`. Normally, you don't bother looking at the bytecode in the `Hotel.class` file. In fact, the compiler doesn't encode the `Hotel.class` file as ordinary text, so you can't examine the bytecode with an ordinary editor. If you try to open `Hotel.class` with Notepad, TextEdit, KWrite, or even Microsoft Word, you'll see nothing but dots, squiggles, and other gobbledygook. To create Listing 2-2, I had to apply yet another tool to my `Hotel.class` file. That tool displays a text-like version of a Java bytecode file. I used Ando Saabas's Java Bytecode Editor (`www.cs.ioc.ee/~ando/jbe`).

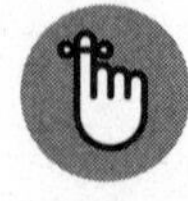
REMEMBER

No one (except for a few crazy programmers in some isolated labs in faraway places) writes Java bytecode. You run software (a compiler) to create Java bytecode. The only reason to look at Listing 2-2 is to understand what a hard worker your computer is.

What is a Java Virtual Machine?

A Java Virtual Machine is a piece of software. A Java Virtual Machine interprets and carries out bytecode instructions.

—*BARRY BURD,* JAVA FOR DUMMIES, *7TH EDITION*

In the preceding "What is a compiler?" section, I make a big fuss about computers following instructions like the ones in Listing 2-2. As fusses go, it's a very nice fuss. But if you don't read every fussy word, you may be misguided. The exact wording is "... computers follow cryptic instructions *like* the ones in Listing 2-2." The instructions in Listing 2-2 are a lot like instructions that a computer can execute, but generally, computers don't execute Java bytecode instructions. Instead, each kind of computer processor has its own set of executable instructions, and each computer operating system uses the processor's instructions in a slightly different way.

Here's a hypothetical situation: The year is 1992 (a few years before Java was made public) and you run the Linux operating system on a computer that has an old Pentium processor. Your friend runs Linux on a computer with a different kind of processor — a PowerPC processor. (In the 1990s, Intel Corporation made Pentium processors, and IBM made PowerPC processors.)

Listing 2-3 contains a set of instructions to display `Hello world!` on the computer screen.* The instructions work on a Pentium processor running the Linux operating system.

LISTING 2-3: A Simple Program for a Pentium Processor

```
.data
msg:
        .ascii  "Hello, world!\n"
        len = . - msg
.text
    .global _start
_start:
        movl    $len,%edx
        movl    $msg,%ecx
        movl    $1,%ebx
        movl    $4,%eax
        int     $0x80

        movl    $0,%ebx
        movl    $1,%eax
        int     $0x80
```

*I paraphrase these Intel instructions from Konstantin Boldyshev's Linux Assembly HOWTO (`http://tldp.org/HOWTO/Assembly-HOWTO/hello.html`).

Listing 2-4 contains another set of instructions to display `Hello world!` on the screen.** The instructions in Listing 2-4 work on a PowerPC processor running Linux.

LISTING 2-4: A Simple Program for a PowerPC Processor

```
.data
msg:
        .string "Hello, world!\n"
        len = . - msg
.text
        .global _start
_start:
        li      0,4
        li      3,1
        lis     4,msg@ha
        addi    4,4,msg@l
        li      5,len
        sc

        li      0,1
        li      3,1
        sc
```

The instructions in Listing 2-3 run smoothly on a Pentium processor. But these instructions mean nothing to a PowerPC processor. Likewise, the instructions in Listing 2-4 run nicely on a PowerPC, but these same instructions are complete gibberish to a computer with a Pentium processor. So your friend's PowerPC software might not be available on your computer. And your Intel computer's software might not run at all on your friend's computer.

Now go to your cousin's house. Your cousin's computer has a Pentium processor (just like yours), but your cousin's computer runs Windows instead of Linux. What does your cousin's computer do when you feed it the Pentium code in Listing 2-3? It screams, "Not a valid Win32 application" or "Windows can't open this file." What a mess!

**I paraphrase the PowerPC code from Hollis Blanchard's PowerPC Assembly page (`www.ibm.com/developerworks/library/l-ppc`). Hollis also reviewed and critiqued this "What is a Java Virtual Machine?" section for me. Thank you, Hollis.

Java bytecode creates order from all this chaos. Unlike the code in Listings 2-3 and 2-4, Java bytecode isn't specific to one kind of processor or to one operating system. Instead, any kind of computer can have a Java Virtual Machine, and Java bytecode instructions run on any computer's Java Virtual Machine. The JVM that runs on a Pentium with Linux translates Java bytecode instructions into the kind of code you see in Listing 2-3. And the JVM that runs on a PowerPC with Linux translates Java bytecode instructions into the kind of code you see in Listing 2-4.

If you write a Java program and compile that Java program into bytecode, then the JVM on your computer can run the bytecode, the JVM on your friend's computer can run the bytecode, the JVM on your grandmother's supercomputer can run the bytecode, and with any luck, the JVM on your cellphone or tablet can run the bytecode.

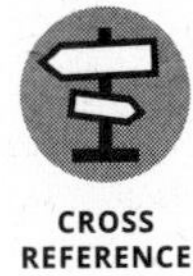
CROSS REFERENCE

For a look at some Java bytecode, see Listing 2-2. But remember: You never have to write or decipher Java bytecode. Writing bytecode is the compiler's job. Deciphering bytecode is the Java Virtual Machine's job.

With Java, you can take a bytecode file that you created with a Windows computer, copy the bytecode to who-knows-what kind of computer, and then run the bytecode with no trouble at all. That's one of the many reasons why Java has become popular so quickly. This outstanding feature, which gives you the ability to run code on many different kinds of computers, is called *portability.*

What makes Java bytecode so versatile? This fantastic universality enjoyed by Java bytecode programs comes from the Java Virtual Machine. The Java Virtual Machine is one of those three tools that you must have on your computer.

Imagine that you're the Windows representative to the United Nations Security Council. (See Figure 2-1.) The Macintosh representative is seated to your right, and the Linux representative is on your left. (Naturally, you don't get along with either of these people. You're always cordial to one another, but you're never sincere. What do you expect? It's politics!) The distinguished representative from Java is at the podium. The Java representative is speaking in bytecode, and neither you nor your fellow ambassadors (Mac and Linux) understand a word of Java bytecode.

But each of you has an interpreter. Your interpreter translates from bytecode to Windows while the Java representative speaks. Another interpreter translates from bytecode to Macintosh-ese. And a third interpreter translates bytecode into Linux-speak.

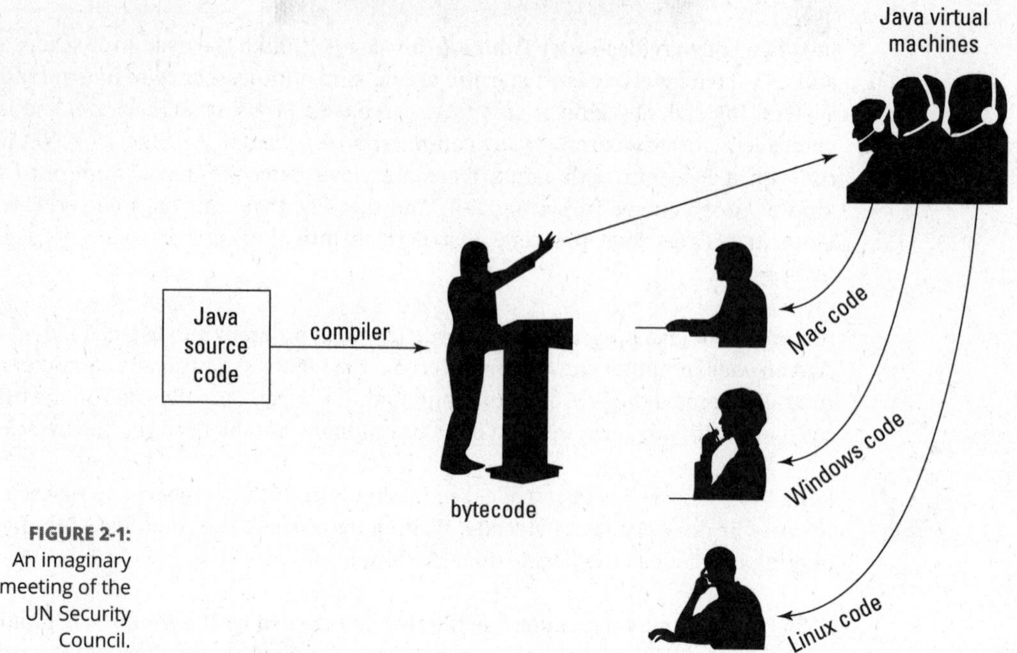

FIGURE 2-1: An imaginary meeting of the UN Security Council.

Think of your interpreter as a virtual ambassador. The interpreter doesn't really represent your country, but the interpreter performs one of the important tasks that a real ambassador performs. The interpreter listens to bytecode on your behalf. The interpreter does what you would do if your native language were Java bytecode. The interpreter pretends to be the Windows ambassador and sits through the boring bytecode speech, taking in every word and processing each word in some way or another.

You have an interpreter — a virtual ambassador. In the same way, a Windows computer runs its own bytecode-interpreting software. That software is the Java Virtual Machine.

A Java Virtual Machine is a proxy, an errand boy, a go-between. The JVM serves as an interpreter between Java's run-anywhere bytecode and your computer's own system. While it runs, the JVM walks your computer through the execution of bytecode instructions. The JVM examines your bytecode, bit by bit, and carries out the instructions described in the bytecode. The JVM interprets bytecode for your Windows system, your Mac, or your Linux box, or for whatever kind of computer you're using. That's a good thing. It's what makes Java programs more portable than programs in any other language.

WHAT ON EARTH IS JAVA 2 STANDARD EDITION 1.2?

If you poke around the web looking for Java tools, you find things with all kinds of strange names. You find the Java Development Kit, the Software Development Kit, the Java Runtime Environment, and other confusing names.

- The names *Java Development Kit* (JDK) and *Software Development Kit* (SDK) stand for different versions of the same toolset — a toolset whose key component is a Java compiler.
- The name *Java Runtime Environment* (JRE) stands for a toolset whose key component is a Java Virtual Machine.

  If you install the JDK on your computer, the JRE comes along with it. You can also get the JRE on its own. In fact, you can have many combinations of the JDK and JRE on your computer. For example, my Windows computer currently has JDK 1.6, JDK 1.8, and JRE 8 in its `c:\program files\Java directory` and has JDK 9 in its `c:\program files (x86)\Java directory`. Only occasionally do I run into any version conflicts. If you suspect that you're experiencing a version conflict, it's best to uninstall all JDK and JRE versions except the latest (for example, JDK 9 and JRE 9).

The numbering of Java versions can be confusing. Instead of "Java 1," "Java 2," and "Java 3," the numbering of Java versions winds through an obstacle course. This sidebar's figure describes the development of new Java versions over time. Each Java version has several names. The *product version* is an official name that's used for the world in general, and the *developer version* is a number that identifies versions so that programmers can keep track of them. (In casual conversation, programmers use all kinds of names for the various Java versions.) The *code name* is a more playful name that identifies a version while it's being created.

The asterisks in the figure mark changes in the formulation of Java product-version names. Back in 1996, the product versions were *Java Development Kit 1.0* and *Java Development Kit 1.1*. In 1998, someone decided to christen the product *Java 2 Standard Edition 1.2*, which confuses everyone to this day. At the time, anyone using the term *Java Development Kit* was asked to use *Software Development Kit* (SDK) instead.

(continued)

(continued)

In 2004 the *1.* business went away from the platform version name, and in 2006 Java platform names lost the *2* and the *.0*.

By far the most significant changes for Java programmers came about in 2004. With the release of J2SE 5.0, the overseers of Java made changes to the language by adding new features — features such as generic types, annotations, and the enhanced `for` statement. (To see Java annotations in action, go to Chapters 8, 9, and 16. For examples of the use of the enhanced `for` statement and generic types, see Chapters 11 and 12.)

Most of the programs in this book run only with Java 5.0 or later. They don't run with any version earlier than Java 5.0. Particularly, they don't run with Java 1.4 or Java 1.4.2. Some of this book's examples don't run with Java 9 or lower. But don't worry too much about Java version numbers. Java 6 or 7 is better than no Java at all. You can learn a lot about Java without having the latest Java version.

	Platform	Codename	Features
1995	(Beta)		
1996	**JDK* 1.0**		
1997	**JDK 1.1**		Inner classes, Java Beans, Reflection
1998	**J2SE* 1.2**	Playground	Swing classes for creation of GUI interfaces
1999			
2000	**J2SE 1.3**	Kestrel	Java Naming and Directory interface (JNDI)
2001			
2002	**J2SE 1.4**	Merlin	New I/O, regular expressions, XML parsing
2003			
2004	**J2SE 5.0**	Tiger	Generic types, annotations, enum types, varargs, enhanced for
2005			statement, static imports, new concurrency classes
2006	**Java SE* 6**	Mustang	Scripting language support, performance enhancements
2007			
2008			
2009			
2010			
2011	**Java SE 7**	Dolphin	Strings in switch statement, catching multiple exceptions
2012			try statement with resources, integration with JavaFX
2013			
2014	**Java SE 8**		Lambda expressions
2015			
2016			
2017	**Java SE 9**		Modularity with Project Jigsaw, interactive coding with JShell

Developing software

All this has happened before, and it will all happen again.
—PETER PAN *(J.M. BARRIE) AND* BATTLESTAR GALACTICA
(2003–2009, NBC UNIVERSAL)

When you create a Java program, you repeat the same steps over and over again. Figure 2-2 illustrates the cycle.

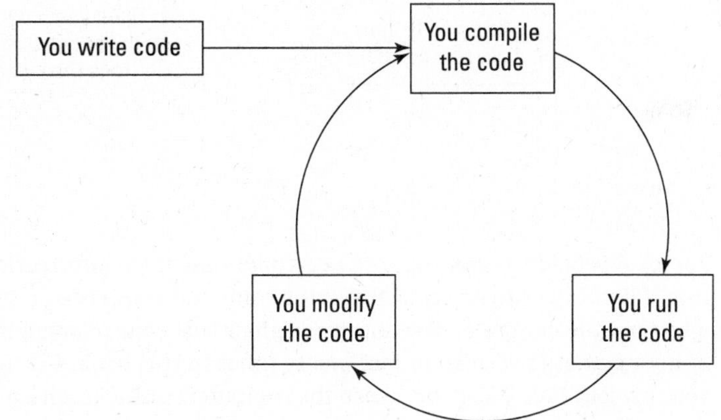

FIGURE 2-2: Developing a Java program.

First, you write a program. After writing the first draft, you repeatedly compile, run, and modify the program. With a little experience, the compile and run steps become very easy. In many cases, one mouse click starts the compilation or the run.

However, writing the first draft and modifying the code are not 1-click tasks. Developing code requires time and concentration.

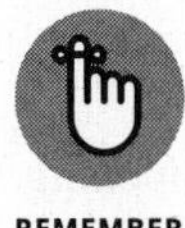
REMEMBER

Never be discouraged when the first draft of your code doesn't work. For that matter, never be discouraged when the 25th draft of your code doesn't work. Rewriting code is one of the most important things you can do (aside from ensuring world peace).

For detailed instructions on compiling and running Java programs, visit this book's website (`www.allmycode.com/JavaForDummies`).

When people talk about writing programs, they use the wording in Figure 2-2. They say, "You compile the code" and "You run the code." But the "you" isn't always accurate, and the "code" differs slightly from one part of the cycle to the next. Figure 2-3 describes the cycle from Figure 2-2 in a bit more detail.

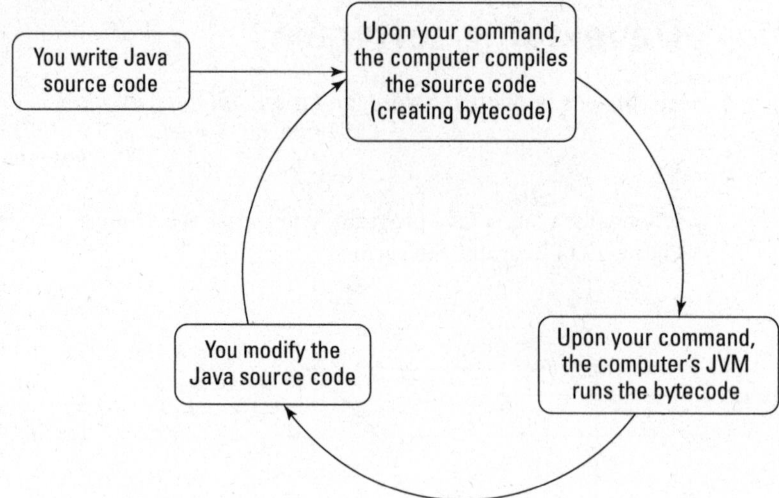

FIGURE 2-3: Who does what with which code?

TIP

For most people's needs, Figure 2-3 contains too much information. If I click a Run icon, I don't have to remember that the computer runs code on my behalf. And for all I care, the computer can run my original Java code or some bytecode knockoff of my original Java code. In fact, many times in this book, I casually write "when you run your Java code," or "when the computer runs your Java program." You can live a very happy life without looking at Figure 2-3. The only use for Figure 2-3 is to help you if the loose wording in Figure 2-2 confuses you. If Figure 2-2 doesn't confuse you, ignore Figure 2-3.

What is an integrated development environment?

"An integrated development environment helps you manage your Java code and provides convenient ways for you to write, compile, and run your code."

—*BARRY BURD,* JAVA FOR DUMMIES, *7TH EDITION*

In the olden days, writing and running a Java program involved opening several windows — a window for typing the program, another window for running the program, and maybe a third window to keep track of all the code you've written. (See Figure 2-4.)

An integrated development environment seamlessly combines all this functionality into one well-organized application. (See Figure 2-5.)

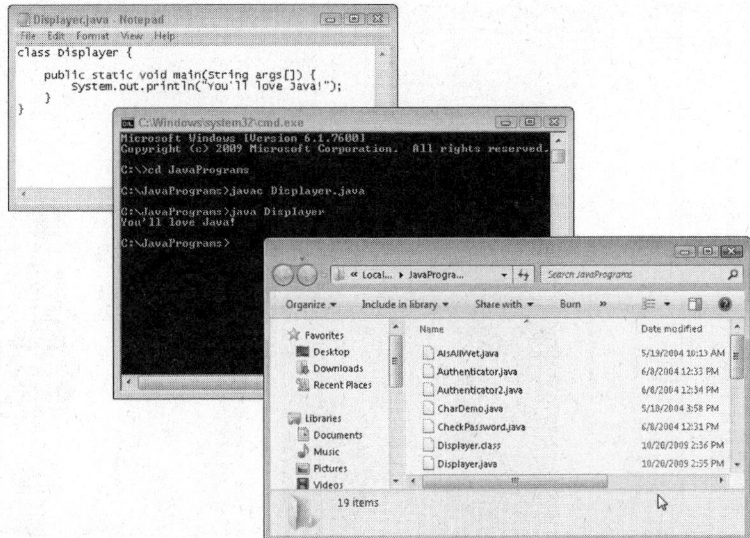

FIGURE 2-4: Developing code without an integrated development environment.

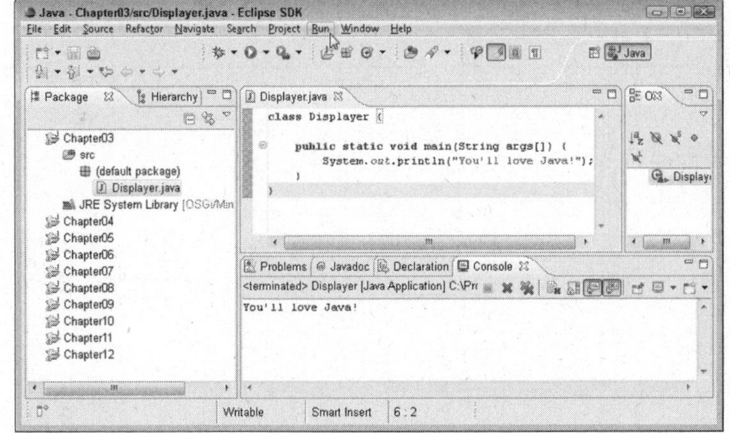

FIGURE 2-5: Developing code with the Eclipse integrated development environment.

Java has its share of integrated development environments such as Eclipse, IntelliJ IDEA, and NetBeans. Many environments have drag-and-drop components so that you can design your graphical interface visually. (See Figure 2-6.)

To run a program, you might click a toolbar button or choose Run from a menu. To compile a program, you might not have to do anything at all. (You might not even have to issue a command. Some IDEs compile your code automatically while you type it.)

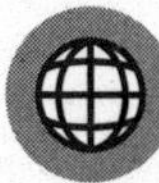

For help with installing and using an integrated development environment, see this book's website (`www.allmycode.com/JavaForDummies`).

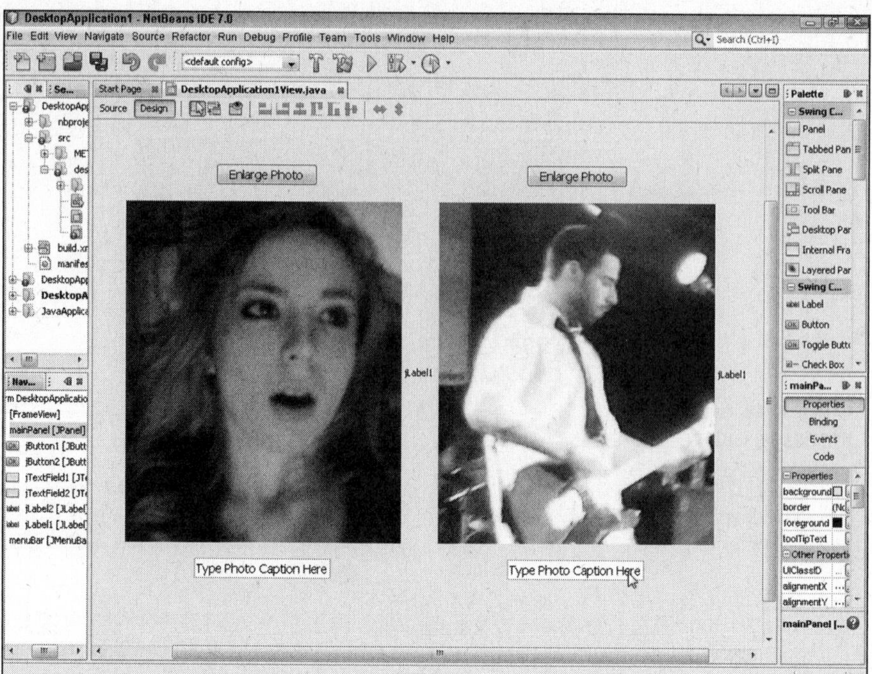

FIGURE 2-6: Using the drag-and-drop Swing GUI Builder in the NetBeans IDE.

- Taking a first glance at Java code
- Understanding the parts of a simple program
- Documenting your code

Chapter 3
Using the Basic Building Blocks

"Все мысли, которые имеют огромные последствия всегда просты. (All great ideas are simple.)"

—LEO TOLSTOY

The quotation applies to all kinds of things — things like life, love, and computer programming. That's why this chapter takes a multilayered approach. In this chapter, you get your first details about Java programming. And in discovering details, you'll see the simplicities.

Speaking the Java Language

If you try to picture in your mind the entire English language, what do you see? Maybe you see words, words, words. (That's what Hamlet saw.) Looking at the language under a microscope, you see one word after another. The bunch-of-words image is fine, but if you step back a bit, you may see two other things:

- The language's grammar
- Thousands of expressions, sayings, idioms, and historical names

The first category (the grammar) includes rules like, "The verb agrees with the noun in number and person." The second category (expressions, sayings, and stuff) includes knowledge like, "Julius Caesar was a famous Roman emperor, so don't name your son Julius Caesar, unless you want him to get beaten up every day after school."

The Java programming language has all the aspects of a spoken language like English. Java has words, grammar, commonly used names, stylistic idioms, and other such elements.

The grammar and the common names

The people at Sun Microsystems who created Java thought of Java as having two parts. Just as English has its grammar and commonly used names, the Java programming language has its specification (its grammar) and its application programming interface (its commonly used names). Whenever I write Java programs, I keep two important pieces of documentation — one for each part of the language — on my desk:

» **The Java Language Specification:** This documentation includes rules like this: "Always put an open parenthesis after the word *for*" and "Use an asterisk to multiply two numbers."

» **The application programming interface:** Java's application programming interface (API) contains thousands of names that were added to Java after the language's grammar was defined. These names range from the commonplace to the exotic. For example, one name — the name *JFrame* — represents a window on your computer's screen. A more razzle-dazzle name — *pow* — helps you raise 5 to the tenth power, or raise whatever to the whatever else power. Other names help you listen for the user's button clicks, query databases, and do all kinds of useful things.

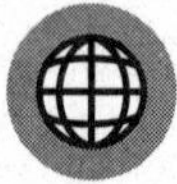

You can download the language specification, the API documents, and all the other Java documentation (or view the documents online) by poking around at `http://docs.oracle.com/javase/specs`.

The first part of Java, the language specification, is relatively small. That doesn't mean you won't take plenty of time finding out how to use the rules in the language specification. Other programming languages, however, have double, triple, or ten times the number of rules.

The second part of Java — the API — can be intimidating because it's so large. The API contains thousands and thousands of names and keeps growing with each new Java language release. Pretty scary, eh? Well, the good news is that you don't have to memorize anything in the API. Nothing. None of it. You can look up the stuff you need to use in the documentation and ignore the stuff you don't need. What you use often, you'll remember. What you don't use often, you'll forget (like any other programmer).

No one knows all there is to know about the Java API. If you're a Java programmer who frequently writes programs that open new windows, you know how to use the API `JFrame` class. If you seldom write programs that open windows, the first few times you need to create a window, you can look up the `JFrame` class in the API documentation. My guess is that if you prevented a typical Java programmer from looking up anything in the API documentation, the programmer would be able to use less than 2 percent of all the names in the Java API.

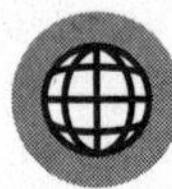

You may love the *For Dummies* style, but unfortunately, Java's official API documentation isn't written that way. The API documentation is both concise and precise. For some help deciphering the API documentation's language and style, see this book's website (`www.allmycode.com/JavaForDummies`).

In a way, nothing about the Java API is special. Whenever you write a Java program — even the smallest, simplest Java program — you create a class that's on par with any of the classes defined in the official Java API. The API is just a set of classes and other names that were created by ordinary programmers who happen to participate in the official Java Community Process (JCP) and in the OpenJDK Project. Unlike the names you create, the names in the API are distributed with every version of Java. (I'm assuming that you, the reader, are not a participant in the Java Community Process or the OpenJDK Project. But, with a fine book like *Java For Dummies*, 7th Edition, one never knows.)

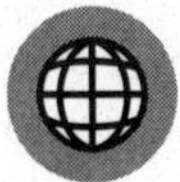

If you're interested in the JCP's activities, visit `www.jcp.org`. If you're interested in the OpenJDK Project, visit `http://openjdk.java.net`.

The folks at the JCP don't keep the Java programs in the official Java API a secret. If you want, you can look at all these programs. When you install Java on your computer, the installation puts a file named `src.zip` on your hard drive. You can open `src.zip` with your favorite unzipping program. There, before your eyes, is all the Java API code.

The words in a Java program

A hard-core Javateer will say that the Java programming language has two kinds of words: keywords and identifiers. This is true. But the bare truth, without any other explanation, is sometimes misleading. So I recommend dressing up the truth a bit and thinking in terms of three kinds of words: keywords, identifiers that ordinary programmers like you and I create, and identifiers from the API.

The differences among these three kinds of words are similar to the differences among words in the English language. In the sentence "Sam is a person," the word *person* is like a Java keyword. No matter who uses the word *person*, the word always means roughly the same thing. (Sure, you can think of bizarre exceptions in English usage, but please don't.)

The word *Sam* is like a Java identifier because Sam is a name for a particular person. Words like *Sam*, *Dinswald*, and *McGillimaroo* aren't prepacked with meaning in the English language. These words apply to different people depending on the context and become names when parents pick one for their newborn kid.

Now consider the sentence "Julius Caesar is a person." If you utter this sentence, you're probably talking about the fellow who ruled Rome until the Ides of March. Although the name *Julius Caesar* isn't hard-wired into the English language, almost everyone uses the name to refer to the same person. If English were a programming language, the name Julius Caesar would be an API identifier.

So here's how I, in my mind, divide the words in a Java program into categories:

- **Keywords:** A *keyword* is a word that has its own special meaning in the Java programming language, and that meaning doesn't change from one program to another. Examples of keywords in Java are `if`, `else`, and `do`.

  The JCP committee members, who have the final say on what constitutes a Java program, have chosen all the Java keywords. If you think about the two parts of Java, which I discuss earlier, in the section "The grammar and the common names," the Java keywords belong solidly to the language specification.

- **Identifiers:** An *identifier* is a name for something. The identifier's meaning can change from one program to another, but some identifiers' meanings tend to change more:

  - *Identifiers created by you and me:* As a Java programmer (yes, even as a novice Java programmer), you create new names for classes and other items you describe in your programs. Of course, you may name something `Prime`, and the guy writing code two cubicles down the hall can name something else `Prime`. That's okay because Java doesn't have a predetermined meaning for `Prime`. In your program, you can make `Prime` stand for the Federal Reserve's prime rate. And the guy down the hall can make `Prime` stand for the "bread, roll, preserves, and prime rib." A conflict doesn't arise, because you and your coworker are writing two different Java programs.

- *Identifiers from the API:* The JCP members have created names for many things and thrown tens of thousands of these names into the Java API. The API comes with each version of Java, so these names are available to anyone who writes a Java program. Examples of such names are `String`, `Integer`, `JWindow`, `JButton`, `JTextField`, and `File`.

Strictly speaking, the meanings of the identifiers in the Java API aren't cast in stone. Although you can make up your own meanings for `JButton` or `JWindow`, this isn't a good idea. If you did, you would confuse the dickens out of other programmers, who are used to the standard API meanings for these familiar identifier names. But even worse, when your code assigns a new meaning to an identifier like `JButton`, you lose any computational power that was created for the identifier in the API code. The programmers at Sun Microsystems, Oracle, the Java Community Process, and the OpenJDK Project did all the work of writing Java code to handle buttons. If you assign your own meaning to `JButton`, you're turning your back on all the progress made in creating the API.

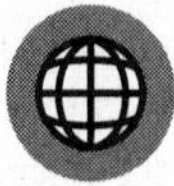

To see the list of Java keywords, visit this book's website: `www.allmycode.com/JavaForDummies`.

Checking Out Java Code for the First Time

The first time you look at somebody else's Java program, you may tend to feel a bit queasy. The realization that you don't understand something (or many things) in the code can make you nervous. I've written hundreds (maybe thousands) of Java programs, but I still feel insecure when I start reading someone else's code.

The truth is that finding out about a Java program is a bootstrapping experience. First, you gawk in awe of the program. Then you run the program to see what it does. Then you stare at the program for a while or read someone's explanation of the program and its parts. Then you gawk a little more and run the program again. Eventually, you come to terms with the program. (Don't believe the wise guys who say they never go through these steps. Even the experienced programmers approach a new project slowly and carefully.)

In Listing 3-1, you get a blast of Java code. (Like all novice programmers, you're expected to gawk humbly at the code.) Hidden in the code, I've placed some important ideas, which I explain in detail in the next section. These ideas include the use of classes, methods, and Java statements.

LISTING 3-1: The Simplest Java Program

```
public class Displayer {

    public static void main(String args[]) {
        System.out.println("You'll love Java!");
    }
}
```

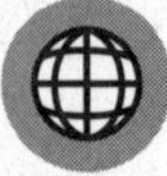

You don't have to type the code in Listing 3-1 (or in any of this book's listings). To download all the code in this book, visit the book's website (`www.allmycode.com/JavaForDummies`).

When you run the program from Listing 3-1, the computer displays `You'll love Java!` (Figure 3-1 shows the output of the Displayer program when you use the Eclipse IDE.) Now, I admit that writing and running a Java program is a lot of work just to get `You'll love Java!` to appear on somebody's computer screen, but every endeavor has to start somewhere.

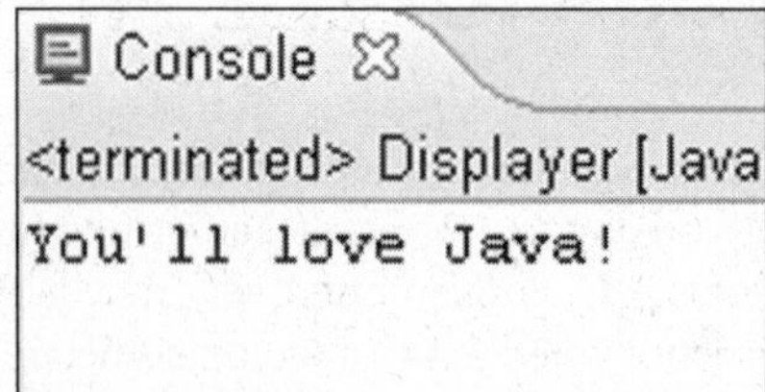

FIGURE 3-1: I use Eclipse to run the program in Listing 3-1.

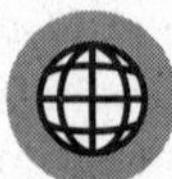

To see how to run the code in Listing 3-1, visit this book's website (`www.allmycode.com/JavaForDummies`).

In the following section, you do more than just admire the program's output. After you read the following section, you actually understand what makes the program in Listing 3-1 work.

Understanding a Simple Java Program

This section presents, explains, analyzes, dissects, and otherwise demystifies the Java program shown previously in Listing 3-1.

The Java class

Because Java is an object-oriented programming language, your primary goal is to describe classes and objects. (If you're not convinced about this, read the sections on object-oriented programming in Chapter 1.)

On those special days when I'm feeling sentimental, I tell people that Java is more pure in its object-orientation than many other so-called object-oriented languages. I say this because, in Java, you can't do anything until you create a class of some kind. It's like being on *Jeopardy!* and hearing Alex Trebek say, "Let's go to a commercial" and then interrupting him by saying, "I'm sorry, Alex. You can't issue an instruction without putting your instruction inside a class."

The code in Listing 3-1 is a Java program, and that program describes a class. I wrote the program, so I get to make up a name for my new class. I chose the name `Displayer` because the program displays a line of text on the computer screen. That's why the first line in Listing 3-1 contains the words `class Displayer`. (See Figure 3-2.)

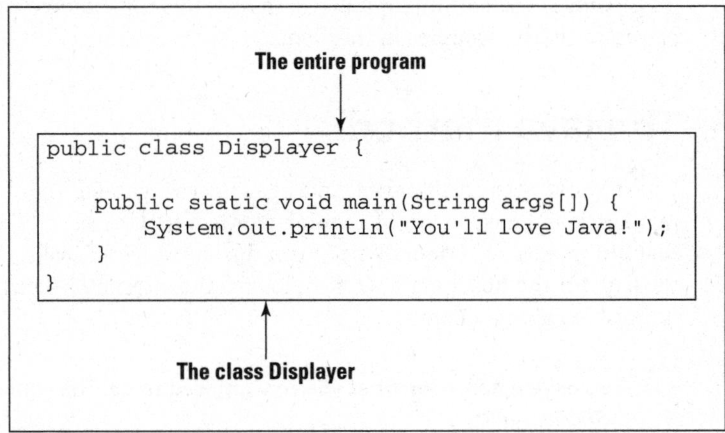
The entire program
public class Displayer {
public static void main(String args[]) {
System.out.println("You'll love Java!");
}
}
The class Displayer

FIGURE 3-2: A Java program is a class.

The first two words in Listing 3-1, `public` and `class`, are Java keywords. (See the section "The words in a Java program," earlier in this chapter.) No matter who writes a Java program, the words `public` and `class` are always used in the same way. On the other hand, `Displayer` in Listing 3-1 is an identifier. I made up the word `Displayer` while I was writing this chapter. `Displayer` is the name of a particular class — the class that I'm creating by writing this program.

This book is filled with talk about classes, but for the best description of a Java class (the reason for using the word `class` in Listing 3-1), visit Chapter 7. The word `public` means that other Java classes (classes other than the `Displayer` class in Listing 3-1) can use the features declared in Listing 3-1. For more details about the meaning of `public` and the use of the word `public` in a Java program, see Chapters 7 and 14.

tHE jAVA PROGRAMMING LANGUAGE IS cASe-sEnsITiVE. If you change a lowercase letter in a word to an UpperCase letter, you can change the word's meaning. cHANGING case can make the entire word go from being meaningful to being meaningless. In the first line of Listing 3-1, you can't replace `class` with `Class`. iF YOU DO, THE WHOLE PROGRAM STOPS WORKING. The same holds true, to some extent, for the name of a file containing a particular class. For example, the name of the class in Listing 3-1 is `Displayer`, starting with an uppercase letter `D`. So it's a good idea to save the code of Listing 3-1 in a file named `Displayer.java`, starting with an uppercase letter `D`.

Normally, if you define a class named DogAndPony, the class's Java code is in a file named `DogAndPony.java`, spelled and capitalized exactly the same way that the class name is spelled and capitalized. In fact, this file-naming convention is mandatory for most examples in this book.

The Java method

You're working as an auto mechanic in an upscale garage. Your boss, who's always in a hurry and has a habit of running words together, says, "fixTheAlternator on that junkyOldFord." Mentally, you run through a list of tasks. "Drive the car into the bay, lift the hood, get a wrench, loosen the alternator belt," and so on. Three things are going on here:

- **You have a name for what you're supposed to do.** The name is *fixTheAlternator.*
- **In your mind, you have a list of tasks associated with the name *fixTheAlternator.*** The list includes "Drive the car into the bay, lift the hood, get a wrench, loosen the alternator belt," and so on.
- **You have a grumpy boss who's telling you to do all this work.** Your boss gets you working by saying, "fixTheAlternator." In other words, your boss gets you working by saying the name of what you're supposed to do.

In this scenario, using the word *method* wouldn't be a big stretch. You have a method for doing something with an alternator. Your boss calls that method into action, and you respond by doing all the things in the list of instructions that you associate with the method.

If you believe all that (and I hope you do), you're ready to read about Java methods. In Java, a *method* is a list of things to do. Every method has a name, and you tell the computer to do the things in the list by using the method's name in your program.

I've never written a program to get a robot to fix an alternator. But, if I did, the program might include a `fixTheAlternator` method. The list of instructions in my `fixTheAlternator` method would look something like the text in Listing 3-2.

WARNING

Don't scrutinize Listings 3-2 and 3-3 too carefully. All the code in Listings 3-2 and 3-3 is fake! I made up this code so that it looks a lot like real Java code, but it's not real. What's more important, the code in Listings 3-2 and 3-3 isn't meant to illustrate all the rules about Java. So, if you have a grain of salt handy, take it with Listings 3-2 and 3-3.

LISTING 3-2: A Method Declaration

```
void fixTheAlternator(onACertainCar) {
   driveInto(car, bay);
   lift(hood);
   get(wrench);
   loosen(alternatorBelt);
   ...
}
```

Somewhere else in my Java code (somewhere outside of Listing 3-2), I need an instruction to call my `fixTheAlternator` method into action. The instruction to call the `fixTheAlternator` method into action may look like the line in Listing 3-3.

LISTING 3-3: A Method Call

```
fixTheAlternator(junkyOldFord);
```

Now that you have a basic understanding of what a method is and how it works, you can dig a little deeper into some useful terminology:

- If I'm being lazy, I refer to the code in Listing 3-2 as a *method.* If I'm not being lazy, I refer to this code as a *method declaration.*
- The method declaration in Listing 3-2 has two parts. The first line (the part with `fixTheAlternator` in it, up to but not including the open curly brace) is

a *method header.* The rest of Listing 3-2 (the part surrounded by curly braces) is a *method body.*

» The term *method declaration* distinguishes the list of instructions in Listing 3-2 from the instruction in Listing 3-3, which is known as a *method call.*

REMEMBER

A *method's declaration* tells the computer what happens if you call the method into action. A *method call* (a separate piece of code) tells the computer to actually call the method into action. A method's declaration and the method's call tend to be in different parts of the Java program.

The main method in a program

Figure 3-3 has a copy of the code from Listing 3-1. The bulk of the code contains the declaration of a method named `main`. (Just look for the word *main* in the code's method header.) For now, don't worry about the other words in the method header: `public`, `static`, `void`, `String`, and `args`. I explain these words in the next several chapters.

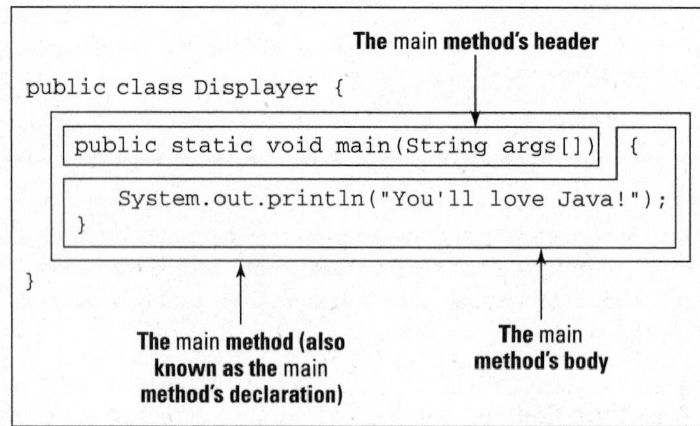
The main method's header
public class Displayer {
public static void main(String args[])
{
System.out.println("You'll love Java!");
}
}
The main method (also known as the main method's declaration)
The main method's body

FIGURE 3-3: The `main` method.

Like any Java method, the `main` method is a recipe:

```
How to make biscuits:
   Heat the oven.
   Roll the dough.
   Bake the rolled dough.
```

or

```
How to follow the main instructions for a Displayer:
    Print "You'll love Java!" on the screen.
```

The word *main* plays a special role in Java. In particular, you never write code that explicitly calls a `main` method into action. The word *main* is the name of the method that is called into action automatically when the program begins running.

Look back at Figure 3-1. When the `Displayer` program runs, the computer automatically finds the program's `main` method and executes any instructions inside the method's body. In the `Displayer` program, the `main` method's body has only one instruction. That instruction tells the computer to print `You'll love Java!` on the screen. So in Figure 3-1, `You'll love Java!` appears on the computer screen.

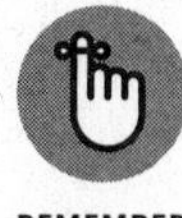

REMEMBER

The instructions in a method aren't executed until the method is called into action. But, if you give a method the name *main*, that method is called into action automatically.

TECHNICAL STUFF

Almost every computer programming language has something akin to Java's methods. If you've worked with other languages, you may remember terms like subprograms, procedures, functions, subroutines, subprocedures, and `PERFORM` statements. Whatever you call it in your favorite programming language, a method is a bunch of instructions collected and given a new name.

How you finally tell the computer to do something

Buried deep in the heart of Listing 3-1 is the single line that actually issues a direct instruction to the computer. The line, which is highlighted in Figure 3-4, tells the computer to display `You'll love Java!` This line is a *statement*. In Java, a statement is a direct instruction that tells the computer to do something (for example, display this text, put 7 in that memory location, make a window appear).

```
public class Displayer {

    public static void main(String args[]) {
        System.out.println("You'll love Java!");
    }
}
```

A statement (a call to the System.out.println method)

FIGURE 3-4: A Java statement.

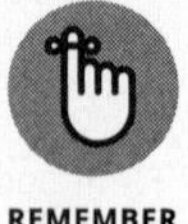

REMEMBER

In `System.out.println`, the next-to-last character is a lowercase letter *l*, not a digit *1*.

Of course, Java has different kinds of statements. A method call, which I introduce in the earlier "The Java method" section, is one of the many kinds of Java statements. Listing 3-3 shows you what a method call looks like, and Figure 3-4 also contains a method call that looks like this:

```
System.out.println("You'll love Java!");
```

When the computer executes this statement, the computer calls a method named `System.out.println` into action. (Yes, in Java, a name can have dots in it. The dots mean something.)

WARNING

I said it already, but it's worth repeating: In `System.out.println`, the next-to-last character is a lowercase letter *l* (*as in the word* line), not a digit *1* (*as in the number* one). If you use a digit *1*, your code won't work. Just think of `println` as a way of saying "print line" and you won't have any problem.

To learn the meaning behind the dots in Java names, see Chapter 7.

Figure 3-5 illustrates the `System.out.println` situation. Actually, two methods play active roles in the running of the `Displayer` program. Here's how they work:

- **There's a declaration for a `main` method.** I wrote the `main` method myself. This `main` method is called automatically whenever I run the `Displayer` program.
- **There's a call to the `System.out.println` method.** The method call for the `System.out.println` method is the only statement in the body of the main method. In other words, calling the `System.out.println` method is the only item on the `main` method's to-do list.

  The declaration for the `System.out.println` method is buried inside the official Java API. For a refresher on the Java API, see the sections "The grammar and the common names" and "The words in a Java program," earlier in this chapter.

TECHNICAL STUFF

When I say things like, "`System.out.println` is buried inside the API," I'm not doing justice to the API. True, you can ignore all the nitty-gritty Java code inside the API. All you need to remember is that `System.out.println` is defined somewhere inside that code. But I'm not being fair when I make the API code sound like something magical. The API is just another bunch of Java code. The statements in the API that tell the computer what it means to carry out a call to `System.out.println` look a lot like the Java code in Listing 3-1.

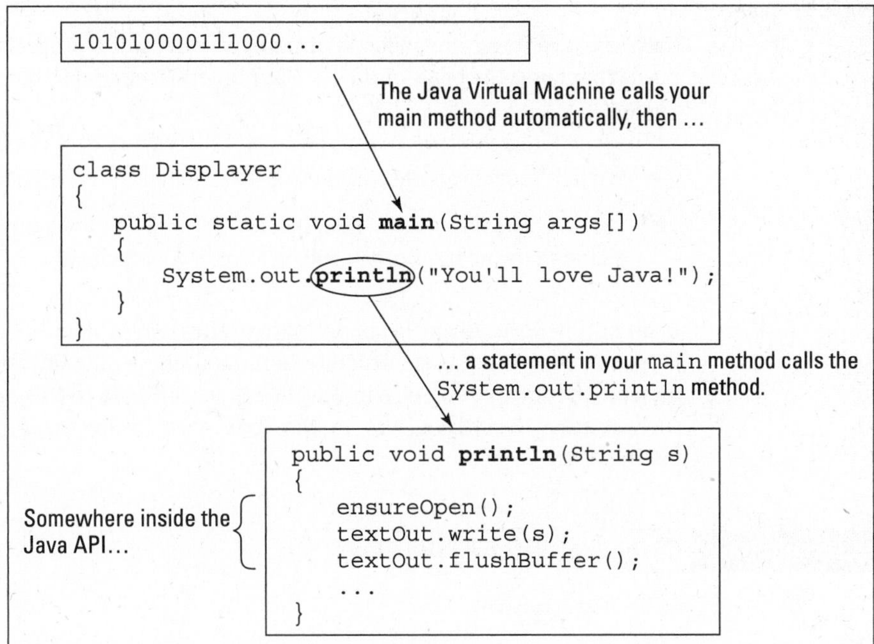

101010000111000...
The Java Virtual Machine calls your main method automatically, then ...
class Displayer
{
public static void main(String args[])
{
System.out.println("You'll love Java!");
}
}
... a statement in your main method calls the System.out.println method.
Somewhere inside the Java API...
public void println(String s)
{
ensureOpen();
textOut.write(s);
textOut.flushBuffer();
...
}

FIGURE 3-5: Calling the `System.out.println` method.

In Java, each statement (like the boxed line in Figure 3-4) ends with a semicolon. Other lines in Figure 3-4 don't end with semicolons, because the other lines in Figure 3-4 aren't statements. For instance, the method header (the line with the word *main* in it) doesn't directly tell the computer to do anything. The method header announces, "Just in case you ever want to do `main`, the next few lines of code tell you how to do it."

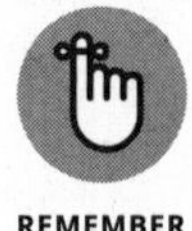

REMEMBER

Every complete Java statement ends with a semicolon.

Curly braces

Long ago, or maybe not so long ago, your schoolteachers told you how useful outlines are. With an outline, you can organize thoughts and ideas, help people see forests instead of trees, and generally show that you're a member of the Tidy Persons Club. Well, a Java program is like an outline. The program in Listing 3-1 starts with a header line that says, "Here comes a class named `Displayer`." After that header, a subheader announces, "Here comes a method named `main`."

Now, if a Java program is like an outline, why doesn't a program *look* like an outline? What takes the place of the Roman numerals, capital letters, and other items? The answer is twofold:

- In a Java program, curly braces enclose meaningful units of code.
- You, the programmer, can (and should) indent lines so that other programmers can see at a glance the outline form of your code.

In an outline, everything is subordinate to the item in Roman numeral *I*. In a Java program, everything is subordinate to the top line — the line with `class` in it. To indicate that everything else in the code is subordinate to this `class` line, you use curly braces. Everything else in the code goes inside these curly braces. (See Listing 3-4.)

LISTING 3-4: Curly Braces for a Java Class

```
public class Displayer {

    public static void main(String args[]) {
        System.out.println("You'll love Java!");
    }
}
```

In an outline, some stuff is subordinate to a capital letter *A* item. In a Java program, some lines are subordinate to the method header. To indicate that something is subordinate to a method header, you use curly braces. (See Listing 3-5.)

LISTING 3-5: Curly Braces for a Java Method

```
public class Displayer {

    public static void main(String args[]) {
        System.out.println("You'll love Java!");
    }
}
```

In an outline, some items are at the bottom of the food chain. In the `Displayer` class, the corresponding line is the line that begins with `System.out.println`. Accordingly, this `System.out.println` line goes inside all the other curly braces and is indented more than any other line.

REMEMBER

Never lose sight of the fact that a Java program is, first and foremost, an outline.

If you put curly braces in the wrong places or omit curly braces where the braces should be, your program probably won't work at all. If your program works, it'll probably work incorrectly.

If you don't indent lines of code in an informative manner, your program will still work correctly, but neither you nor any other programmer will be able to figure out what you were thinking when you wrote the code.

If you're a visual thinker, you can picture outlines of Java programs in your head. One friend of mine visualizes an actual numbered outline morphing into a Java program. (See Figure 3-6.) Another person, who shall remain nameless, uses more bizarre imagery. (See Figure 3-7.)

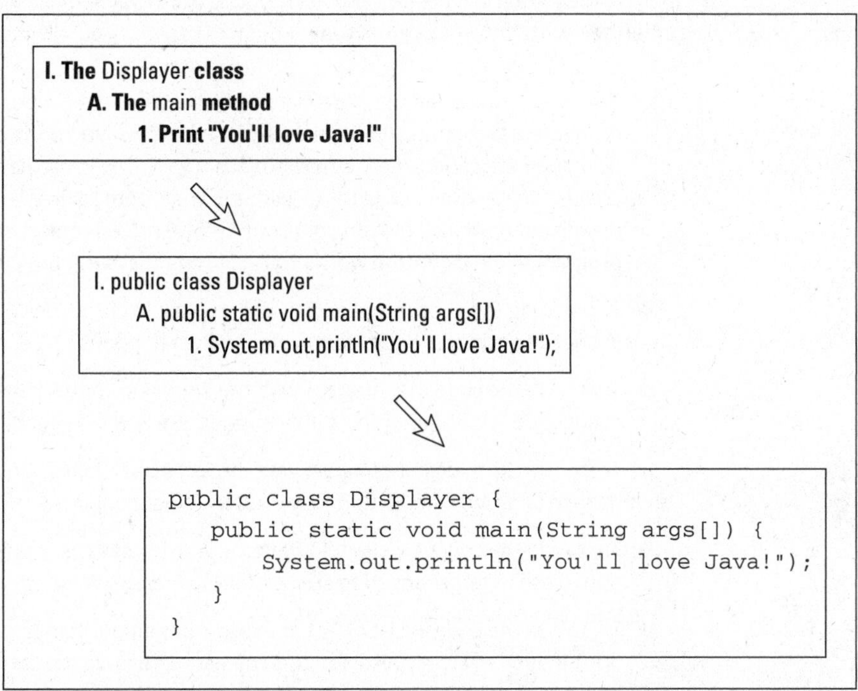
I. The Displayer class
A. The main method
1. Print "You'll love Java!"
I. public class Displayer
A. public static void main(String args[])
1. System.out.println("You'll love Java!");
public class Displayer {
public static void main(String args[]) {
System.out.println("You'll love Java!");
}
}

FIGURE 3-6: An outline turns into a Java program.

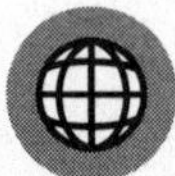

I appreciate a good excuse as much as the next guy, but failing to indent your Java code is inexcusable. In fact, many Java IDEs have tools to indent your code automatically. Visit this book's website (`www.allmycode.com/JavaForDummies`) for more information.

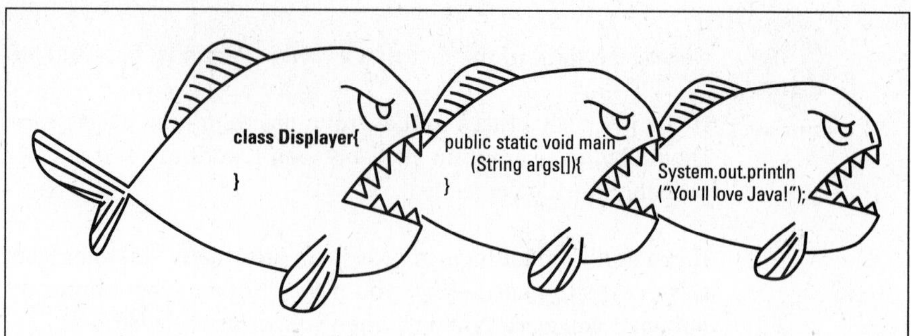

FIGURE 3-7: A class is bigger than a method; a method is bigger than a statement.

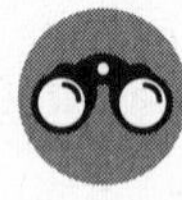

TRY IT OUT

Here are some things for you to try to help you understand the material in this section. If trying these things builds your confidence, that's good. If trying these things makes you question what you've read, that's good too. If trying these things makes you nervous, don't be discouraged. You can find answers and other help at this book's website (`www.allmycode.com/JavaForDummies`). You can also email me with your questions (`JavaForDummies@allmycode.com`).

- If you've downloaded the code from this book's website, import Listing 3-1 (from the downloaded 03-01 folder) into your IDE. If you don't plan to download the code, create a new project in your IDE. In the new project, create a class named `Displayer` with the code from Listing 3-1. With the downloaded project, or with your own, newly created project, run the program and look for the words `You'll love Java!` in the output.
- Try running the code in Listing 3-1 with the text `"You'll love Java!"` changed to `"No more baked beans!"`. What happens?
- Try to run the code in Listing 3-1 with the word `public` (all lowercase) changed to `Public` (starting with an uppercase letter). What happens?
- Try to run the code in Listing 3-1 with the word `main` (all lowercase) changed to `Main` (starting with an uppercase letter). What happens?
- Try to run the code in Listing 3-1 with the word `System` (starting with an uppercase letter) changed to `system` (all lowercase). What happens?
- Try to run the code in Listing 3-1 with the indentation changed. For example, don't indent any lines. Also, for good measure, remove the line breaks between the first curly brace and the word `public` (so that the code reads `public class Displayer { public ...`). What happens?
- Try to run the code in Listing 3-1 with the word `println` changed to `print1n` (with the digit `1` near the end). What happens?
- Try to run the code in Listing 3-1 with the semicolon missing. What happens?

» Try to run the code in Listing 3-1 with additional semicolons added at the ends of some of the lines. What happens?

» Try to run the code in Listing 3-1 with the text `"You'll love Java!"` changed to `" Use a straight quote \", not a curly quote \u201D"`. What happens?

And Now, a Few Comments

People gather around campfires to hear the old legend about a programmer whose laziness got her into trouble. To maintain this programmer's anonymity, I call her Jane Pro. Jane worked many months to create the holy grail of computing: a program that thinks on its own. If completed, this program could work independently, learning new things without human intervention. Day after day, night after night, Jane Pro labored to give the program that spark of creative, independent thought.

One day, when she was almost finished with the project, she received a disturbing piece of paper mail from her health insurance company. No, the mail wasn't about a serious illness. It was about a routine office visit. The insurance company's claim form had a place for Jane's date of birth, as if her date of birth had changed since the last time she sent in a claim. She had absentmindedly scribbled 2016 as her year of birth, so the insurance company refused to pay the bill.

Jane dialed the insurance company's phone number. Within 20 minutes, she was talking to a live person. "I'm sorry," said the live person. "To resolve this issue, you must dial a different number." Well, you can guess what happened next. "I'm sorry. The other operator gave you the wrong number." And then, "I'm sorry. You must call back the original phone number."

Five months later, Jane's ear ached, but after 800 hours on the phone, she had finally gotten a tentative promise that the insurance company would eventually reprocess the claim. Elated as she was, she was anxious to get back to her programming project. Could she remember what all those lines of code were supposed to be doing?

No, she couldn't. Jane stared and stared at her own work and, like a dream that doesn't make sense the next morning, the code was completely meaningless to her. She had written a million lines of code, and not one line was accompanied by an informative explanatory comment. She had left no clues to help her understand what she'd been thinking, so in frustration, she abandoned the whole project.

Adding comments to your code

Listing 3-6 has an enhanced version of this chapter's sample program. In addition to all the keywords, identifiers, and punctuation, Listing 3-6 has text that's meant for human beings to read.

LISTING 3-6: Three Kinds of Comments

```
/*
 * Listing 3-6 in "Java For Dummies, 7th Edition"
 *
 * Copyright 2017 Wiley Publishing, Inc.
 * All rights reserved.
 */

/**
 * The Displayer class displays text
 * on the computer screen.
 *
 * @author  Barry Burd
 * @version 1.0 1/24/17
 * @see     java.lang.System
 */
public class Displayer {

    /**
     * The main method is where
     * execution of the code begins.
     *
     * @param  args   (See Chapter 11.)
     */
    public static void main(String args[]) {
        System.out.println("I love Java!");  //I? You?
    }
}
```

A *comment* is a special section of text, inside a program, whose purpose is to help people understand the program. A comment is part of a good program's documentation.

The Java programming language has three kinds of comments:

- **Traditional comments:** The first five lines of Listing 3-6 form one *traditional* comment. The comment begins with `/*` and ends with `*/`. Everything between the opening `/*` and the closing `*/` is for human eyes only. No information about `"Java For Dummies, 7th Edition"` or `Wiley Publishing, Inc.` is translated by the compiler.

  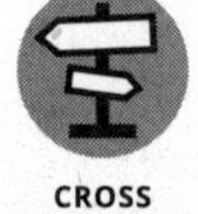

  CROSS REFERENCE

  To read about compilers, see Chapter 2.

  The second, third, fourth, and fifth lines in Listing 3-6 have extra asterisks (`*`). I call them extra because these asterisks aren't required when you create a comment. They just make the comment look pretty. I include them in Listing 3-6 because, for some reason that I don't entirely understand, most Java programmers add these extra asterisks.

- **End-of-line comments:** The text `//I? You?` in Listing 3-6 is an end-of-line comment. An *end-of-line* comment starts with two slashes and goes to the end of a line of type. Once again, the compiler doesn't translate the text inside the end-of-line comment.

- **Javadoc comments:** A *javadoc* comment begins with a slash and two asterisks (/**). Listing 3-6 has two javadoc comments: one with the text `The Displayer class ...` and another with the text `The main method is where ....`

  A *javadoc* comment, which is a special kind of traditional comment, is meant to be read by people who never even look at the Java code. But that doesn't make sense. How can you see the javadoc comments in Listing 3-6 if you never look at Listing 3-6?

- Well, a certain program called *javadoc* (what else?) can find all the javadoc comments in Listing 3-6 and turn these comments into a nice-looking web page. Figure 3-8 shows the page.

Javadoc comments are great. Here are several great things about them:

- The only person who has to look at a piece of Java code is the programmer who writes the code. Other people who use the code can find out what the code does by viewing the automatically generated web page.
- Because other people don't look at the Java code, other people don't make changes to the Java code. (In other words, other people don't introduce errors into the existing Java code.)
- Because other people don't look at the Java code, other people don't have to decipher the inner workings of the Java code. All these people need to know about the code is what they read on the code's web page.

- The programmer doesn't create two separate files — some Java code over here and some documentation about the code over there. Instead, the programmer creates one piece of Java code and embeds the documentation (in the form of javadoc comments) right inside the code.
- Best of all, the generation of web pages from javadoc comments is automatic. So everyone's documentation has the same format. No matter whose Java code you use, you find out about that code by reading a page like the one in Figure 3-8. That's good because the format in Figure 3-8 is familiar to anyone who uses Java.

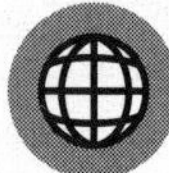

You can generate your own web pages from the javadoc comments that you put in your code. To discover how, visit this book's website (`www.allmycode.com/JavaForDummies`).

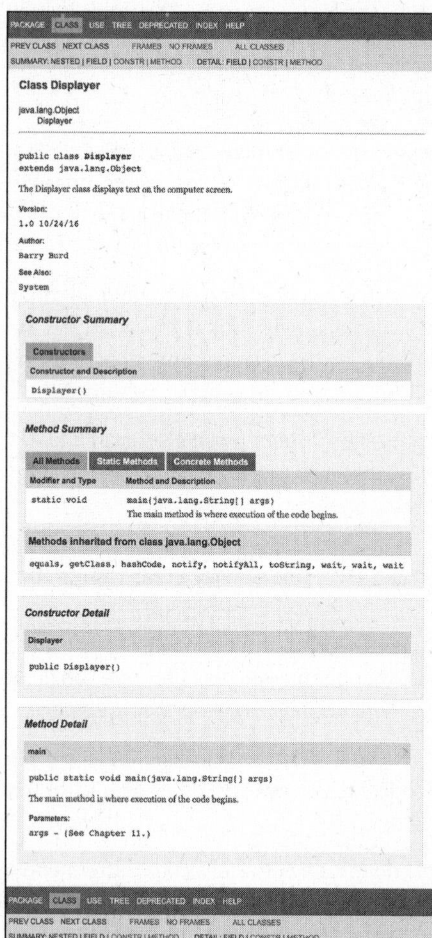

PACKAGE CLASS USE TREE DEPRECATED INDEX HELP
PREV CLASS NEXT CLASS FRAMES NO FRAMES ALL CLASSES
SUMMARY: NESTED | FIELD | CONSTR | METHOD DETAIL: FIELD | CONSTR | METHOD
Class Displayer
java.lang.Object
Displayer
public class Displayer
extends java.lang.Object
The Displayer class displays text on the computer screen.
Version:
1.0 10/24/16
Author:
Barry Burd
See Also:
System
Constructor Summary
Constructors
Constructor and Description
Displayer()
Method Summary
All Methods Static Methods Concrete Methods
Modifier and Type Method and Description
static void main(java.lang.String[] args)
The main method is where execution of the code begins.
Methods inherited from class java.lang.Object
equals, getClass, hashCode, notify, notifyAll, toString, wait, wait, wait
Constructor Detail
Displayer
public Displayer()
Method Detail
main
public static void main(java.lang.String[] args)
The main method is where execution of the code begins.
Parameters:
args - (See Chapter 11.)
PACKAGE CLASS USE TREE DEPRECATED INDEX HELP
PREV CLASS NEXT CLASS FRAMES NO FRAMES ALL CLASSES
SUMMARY: NESTED | FIELD | CONSTR | METHOD DETAIL: FIELD | CONSTR | METHOD

FIGURE 3-8: The javadoc page generated from the code in Listing 3-6.

What's Barry's excuse?

For years I've been telling my students to put comments in their code, and for years I've been creating sample code (like the code in Listing 3-1) with no comments in it. Why?

Three little words: *Know your audience.* When you write complicated, real-life code, your audience is other programmers, information technology managers, and people who need help deciphering what you've done. When I write simple samples of code for this book, my audience is you — the novice Java programmer. Instead of reading my comments, your best strategy is to stare at my Java statements — the statements that Java's compiler deciphers. That's why I put so few comments in this book's listings.

Besides, I'm a little lazy.

Using comments to experiment with your code

You may hear programmers talk about *commenting out* certain parts of their code. When you're writing a program and something's not working correctly, it often helps to try removing some of the code. If nothing else, you find out what happens when that suspicious code is removed. Of course, you may not like what happens when the code is removed, so you don't want to delete the code completely. Instead, you turn your ordinary Java statements into comments. For instance, you turn the statement

```
System.out.println("I love Java!");
```

into the comment

```
// System.out.println("I love Java!");
```

This change keeps the Java compiler from seeing the code while you try to figure out what's wrong with your program.

Traditional comments aren't very useful for commenting out code. The big problem is that you can't put one traditional comment inside of another. Suppose that you want to comment out the following statements:

```
System.out.println("Parents,");
System.out.println("pick your");
/*
```

```
 * Intentionally displays on four separate lines
 */
System.out.println("battles");
System.out.println("carefully!");
```

If you try to turn this code into one traditional comment, you get the following mess:

```
/*
  System.out.println("Parents,");
  System.out.println("pick your");
  /*
   * Intentionally displays on four separate lines
   */
  System.out.println("battles");
  System.out.println("carefully!");
*/
```

The first `*/` (after `Intentionally displays`) ends the traditional comment prematurely. Then the `battles` and `carefully` statements aren't commented out, and the last `*/` chokes the compiler. You can't nest traditional comments inside one another. Because of this, I recommend end-of-line comments as tools for experimenting with your code.

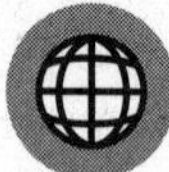

Most IDEs can comment out sections of your code for you automatically. For details, visit this book's website (`www.allmycode.com/JavaForDummies`).

2

Writing Your Own Java Programs

IN THIS PART . . .

Create new values and modify existing values.

Put decision-making into your application's logic.

Repeat things as needed when your program runs.

» **Making things store certain types of values**

» **Applying operators to get new values**

Chapter 4
Making the Most of Variables and Their Values

The following conversation between Mr. Van Doren and Mr. Barasch never took place:

> *Charles:* A sea squirt eats its brain, turning itself from an animal into a plant.
>
> *Jack:* Is that your final answer, Charles?
>
> *Charles:* Yes, it is.
>
> *Jack:* How much money do you have in your account today, Charles?
>
> *Charles:* I have fifty dollars and twenty-two cents in my checking account.
>
> *Jack:* Well, you better call the IRS, because your sea squirt answer is correct. You just won a million dollars to add to your checking account. What do you think of that, Charles?
>
> *Charles:* I owe it all to honesty, diligence, and hard work, Jack.

Some aspects of this dialogue can be represented in Java by a few lines of code.

Varying a Variable

No matter how you acquire your million dollars, you can use a variable to tally your wealth. Listing 4-1 shows the code.

LISTING 4-1: Using a Variable

```
amountInAccount = 50.22;
amountInAccount = amountInAccount + 1000000.00;
```

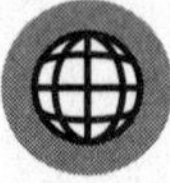

You don't have to type the code in Listing 4-1 (or in any of this book's listings). To download all the code in this book, visit the book's website (`www.allmycode.com/JavaForDummies`).

The code in Listing 4-1 makes use of the `amountInAccount` variable. A *variable* is a placeholder. You can stick a number like 50.22 into a variable. After you place a number in the variable, you can change your mind and put a different number into the variable. (That's what varies in a variable.) Of course, when you put a new number in a variable, the old number is no longer there. If you didn't save the old number somewhere else, the old number is gone.

Figure 4-1 gives a before-and-after picture of the code in Listing 4-1. After the first statement in Listing 4-1 is executed, the variable `amountInAccount` has the number 50.22 in it. Then, after the second statement of Listing 4-1 is executed, the `amountInAccount` variable suddenly has 1000050.22 in it. When you think about a variable, picture a place in the computer's memory where wires and transistors store 50.22, 1000050.22, or whatever. On the left side of Figure 4-1, imagine that the box with 50.22 in it is surrounded by millions of other such boxes.

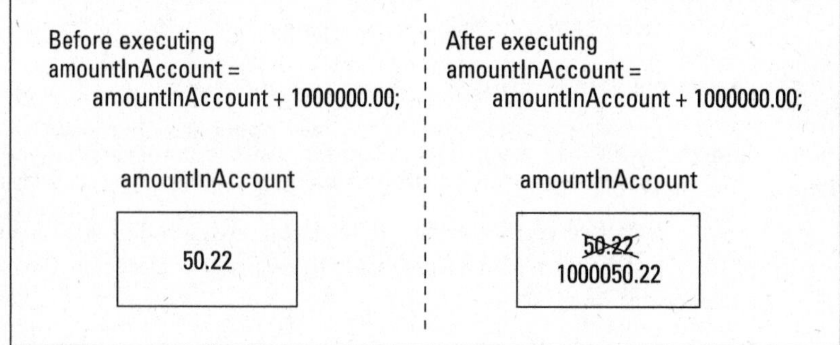

FIGURE 4-1: A variable (before and after).

Now you need some terminology. The thing stored in a variable is a *value*. A variable's value can change during the run of a program (when Jack gives you a million bucks, for instance). The value that's stored in a variable isn't necessarily a number. (For instance, you can create a variable that always stores a letter.) The kind of value that's stored in a variable is a variable's *type*.

You can read more about types in the section "The types of values that variables may have," later in this chapter.

TECHNICAL STUFF

A subtle, almost unnoticeable difference exists between a variable and a variable's *name*. Even in formal writing, I often use the word *variable* when I mean *variable name*. Strictly speaking, `amountInAccount` is a variable name, and all the memory storage associated with `amountInAccount` (including the type that `amountInAccount` has and whatever value `amountInAccount` currently represents) is the variable itself. If you think this distinction between *variable* and *variable name* is too subtle for you to worry about, join the club.

Every variable name is an identifier — a name that you can make up in your own code. In preparing Listing 4-1, I made up the name *amountInAccount*.

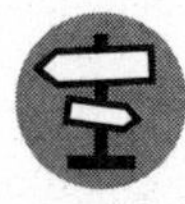

CROSS REFERENCE

For more information on the kinds of names in a Java program, see Chapter 3.

Before the sun sets on Listing 4-1, you need to notice one more part of the listing. The listing has `50.22` and `1000000.00` in it. Anybody in his or her right mind would call these things *numbers*, but in a Java program it helps to call these things *literals*.

And what's so literal about `50.22` and `1000000.00`? Well, think about the variable `amountInAccount` in Listing 4-1. The variable `amountInAccount` stands for 50.22 some of the time, but it stands for 1000050.22 the rest of the time. You could use the word *number* to talk about `amountInAccount`. But really, what `amountInAccount` stands for depends on the fashion of the moment. On the other hand, 50.22 literally stands for the value 50 22/100.

REMEMBER

A variable's value changes; a literal's value doesn't.

TIP

Starting with Java 7, you can add underscores to numeric literals. Instead of using the plain old `1000000.00` in Listing 4-1, you can write `amountInAccount = amountInAccount + 1_000_000.00`. Unfortunately, you can't easily do what you're most tempted to do. You can't write `1,000,000.00` (as you would in the United States), nor can you write `1.000.000,00` (as you would in Germany). If you want to display a number such as `1,000,000.00` in the program's output, you have to use some fancy formatting tricks. For more information about formatting, check Chapters 10 and 11.

Assignment statements

Statements like the ones in Listing 4-1 are called *assignment statements.* In an assignment statement, you assign a value to something. In many cases, this something is a variable.

I recommend getting into the habit of reading assignment statements from right to left. Figure 4-2 illustrates the action of the first line in Listing 4-1.

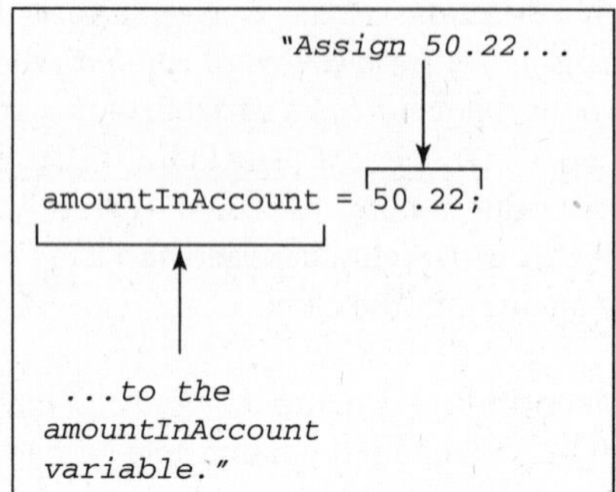

FIGURE 4-2: The action of the first line in Listing 4-1.

The second line in Listing 4-1 is just a bit more complicated. Figure 4-3 illustrates the action of the second line in Listing 4-1.

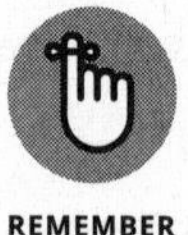

REMEMBER

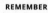

In an assignment statement, the thing being assigned a value is always on the left side of the equal sign.

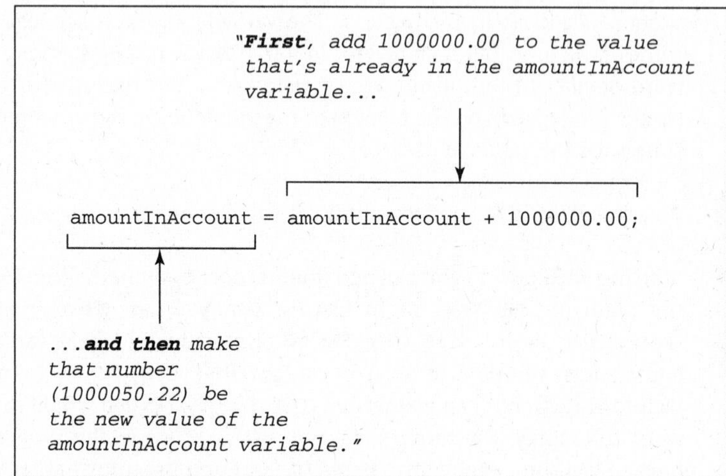

FIGURE 4-3: The action of the second line in Listing 4-1.

The types of values that variables may have

Have you seen the TV commercials that make you think you're flying among the circuits inside a computer? Pretty cool, eh? These commercials show 0s (zeros) and 1s (ones) sailing by because 0s and 1s are the only things that computers can deal with. When you think a computer is storing the letter *J*, the computer is really storing 01001010. Everything inside the computer is a sequence of 0s and 1s. As every computer geek knows, a 0 or 1 is called a *bit*.

As it turns out, the sequence 01001010, which stands for the letter *J*, can also stand for the number 74. The same sequence can also stand for $1.0369608636003646 \times 10^{-43}$. In fact, if the bits are interpreted as screen pixels, the same sequence can be used to represent the dots shown in Figure 4-4. The meaning of 01001010 depends on the way the software interprets this sequence of 0s and 1s.

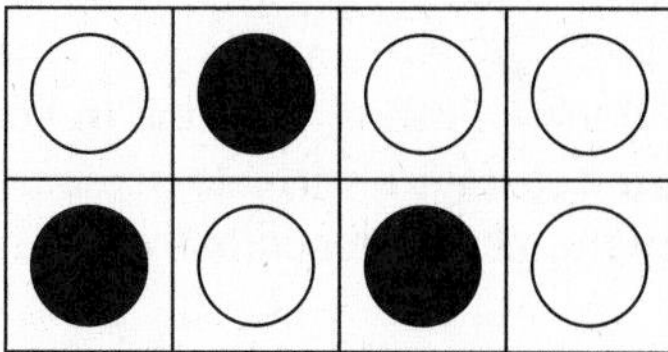

FIGURE 4-4: An extreme close-up of eight black and white screen pixels.

How do you tell the computer what 01001010 stands for? The answer is in the concept of type. The *type* of a variable is the range of values that the variable is permitted to store.

I copied the lines from Listing 4-1 and put them into a complete Java program. The program is in Listing 4-2. When I run the program in Listing 4-2, I get the output shown in Figure 4-5.

LISTING 4-2: A Program Uses amountInAccount

```
public class Millionaire {

    public static void main(String args[]) {
        double amountInAccount;

        amountInAccount = 50.22;
        amountInAccount = amountInAccount + 1000000.00;
```

(continued)

LISTING 4-2: (continued)

```
        System.out.print("You have $");
        System.out.print(amountInAccount);
        System.out.println(" in your account.");
    }
}
```

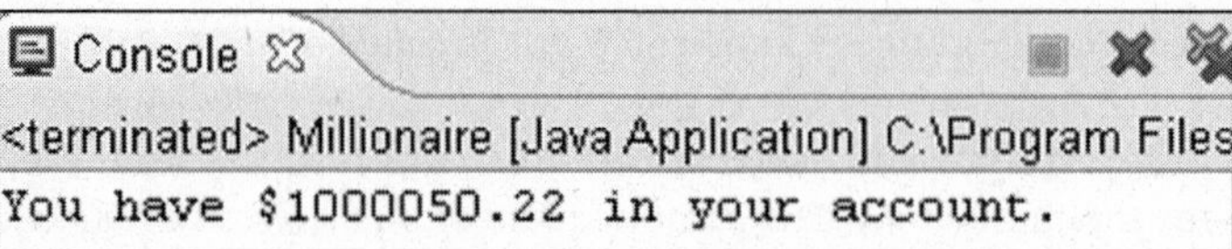

Console
<terminated> Millionaire [Java Application] C:\Program Files
You have $1000050.22 in your account.

FIGURE 4-5: Running the program in Listing 4-2.

In Listing 4-2, look at the first line in the body of the `main` method:

```
double amountInAccount;
```

This line is called a *variable declaration.* Putting this line in your program is like saying, "I'm declaring my intention to have a variable named *amountInAccount* in my program." This line reserves the name *amountInAccount* for your use in the program.

In this variable declaration, the word *double* is a Java keyword. This word *double* tells the computer what kinds of values you intend to store in `amountInAccount`. In particular, the word *double* stands for numbers between -1.8×10^{308} and 1.8×10^{308}. (These are enormous numbers with 308 zeros before the decimal point. Only the world's richest people write checks with 308 zeros in them. The second of these numbers is one-point-eight gazazzo-zillion-kaskillion. The number 1.8×10^{308}, a constant defined by the International Bureau of Weights and Measures, is the number of eccentric computer programmers between Sunnyvale, California, and the M31 Andromeda Galaxy.)

More important than the humongous range of the `double` keyword's numbers is the fact that a `double` value can have digits beyond the decimal point. After you declare `amountInAccount` to be of type `double`, you can store all sorts of numbers in `amountInAccount`. You can store `50.22`, `0.02398479`, or `-3.0`. In Listing 4-2, if I hadn't declared `amountInAccount` to be of type `double`, I may not have been able to store `50.22`. Instead, I would have had to store plain old `50`, without any digits beyond the decimal point.

Another type — type `float` — also allows you to have digits beyond the decimal point. But `float` values aren't as accurate as `double` values.

DIGITS BEYOND THE DECIMAL POINT

Java has two different types that have digits beyond the decimal point: type `double` and type `float`. So what's the difference? When you declare a variable to be of type `double`, you're telling the computer to keep track of 64 bits when it stores the variable's values. When you declare a variable to be of type `float`, the computer keeps track of only 32 bits.

You could change Listing 4-2 and declare `amountInAccount` to be of type `float`.

```
float amountInAccount;
```

Surely, 32 bits are enough to store a small number like 50.22, right? Well, they are and they aren't. You could easily store 50.00 with only 32 bits. Heck, you could store 50.00 with only 6 bits. The size of the number doesn't matter. The accuracy matters. In a 64-bit double variable, you're using most of the bits to store stuff beyond the decimal point. To store the .22 part of 50.22, you need more than the measly 32 bits that you get with type `float`.

Do you really believe what you just read — that it takes more than 32 bits to store .22? To help convince you, I made a few changes to the code in Listing 4-2. I made `amountInAccount` be of type `float`. Then I changed the first three statements inside the main method as follows:

```
float amountInAccount;

amountInAccount = 50.22F;
amountInAccount = amountInAccount + 1000000.00F;
```

(To understand why I used the letter F in `50.22F` and `1000000.00F`, see Table 4-1, later in this chapter.) The output I got was

```
You have $1000050.25 in your account.
```

Compare this with the output in Figure 4-5. When I switch from type `double` to type `float`, Charles has an extra three cents in his account. By changing to the 32-bit `float` type, I've clobbered the accuracy in the `amountInAccount` variable's hundredths place. That's bad.

Another difficulty with `float` values is purely cosmetic. Look again at the literals, `50.22` and `1000000.00`, in Listing 4-2. The Laws of Java say that literals like these take up 64 bits each. So, if you declare `amountInAccount` to be of type `float`, you'll run into trouble. You'll have trouble stuffing those 64-bit literals into your little 32-bit

(continued)

(continued)

amountInAccount variable. To compensate, you can switch from double literals to float literals by adding an F to each double literal, but a number with an extra F at the end looks funny.

```
float amountInAccount;
amountInAccount = 50.22F;
amountInAccount = amountInAccount + 1000000.00F;
```

To experiment with numbers, visit http://babbage.cs.qc.cuny.edu/IEEE-754.old/Decimal.html. The page takes any number you enter and shows you how the number would be represented as 32 bits and as 64 bits.

TIP

In many situations, you have a choice. You can declare certain values to be either float values or double values. But don't sweat the choice between float and double. For most programs, just use double. With today's fancy processors, the space you save using the float type is almost never worth the loss of accuracy. (For more details, see the nearby sidebar, "Digits beyond the decimal point.")

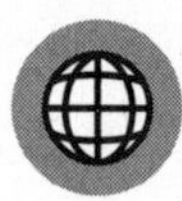

The big million-dollar jackpot in Listing 4-2 is impressive. But Listing 4-2 doesn't illustrate the best way to deal with dollar amounts. In a Java program, the best way to represent currency is to shun the double and float types and opt instead for a type named BigDecimal. For more information, see this book's website (www.allmycode.com/JavaForDummies).

Displaying text

The last three statements in Listing 4-2 use a neat formatting trick. You want to display several different items on a single line on the screen. You put these items in separate statements. All but the last of the statements are calls to System.out.print. (The last statement is a call to System.out.println.) Calls to System.out.print display text on part of a line and then leave the cursor at the end of the current line. After executing System.out.print, the cursor is still at the end of the same line, so the next System.out.*whatever* can continue printing on that same line. With several calls to print capped off by a single call to println, the result is just one nice-looking line of output. (Refer to Figure 4-5.)

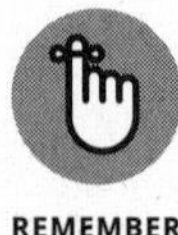

REMEMBER

A call to System.out.print writes some things and leaves the cursor sitting at the end of the line of output. A call to System.out.println writes things and then finishes the job by moving the cursor to the start of a brand-new line of output.

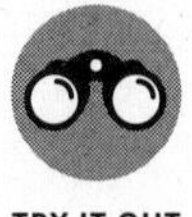

TRY IT OUT

Run the code in Listing 4-2 to make sure that it runs correctly on your computer. Then see what happens when you make the following changes:

- Add thousands-separators to the number `1000000.00` in the code. For example, if you live in the United States, where the thousands-separator is a comma, change the number to `1,000,000.00` and see what happens. (***Hint:*** Nothing good happens.)
- Try using underscores as thousands-separators in the code. That is, change `1000000.00` to `1_000_000.00` and see what happens.
- Add a currency symbol to the number `50.22` in the code. For example, if you live in the United States, where the currency symbol is $, see what happens when you change the first assignment statement to `amountInAccount = $50.22`.
- Listing 4-2 has two `System.out.print` statements and one `System.out.println` statement. Change all three to `System.out.println` statements and then run the program.
- The code in Listing 4-2 displays one line of text in its output. Using the `amountInAccount` variable, add statements to the program so that it displays a second line of text. Have the second line of text be "Now you have even more! You have 2000000.00 in your account."

Numbers without decimal points

"In 1995, the average family had 2.3 children."

At this point, a wise guy always remarks that no real family has exactly 2.3 children. Clearly, whole numbers have a role in this world. Therefore, in Java, you can declare a variable to store nothing but whole numbers. Listing 4-3 shows a program that uses whole number variables.

LISTING 4-3: Using the int Type

```
public class ElevatorFitter {

    public static void main(String args[]) {
        int weightOfAPerson;
        int elevatorWeightLimit;
        int numberOfPeople;
```

(continued)

LISTING 4-3: (continued)

```
        weightOfAPerson = 150;
        elevatorWeightLimit = 1400;
        numberOfPeople = elevatorWeightLimit / weightOfAPerson;

        System.out.print("You can fit ");
        System.out.print(numberOfPeople);
        System.out.println(" people on the elevator.");
    }
}
```

The story behind the program in Listing 4-3 takes some heavy-duty explaining. Here goes:

You have a hotel elevator whose weight capacity is 1,400 pounds. One weekend the hotel hosts the Brickenchicker family reunion. A certain branch of the Brickenchicker family has been blessed with identical dectuplets (ten siblings, all with the same physical characteristics). Normally, each of the Brickenchicker dectuplets weighs exactly 145 pounds. But on Saturday the family has a big catered lunch, and, because lunch included strawberry shortcake, each of the Brickenchicker dectuplets now weighs 150 pounds. Immediately after lunch, all ten of the Brickenchicker dectuplets arrive at the elevator at exactly the same time. (Why not? All ten of them think alike.) So, the question is, how many of the dectuplets can fit on the elevator?

Now remember, if you put one ounce more than 1,400 pounds of weight on the elevator, the elevator cable breaks, plunging all dectuplets on the elevator to their sudden (and costly) deaths.

The answer to the Brickenchicker riddle (the output of the program of Listing 4-3) is shown in Figure 4-6.

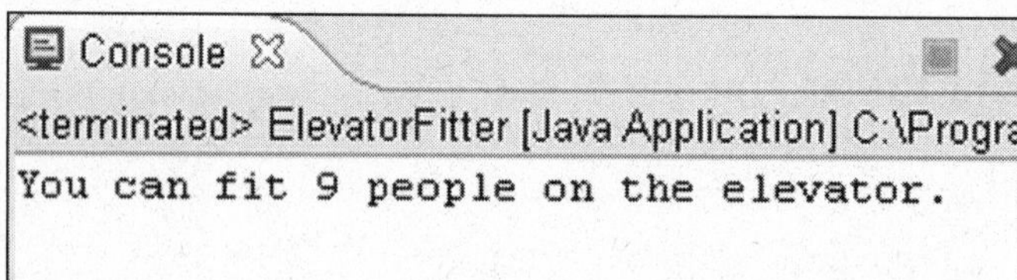
Console
<terminated> ElevatorFitter [Java Application] C:\Progra
You can fit 9 people on the elevator.

FIGURE 4-6: Save the Brickenchickers.

At the core of the Brickenchicker elevator problem, you have whole numbers — numbers with no digits beyond the decimal point. When you divide 1,400 by 150, you get 9⅓, but you shouldn't take the ⅓ seriously. No matter how hard you try, you can't squeeze an extra 50 pounds' worth of Brickenchicker dectuplet onto the elevator. This fact is reflected nicely in Java. In Listing 4-3, all three variables (weightOfAPerson, elevatorWeightLimit, and numberOfPeople) are of type int. An int value is a whole number. When you divide one int value by another (as you do with the slash in Listing 4-3), you get another int. When you divide 1,400 by 150, you get 9 — not 9⅓. You see this in Figure 4-6. Taken together, the following statements display 9 onscreen:

```
numberOfPeople = elevatorWeightLimit / weightOfAPerson;

System.out.print(numberOfPeople);
```

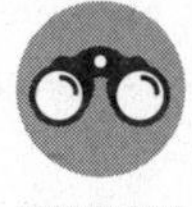

TRY IT OUT

My wife and I were married on February 29, so we have one anniversary every four years. Write a program with a variable named years. Based on the value of the years variable, the program displays the number of anniversaries we've had. For example, if the value of years is 4, the program displays the sentence Number of anniversaries: 1. If the value of years is 7, the program still displays Number of anniversaries: 1. But if the value of years is 8, the program displays Number of anniversaries: 2.

Combining declarations and initializing variables

Look back at Listing 4-3. In that listing, you see three variable declarations — one for each of the program's three int variables. I could have done the same thing with just one declaration:

```
int weightOfAPerson, elevatorWeightLimit, numberOfPeople;
```

FOUR WAYS TO STORE WHOLE NUMBERS

Java has four types of whole numbers. The types are byte, short, int, and long. Unlike the complicated story about the accuracy of types float and double, the only thing that matters when you choose among the whole number types is the size of the number you're trying to store. If you want to use numbers larger than 127, don't use byte. To store numbers larger than 32767, don't use short.

Most of the time, you'll use int. But if you need to store numbers larger than 2147483647, forsake int in favor of long. (A long number can be as big as 9223372036854775807.) For the whole story, see Table 4-1, a little later in this chapter.

WARNING

If two variables have completely different types, you can't create both variables in the same declaration. For instance, to create an `int` variable named *weightOfFred* and a `double` variable named *amountInFredsAccount*, you need two separate variable declarations.

You can give variables their starting values in a declaration. In Listing 4-3, for instance, one declaration can replace several lines in the `main` method (all but the calls to `print` and `println`):

```
int weightOfAPerson = 150, elevatorWeightLimit = 1400,
  numberOfPeople = elevatorWeightLimit/weightOfAPerson;
```

When you do this, you don't say that you're assigning values to variables. The pieces of the declarations with equal signs in them aren't really called assignment statements. Instead, you say that you're *initializing* the variables. Believe it or not, keeping this distinction in mind is helpful.

Like everything else in life, initializing a variable has advantages and disadvantages:

- **When you combine six lines of Listing 4-3 into just one declaration, the code becomes more concise.** Sometimes concise code is easier to read. Sometimes it's not. As a programmer, it's your judgment call.
- **By initializing a variable, you might automatically avoid certain programming errors.** For an example, see Chapter 7.
- **In some situations, you have no choice. The nature of your code forces you either to initialize or not to initialize.** For an example that doesn't lend itself to variable initialization, see the deleting-evidence program in Chapter 6.

Experimenting with JShell

The programs in Listings 4-2 and 4-3 both begin with the same old, tiresome refrain:

```
public class SomethingOrOther {

    public static void main(String args[]) {
```

A Java program requires this verbose introduction because

- » In Java the entire program is a class.
- » The `main` method is called into action automatically when the program begins running.

I explain all of this in Chapter 3.

Anyway, retyping this boilerplate code into an editor window can be annoying, especially when your goal is to test the effect of executing a few simple statements. To fix this problem, the stewards of Java came up with a new tool in Java 9. They call it *JShell*.

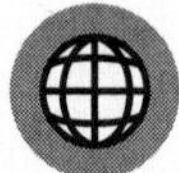

Instructions for launching JShell differ from one computer to the next. For instructions that work on your computer, visit this book's website (`www.allmycode.com/JavaForDummies`).

When you use JShell, you hardly ever type an entire program. Instead, you type a Java statement, and then JShell responds to your statement, and then you type a second statement, and then JShell responds to your second statement, and then you type a third statement, and so on. A single statement is enough to get a response from JShell.

JShell is only one example of a language's *Read Evaluate Print Loop* (REPL). Many programming languages have REPLs and, with Java 9, the Java language finally has a REPL of its own.

In Figure 4-7, I use JShell to find out how Java responds to the assignment statements in Listings 4-2 and 4-3.

When you run JShell, the dialogue goes something like this:

```
jshell> You type a statement
JShell responds

jshell> You type another statement
JShell responds
```

For example, in Figure 4-7, I type `double amountInAccount` and then press Enter. JShell responds by displaying

```
amountInAccount ==> 0.0
```

```
jshell> double amountInAccount
amountInAccount ==> 0.0

jshell> amountInAccount = 50.22
amountInAccount ==> 50.22

jshell> amountInAccount = amountInAccount + 1000000.00
amountInAccount ==> 1000050.22

jshell> int weightOfAPerson, elevatorWeightLimit
weightOfAPerson ==> 0
elevatorWeightLimit ==> 0

jshell> weightOfAPerson = 150;
weightOfAPerson ==> 150

jshell> elevatorWeightLimit = 1400
elevatorWeightLimit ==> 1400

jshell> elevatorWeightLimit / weightOfAPerson
$8 ==> 9

jshell> $8 + 1
$9 ==> 10

jshell> 42 + 7
$10 ==> 49

jshell>
```

FIGURE 4-7: An intimate conversation between me and JShell.

Here are a few things to notice about JShell:

- **You don't have to type an entire Java program.**

  Typing a few statements such as

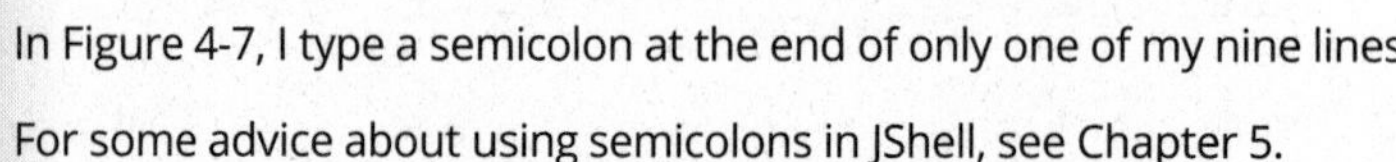

```
double amountInAccount
amountInAccount = 50.22
amountInAccount = amountInAccount + 1000000.00
```

  does the trick. It's like running the code snippet in Listing 4-1 (except that Listing 4-1 doesn't declare `amountInAccount` to be a `double`).

- **In JShell, semicolons are (to a large extent) optional.**

  In Figure 4-7, I type a semicolon at the end of only one of my nine lines.

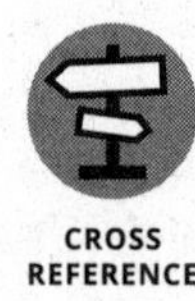

CROSS REFERENCE

  For some advice about using semicolons in JShell, see Chapter 5.

- **JShell responds immediately after you type each line.**

  After I declare `amountInAccount` to be `double`, JShell responds by telling me that the `amountInAccount` variable has the value 0.0. After I type `amountInAccount = amountInAccount + 1000000.00`, JShell tells me that the new value of `amountInAccount` is 1000050.22.

* **You can mix statements from many different Java programs.**

  In Figure 4-7, I mix statements from the programs in Listings 4-2 and 4-3. JShell doesn't care.

* **You can ask JShell for the value of an expression.**

  You don't have to assign the expression's value to a variable. For example, in Figure 4-7, I type

  ```
  elevatorWeightLimit / weightOfAPerson
  ```

  JShell responds by telling me that the value of `elevatorWeightLimit / weightOfAPerson` is 9. JShell makes up a temporary name for that value. In Figure 4-7, the name happens to be $8. So, on the next line in Figure 4-7, I ask for the value of `$8 +1`, and JShell gives me the answer 10.

* **You can even get answers from JShell without using variables.**

  On the last line in Figure 4-7, I ask for the value of 42 + 7, and JShell generously answers with the value 49.

TIP

While you're running JShell, you don't have to retype commands that you've already typed. If you press the up-arrow key once, JShell shows you the command that you typed most recently. If you press the up-arrow key twice, JShell shows you the next-to-last command that you typed. And so on. When JShell shows you a command, you can use your left- and right-arrow keys to move to any character in the middle of the command. You can modify characters in the command. Finally, when you press Enter, JShell executes your newly modified command.

To end your run of JShell, you type **/exit** (starting with a slash). But `/exit` is only one of many commands you can give to JShell. To ask JShell what other kinds of commands you can use, type **/help**.

With JShell, you can test your statements before you put them into a full-blown Java program. That makes JShell a truly useful tool.

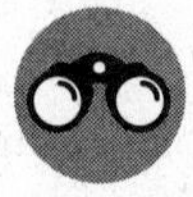

TRY IT OUT

Visit this book's website (`www.allmycode.com/JavaForDummies`) for instructions on launching JShell on your computer. After launching JShell, type a few lines of code from Figure 4-7. See what happens when you type some slightly different lines.

What Happened to All the Cool Visual Effects?

The programs in Listings 4-2 and 4-3 are text-based. A *text-based* program has no windows, no dialog boxes — nothing of that kind. All you see is line after line of plain, unformatted text. The user types something, and the computer displays a response beneath each line of input.

The opposite of a text-based program is a *graphical user interface* (GUI) program. A GUI program has windows, text fields, buttons, and other visual goodies.

As visually unexciting as text-based programs are, they contain the basic concepts for all computer programming. Also, text-based programs are easier for the novice programmer to read, write, and understand than the corresponding GUI programs. So, in this book I take a three-pronged approach:

- **Text-based examples:** I introduce most of the new concepts with these examples.
- **The `DummiesFrame` class:** Alongside the text-based examples, I present GUI versions using the `DummiesFrame` class, which I created especially for this book. (I introduce the `DummiesFrame` class in Chapter 7.)
- **GUI programming techniques:** I describe some of the well-known techniques in Chapters 9, 10, 14, and 16. I even have a tiny GUI example in this chapter. (See the later section "The Molecules and Compounds: Reference Types.")

With this careful balance of drab programs and sparkly programs, you're sure to learn Java.

The Atoms: Java's Primitive Types

The words *int* and *double* that I describe in the previous sections are examples of *primitive types* (also known as *simple* types) in Java. The Java language has exactly eight primitive types. As a newcomer to Java, you can pretty much ignore all but four of these types. (As programming languages go, Java is nice and compact that way.) Table 4-1 shows the complete list of primitive types.

TABLE 4-1: Java's Primitive Types

Type Name	What a Literal Looks Like	Range of Values
Whole number types		
`byte`	`(byte)42`	–128 to 127
`short`	`(short)42`	–32768 to 32767
`int`	`42`	–2147483648 to 2147483647
`long`	`42L`	–9223372036854775808 to 9223372036854775807
Decimal number types		
`float`	`42.0F`	-3.4×10^{38} to 3.4×10^{38}
`double`	`42.0`	-1.8×10^{308} to 1.8×10^{308}
Character type		
`char`	`'A'`	Thousands of characters, glyphs, and symbols
Logical type		
`boolean`	`true`	true, false

The types that you shouldn't ignore are `int`, `double`, `char`, and `boolean`. Previous sections in this chapter cover the `int` and `double` types. So the next two sections cover `char` and `boolean` types.

The char type

Several decades ago, people thought computers existed only for doing big number-crunching calculations. Nowadays, nobody thinks that way. So, if you haven't been in a cryogenic freezing chamber for the past 20 years, you know that computers store letters, punctuation symbols, and other characters.

The Java type that's used to store characters is called *char.* Listing 4-4 has a simple program that uses the `char` type. Figure 4-8 shows the output of the program in Listing 4-4.

LISTING 4-4: Using the char Type

```
public class CharDemo {

  public static void main(String args[]) {
     char myLittleChar = 'b';
     char myBigChar = Character.toUpperCase(myLittleChar);
     System.out.println(myBigChar);
  }
}
```

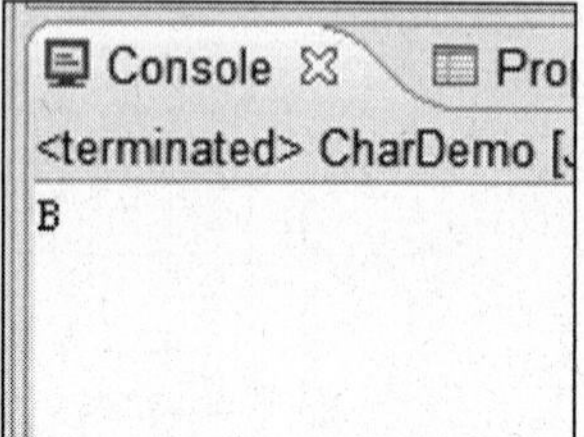

FIGURE 4-8: An exciting run of the program of Listing 4-4 as it appears in the Eclipse Console view.

In Listing 4-4, the first initialization stores the letter *b* in the variable `myLittleChar`. In the initialization, notice how *b* is surrounded by single quote marks. In Java, every `char` literal starts and ends with a single quote mark.

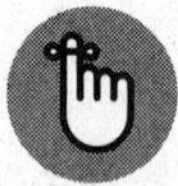

REMEMBER

In a Java program, single quote marks surround the letter in a `char` literal.

If you need help sorting out the terms *assignment*, *declaration*, and *initialization*, see the "Combining declarations and initializing variables" section, earlier in this chapter.

In the second initialization of Listing 4-4, the program calls an API method whose name is *Character.toUpperCase*. The `Character.toUpperCase` method does just what its name suggests — the method produces the uppercase equivalent of the letter *b*. This uppercase equivalent (the letter *B*) is assigned to the `myBigChar` variable, and the *B* that's in `myBigChar` prints onscreen.

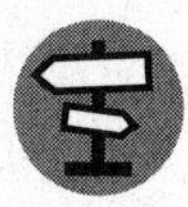

CROSS REFERENCE

For an introduction to the Java application programming interface (API), see Chapter 3.

If you're tempted to write the following statement,

```
char myLittleChars = 'barry';  //Don't do this
```

please resist the temptation. You can't store more than one letter at a time in a `char` variable, and you can't put more than one letter between a pair of single quotes. If you're trying to store words or sentences (not just single letters), you need to use something called a String.

For a look at Java's `String` type, see the section "The Molecules and Compounds: Reference Types," later in this chapter.

WARNING

If you're used to writing programs in other languages, you may be aware of something called ASCII character encoding. Most languages use ASCII; Java uses Unicode. In the old ASCII representation, each character takes up only 8 bits, but in Unicode, each character takes up 8, 16, or 32 bits. Whereas ASCII stores the letters of the Roman (English) alphabet, Unicode has room for characters from most of the world's commonly spoken languages. The only problem is that some of the Java API methods are geared specially toward 16-bit Unicode. Occasionally, this bites you in the back (or it bytes you in the back, as the case may be). If you're using a method to write `Hello` on the screen and `H e l l o` shows up instead, check the method's documentation for mention of Unicode characters.

It's worth noticing that the two methods, `Character.toUpperCase` and `System.out.println`, are used quite differently in Listing 4-4. The method `Character.toUpperCase` is called as part of an initialization or an assignment statement, but the method `System.out.println` is called on its own. To find out more about this topic, see the explanation of return values in Chapter 7.

The boolean type

A variable of type `boolean` stores one of two values: `true` or `false`. Listing 4-5 demonstrates the use of a `boolean` variable. Figure 4-9 shows the output of the program in Listing 4-5.

LISTING 4-5: Using the boolean Type

```
public class ElevatorFitter2 {

    public static void main(String args[]) {
        System.out.println("True or False?");
        System.out.println("You can fit all ten of the");
        System.out.println("Brickenchicker dectuplets");
        System.out.println("on the elevator:");
        System.out.println();

        int weightOfAPerson = 150;
```

(continued)

LISTING 4-5: (continued)

```
        int elevatorWeightLimit = 1400;
        int numberOfPeople = elevatorWeightLimit / weightOfAPerson;

        boolean allTenOkay = numberOfPeople >= 10;

        System.out.println(allTenOkay);
    }
}
```

```
True or False?
You can fit all ten of the
Brickenchicker dectuplets
on the elevator:

false
```

FIGURE 4-9: The Brickenchicker dectuplets strike again.

In Listing 4-5, the `allTenOkay` variable is of type `boolean`. To find a value for the `allTenOkay` variable, the program checks to see whether `numberOfPeople` is greater than or equal to ten. (The symbols `>=` stand for *greater than or equal to.*)

At this point, it pays to be fussy about terminology. Any part of a Java program that has a value is an *expression.* If you write

```
weightOfAPerson = 150;
```

then `150` is an expression (an expression whose value is the quantity `150`). If you write

```
numberOfEggs = 2 + 2;
```

then `2 + 2` is an expression (because `2 + 2` has the value `4`). If you write

```
int numberOfPeople = elevatorWeightLimit / weightOfAPerson;
```

then `elevatorWeightLimit / weightOfAPerson` is an expression. (The value of the expression `elevatorWeightLimit / weightOfAPerson` depends on whatever values the variables `elevatorWeightLimit` and `weightOfAPerson` have when the code containing the expression is executed.)

REMEMBER

Any part of a Java program that has a value is an *expression.*

In Listing 4-5, the code `numberOfPeople >= 10` is an expression. The expression's value depends on the value stored in the `numberOfPeople` variable. But, as you know from seeing the strawberry shortcake at the Brickenchicker family's catered lunch, the value of `numberOfPeople` isn't greater than or equal to ten. As a result, the value of `numberOfPeople >= 10` is `false`. So, in the statement in Listing 4-5, in which `allTenOkay` is assigned a value, the `allTenOkay` variable is assigned a `false` value.

TIP

In Listing 4-5, I call `System.out.println()` with nothing inside the parentheses. When I do this, Java adds a line break to the program's output. In Listing 4-5, `System.out.println()` tells the program to display a blank line.

The Molecules and Compounds: Reference Types

By combining simple things, you get more complicated things. That's the way things always go. Take some of Java's primitive types, whip them together to make a primitive type stew, and what do you get? A more complicated type called a *reference type.*

The program in Listing 4-6 uses reference types. Figure 4-10 shows you what happens when you run the program in Listing 4-6.

LISTING 4-6: Using Reference Types

```
import javax.swing.JFrame;

public class ShowAFrame {

    public static void main(String args[]) {
        JFrame myFrame = new JFrame();
        String myTitle = "Blank Frame";

        myFrame.setTitle(myTitle);
        myFrame.setSize(300, 200);
        myFrame.setDefaultCloseOperation(JFrame.EXIT_ON_CLOSE);
        myFrame.setVisible(true);
    }
}
```

The program in Listing 4-6 uses two references types. Both types are defined in the Java API. One of the types (the one that you'll use all the time) is called *String*. The other type (the one that you can use to create GUIs) is called *JFrame*.

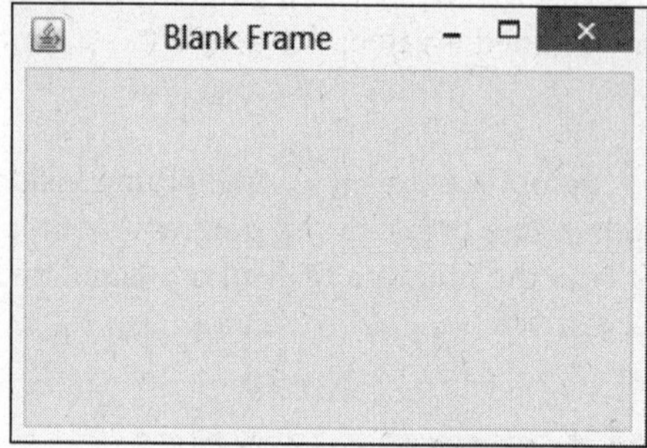

FIGURE 4-10: An empty frame.

A `String` is a bunch of characters. It's like having several `char` values in a row. So, with the `myTitle` variable declared to be of type `String`, assigning `"Blank Frame"` to the `myTitle` variable makes sense in Listing 4-6. The `String` class is declared in the Java API.

REMEMBER

In a Java program, double quote marks surround the letters in a `String` literal.

A Java *JFrame* is a lot like a window. (The only difference is that you call it a JFrame instead of a window.) To keep Listing 4-6 short and sweet, I decided not to put anything in my frame — no buttons, no fields, nothing.

Even with a completely empty frame, Listing 4-6 uses tricks that I don't describe until later in this book. So don't try reading and interpreting every word of Listing 4-6. The big thing to get from Listing 4-6 is that the program has two variable declarations. In writing the program, I made up two variable names: `myTitle` and `myFrame`. According to the declarations, `myTitle` is of type `String`, and `myFrame` is of type `JFrame`.

You can look up `String` and `JFrame` in Java's API documentation. But, even before you do, I can tell you what you'll find. You'll find that `String` and `JFrame` are the names of Java classes. So that's the big news. Every class is the name of a reference type. You can reserve `amountInAccount` for `double` values by writing

```
double amountInAccount;
```

or by writing

```
double amountInAccount = 50.22;
```

You can also reserve `myFrame` for a `JFrame` value by writing

```
JFrame myFrame;
```

or by writing

```
JFrame myFrame = new JFrame();
```

To review the notion of a Java class, see the sections on object-oriented programming (OOP) in Chapter 1.

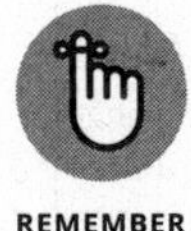
REMEMBER

Every Java class is a reference type. If you declare a variable to have some type that's not a primitive type, the variable's type is (most of the time) the name of a Java class.

Now, when you declare a variable to have type `int`, you can visualize what that declaration means in a fairly straightforward way. It means that, somewhere inside the computer's memory, a storage location is reserved for that variable's value. In the storage location is a bunch of bits. The arrangement of the bits ensures that a certain whole number is represented.

That explanation is fine for primitive types like `int` or `double`, but what does it mean when you declare a variable to have a reference type? What does it mean to declare variable `myFrame` to be of type `JFrame`?

Well, what does it mean to declare *i thank You God* to be an E. E. Cummings poem? What would it mean to write the following declaration?

```
EECummingsPoem ithankYouGod;
```

It means that a class of things is `EECummingsPoem`, and `ithankYouGod` refers to an instance of that class. In other words, `ithankYouGod` is an object belonging to the `EECummingsPoem` class.

Because `JFrame` is a class, you can create objects from that class. (If you don't believe me, read some of my paragraphs about classes and objects in Chapter 1.) Each object (each instance of the `JFrame` class) is an actual frame — a window that appears on the screen when you run the code in Listing 4-6. By declaring the variable `myFrame` to be of type `JFrame`, you're reserving the use of the name `myFrame`. This reservation tells the computer that `myFrame` can refer to an actual `JFrame`-type object. In other words, `myFrame` can become a nickname for one of the windows that appears on the computer screen. Figure 4-11 illustrates the situation.

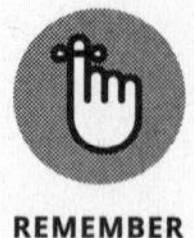

REMEMBER

When you declare *ClassName variableName;*, you're saying that a certain variable can refer to an instance of a particular class.

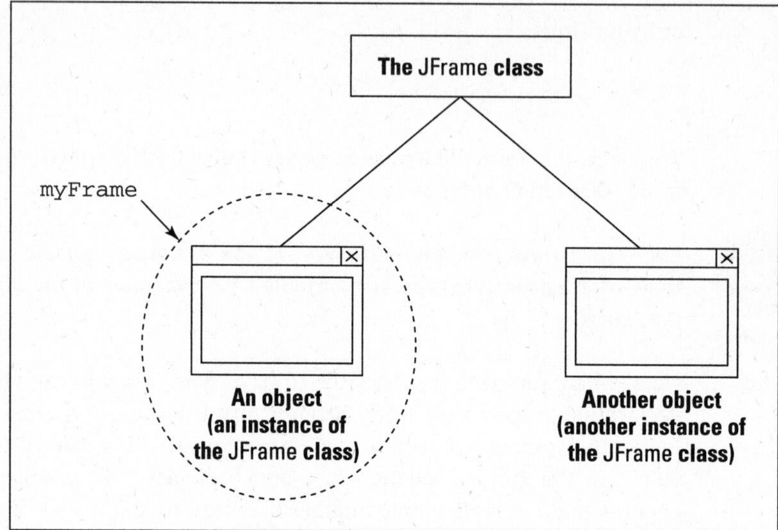

FIGURE 4-11: The variable myFrame refers to an instance of the JFrame class.

TECHNICAL STUFF

In Listing 4-6, the phrase JFrame myFrame reserves the use of the name myFrame. On that same line of code, the phrase new JFrame() creates a new object (an instance of the JFrame class). Finally, that line's equal sign makes myFrame refer to the new object. Knowing that the two words new JFrame() create an object can be very important. For a more thorough explanation of objects, see Chapter 7.

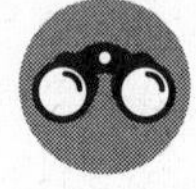

TRY IT OUT

Try these things:

- Run the code in Listing 4-6 on your computer.
- Before running the code in Listing 4-6, comment out the myFrame.setVisible(true) statement by putting two forward slashes (//) immediately to the left of the statement. Does anything happen when you run the modified code?
- Experiment with the code in Listing 4-6 by changing the order of the statements inside the body of the main method. What rearrangements of these statements are okay, and which aren't?

PRIMITIVE TYPE STEW

While I'm on the subject of frames, what's a frame, anyway? A *frame* is a window that has a certain height and width and a certain location on your computer's screen. Therefore, deep inside the declaration of the `Frame` class, you can find variable declarations that look something like this:

```
int width;
int height;
int x;
int y;
```

Here's another example — `Time`. An instance of the `Time` class may have an hour (a number from 1 to 12), a number of minutes (from 0 to 59), and a letter (*a* for a.m.; *p* for p.m.).

```
int hour;
int minutes;
char amOrPm;
```

Notice that this high-and-mighty thing called a Java API class is neither high nor mighty. A class is just a collection of declarations. Some of those declarations are the declarations of variables. Some of those variable declarations use primitive types, and other variable declarations use reference types. These reference types, however, come from other classes, and the declarations of those classes have variables. The chain goes on and on. Ultimately, everything comes, in one way or another, from the primitive types.

An Import Declaration

It's always good to announce your intentions up front. Consider the following classroom lecture:

> *Today, in our History of Film course, we'll be discussing the career of actor* ***Lionel Herbert Blythe Barrymore****.*
>
> *Born in Philadelphia,* ***Barrymore*** *appeared in more than 200 films, including* It's a Wonderful Life, Key Largo, and Dr. Kildare's Wedding Day. *In addition,* ***Barrymore*** *was a writer, composer, and director. Barrymore did the voice of Ebenezer Scrooge every year on radio . . . .*

Interesting stuff, heh? Now compare these paragraphs with a lecture in which the instructor doesn't begin by introducing the subject:

> *Welcome once again to the History of Film.*
>
> *Born in Philadelphia,* ***Lionel Barrymore*** *appeared in more than 200 films, including* It's a Wonderful Life, Key Largo, *and* Dr. Kildare's Wedding Day. *In addition,* ***Barrymore (not Ethel, John, or Drew)*** *was a writer, composer, and director.* ***Lionel Barrymore*** *did the voice of Ebenezer Scrooge every year on radio . . . .*

Without a proper introduction, a speaker may have to remind you constantly that the discussion is about Lionel Barrymore and not about any other Barrymore. The same is true in a Java program. Look again at Listing 4-6:

```
import javax.swing.JFrame;

public class ShowAFrame {

    public static void main(String args[]) {
        JFrame myFrame = new JFrame();
```

In Listing 4-6, you announce in the introduction (in the import declaration) that you're using `JFrame` in your Java class. You clarify what you mean by `JFrame` with the full name `javax.swing.JFrame`. (Hey! Didn't the first lecturer clarify with the full name "Lionel Herbert Blythe Barrymore"?) After announcing your intentions in the import declaration, you can use the abbreviated name *JFrame* in your Java class code.

If you don't use an import declaration, you have to repeat the full `javax.swing.JFrame` name wherever you use the name *JFrame* in your code. For example, without an import declaration, the code of Listing 4-6 would look like this:

```
public class ShowAFrame {

    public static void main(String args[]) {
        javax.swing.JFrame myFrame = new javax.swing.JFrame();
        String myTitle = "Blank Frame";

        myFrame.setTitle(myTitle);
        myFrame.setSize(3200, 200);
        myFrame.setDefaultCloseOperation(javax.swing.JFrame.EXIT_ON_CLOSE);
        myFrame.setVisible(true);
    }
}
```

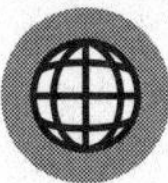

The details of this import stuff can be pretty nasty. But fortunately, many IDEs have convenient helper features for import declarations. For details, see this book's website (`www.allmycode.com/JavaForDummies`).

No single section in this book can present the entire story about import declarations. To begin untangling some of the import declaration's subtleties, see Chapters 5, 9, and 10.

Creating New Values by Applying Operators

What could be more comforting than your old friend the plus sign? It was the first topic you learned about in elementary school math. Almost everybody knows how to add 2 and 2. In fact, in English usage, adding 2 and 2 is a metaphor for something that's easy to do. Whenever you see a plus sign, a cell in your brain says, "Thank goodness — it could be something much more complicated."

Java has a plus sign. You can use it for several purposes. You can use the plus sign to add two numbers, like this:

```
int apples, oranges, fruit;
apples = 5;
oranges = 16;
fruit = apples + oranges;
```

You can also use the plus sign to paste `String` values together:

```
String startOfChapter =
    "It's three in the morning. I'm dreaming about the"+
    "history course that I failed in high school.";
System.out.println(startOfChapter);
```

This can be handy because in Java, you're not allowed to make a `String` straddle from one line to another. In other words, the following code wouldn't work:

```
String thisIsBadCode =
    "It's three in the morning. I'm dreaming about the
     history course that I failed in high school.";
System.out.println(thisIsBadCode);
```

TECHNICAL STUFF

The correct way to say that you're pasting `String` values together is to say that you're *concatenating* `String` values.

You can even use the plus sign to paste numbers next to `String` values:

```
int apples, oranges, fruit;
apples = 5;
oranges = 16;
fruit = apples + oranges;
System.out.println("You have" + fruit + "pieces of fruit.");
```

Of course, the old minus sign is available, too (but not for `String` values):

```
apples = fruit - oranges;
```

Use an asterisk (*) for multiplication and a slash (/) for division:

```
double rate, pay;
int hours;

rate = 6.25;
hours = 35;
pay = rate * hours;
System.out.println(pay);
```

For an example using division, refer to Listing 4-3.

WARNING

When you divide an `int` value by another `int` value, you get an `int` value. The computer doesn't round. Instead, the computer chops off any remainder. If you put `System.out.println(11 / 4)` in your program, the computer prints `2`, not `2.75`. To get past this, make either (or both) of the numbers you're dividing `double` values. If you put `System.out.println(11.0 / 4)` in your program, the computer prints `2.75`.

Another useful arithmetic operator is called the *remainder* operator. The symbol for the remainder operator is the percent sign (%). When you put `System.out.println(11 % 4)` in your program, the computer prints `3`. It does this because 4 goes into 11 who-cares-how-many times with a remainder of 3. The remainder operator turns out to be fairly useful. Listing 4-7 has an example.

LISTING 4-7: **Making Change**

```
import static java.lang.System.out;

public class MakeChange {

    public static void main(String args[]) {
        int total = 248;
        int quarters = total / 25;
        int whatsLeft = total % 25;

        int dimes = whatsLeft / 10;
        whatsLeft = whatsLeft % 10;

        int nickels = whatsLeft / 5;
        whatsLeft = whatsLeft % 5;

        int cents = whatsLeft;

        out.println("From " + total + " cents you get");
        out.println(quarters + " quarters");
        out.println(dimes + " dimes");
        out.println(nickels + " nickels");
        out.println(cents + " cents");
    }
}
```

Figure 4-12 shows a run of the code in Listing 4-7. You start with a total of 248 cents. Then

```
quarters = total / 25
```

divides 248 by 25, giving 9. That means you can make 9 quarters from 248 cents. Next,

```
whatsLeft = total % 25
```

divides 248 by 25 again and puts only the remainder, 23, into `whatsLeft`. Now you're ready for the next step, which is to take as many dimes as you can out of cents.

```
From 248 cents you get
9 quarters
2 dimes
0 nickels
3 cents
```

FIGURE 4-12: Change for $2.48.

The code in Listing 4-7 makes change in U.S. currency with the following coin denominations: 1 cent, 5 cents (one nickel), 10 cents (one dime), and 25 cents (one quarter). With these denominations, the `MakeChange` class gives you more than simply a set of coins adding up to 248 cents. The `MakeChange` class gives you the *smallest number of coins* that add up to 248 cents. With some minor tweaking, you can make the code work in any country's coinage. You can always get a set of coins adding up to a total. But, for the denominations of coins in some countries, you won't always get the *smallest number of coins* that add up to a total. In fact, I'm looking for examples. If your country's coinage prevents `MakeChange` from always giving the best answer, please, send me an email (`JavaForDummies@allmycode.com`).

IMPORT DECLARATIONS: THE UGLY TRUTH

Notice the import declaration at the top of Listing 4-7:

```
import static java.lang.System.out;
```

Compare this with the import declaration at the top of Listing 4-6:

```
import javax.swing.JFrame;
```

By adding the `import static java.lang.System.out;` line to Listing 4-7, I can make the rest of the code a bit easier to read, and I can avoid having long Java statements that start on one line and continue on another. But you never have to do that. If you remove the `import static java.lang.System.out;` line and pepper the code liberally with `System.out.println`, the code works just fine.

Here's a question: Why does one declaration include the word *static* and the other declaration doesn't? Well, to be honest, I wish I hadn't asked!

For the real story about *static*, you have to read part of Chapter 10. And frankly, I don't recommend skipping ahead to that chapter's *static* section if you take medicine for a heart condition, if you're pregnant or nursing, or if you have no previous experience with object-oriented programming. For now, rest assured that Chapter 10 is easy to read after you've made the journey through Part 3 of this book. And when you have to decide whether to use the word *static* in an import declaration, remember these hints:

- The vast majority of import declarations in Java program do not use the word *static*.
- In this book, I never use *import static* to import anything except `System.out`. (Well, almost never . . . .)
- Most import declarations don't use the word *static* because most declarations import classes. Unfortunately, `System.out` is not the name of a class.

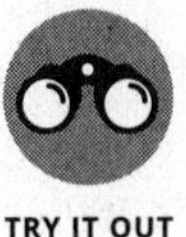

Find the values of the following expressions by typing each expression in JShell (if you have trouble launching JShell, create a Java program that displays the value of each of these expressions):

» 5 / 4

» 5 / 4.0

» 5.0 / 4

» 5.0 / 4.0

» "5" + "4"

» 5 + 4

» " " + 5 + 4

Initialize once, assign often

Listing 4-7 has three lines that put values into the variable `whatsLeft`:

```
int whatsLeft = total % 25;

whatsLeft = whatsLeft % 10;

whatsLeft = whatsLeft % 5;
```

Only one of these lines is a declaration. The other two lines are assignment statements. That's good because you can't declare the same variable more than once (not without creating something called a *block*). If you goof and write

```
int whatsLeft = total % 25;

int whatsLeft = whatsLeft % 10;
```

in Listing 4-7, you see an error message (such as `Duplicate variable whatsLeft` or `Variable 'whatsLeft' is already defined`) when you try to compile your code.

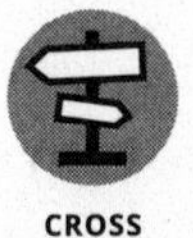

To find out what a block is, see Chapter 5. Then, for some honest talk about redeclaring variables, see Chapter 10.

The increment and decrement operators

Java has some neat little operators that make life easier (for the computer's processor, for your brain, and for your fingers). Altogether, four such operators exist — two increment operators and two decrement operators. The increment operators add 1, and the decrement operators subtract 1. The increment operators use double plus signs (++), and the decrement operators use double minus signs (--). To see how they work, you need some examples. The first example is shown in Figure 4-13.

Figure 4-14 shows a run of the program in Figure 4-13. In this horribly uneventful run, the count of bunnies prints three times.

The double plus signs go by two names, depending on where you put them. When you put the ++ before a variable, the ++ is called the *preincrement* operator. (The *pre* stands for *before*.)

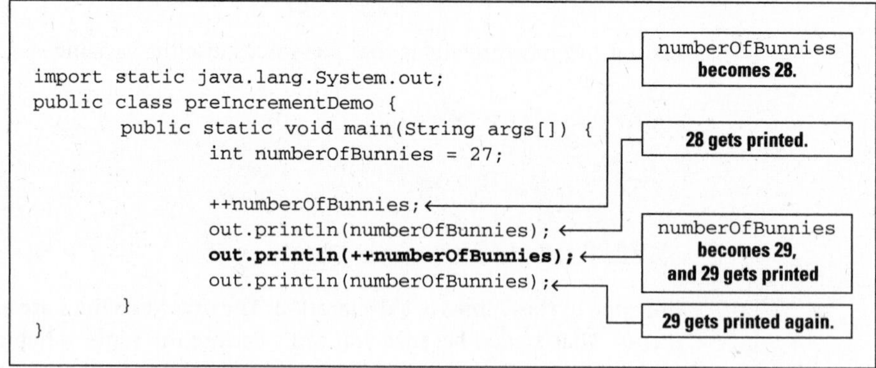

```
import static java.lang.System.out;
public class preIncrementDemo {
        public static void main(String args[]) {
                int numberOfBunnies = 27;

                ++numberOfBunnies;
                out.println(numberOfBunnies);
                out.println(++numberOfBunnies);
                out.println(numberOfBunnies);
        }
}
```


FIGURE 4-13: Using preincrement.

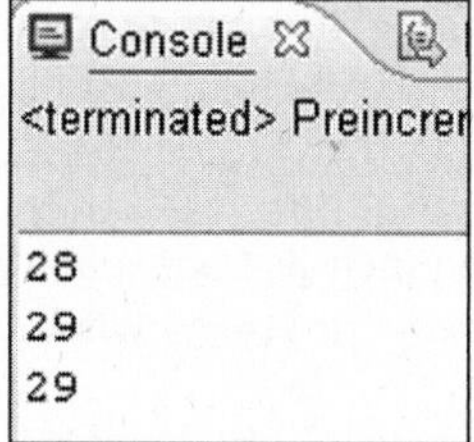

FIGURE 4-14: A run of the code in Figure 4-13.

The word *before* has two meanings:

- » You put ++ before the variable.
- » The computer adds 1 to the variable's value before the variable is used in any other part of the statement.

To understand this, look at the bold line in Figure 4-13. The computer adds 1 to numberOfBunnies (raising the value of numberOfBunnies to 29) and then prints 29 onscreen.

REMEMBER

With out.println(++numberOfBunnies), the computer adds 1 to numberOfBunnies before printing the new value of numberOfBunnies onscreen.

An alternative to preincrement is *postincrement.* (The *post* stands for *after.*) The word *after* has two different meanings:

- You put ++ after the variable.
- The computer adds 1 to the variable's value after the variable is used in any other part of the statement.

To see more clearly how postincrement works, look at the bold line in Figure 4-15. The computer prints the old value of numberOfBunnies (which is 28) on the screen, and then the computer adds 1 to numberOfBunnies, which raises the value of numberOfBunnies to 29.

REMEMBER

With out.println(numberOfBunnies++), the computer adds 1 to numberOfBunnies after printing the old value that numberOfBunnies already had.

Figure 4-16 shows a run of the code in Figure 4-15. Compare Figure 4-16 with the run in Figure 4-14:

- With preincrement in Figure 4-14, the second number is 29.
- With postincrement in Figure 4-16, the second number is 28.

  In Figure 4-16, 29 doesn't show onscreen until the end of the run, when the computer executes one last out.println(numberOfBunnies).

```
import static java.lang.System.out;
public class postIncrementDemo {
       public static void main(String args[]) {
              int numberOfBunnies = 27;

              numberOfBunnies++;
              out.println(numberOfBunnies);
              out.println(numberOfBunnies++);
              out.println(numberOfBunnies);
       }
}
```

numberOfBunnies becomes 28.
28 gets printed.
28 gets printed, and then numberOfBunnies becomes 29.
29 gets printed.

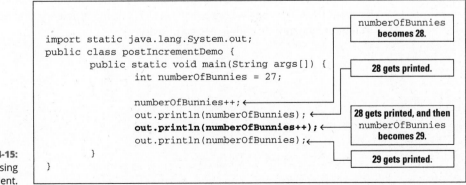

FIGURE 4-15: Using postincrement.

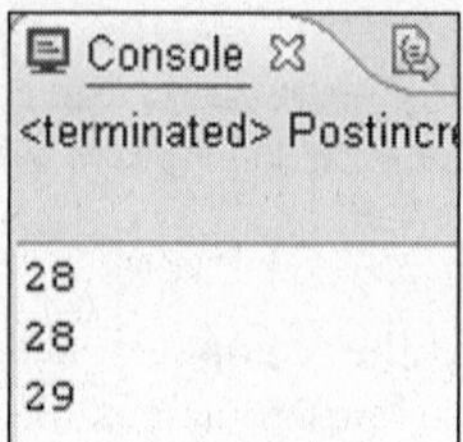

FIGURE 4-16: A run of the code in Figure 4-15.

TIP

Are you trying to decide between using preincrement or postincrement? Try no longer. Most programmers use postincrement. In a typical Java program, you often see things like `numberOfBunnies++`. You seldom see things like `++numberOfBunnies`.

In addition to preincrement and postincrement, Java has two operators that use `--`. These operators are called *predecrement* and *postdecrement:*

- With predecrement (`--numberOfBunnies`), the computer subtracts 1 from the variable's value before the variable is used in the rest of the statement.
- With postdecrement (`numberOfBunnies--`), the computer subtracts 1 from the variable's value after the variable is used in the rest of the statement.

TECHNICAL STUFF

Instead of writing `++numberOfBunnies`, you could achieve the same effect by writing `numberOfBunnies = numberOfBunnies + 1`. So some people conclude that Java's `++` and `--` operators are for saving keystrokes — to keep those poor fingers from overworking themselves. This is entirely incorrect. The best reason for using `++` is to avoid the inefficient and error-prone practice of writing the same variable name, such as `numberOfBunnies`, twice in the same statement. If you write `numberOfBunnies` only once (as you do when you use `++` or `--`), the computer has to figure out what `numberOfBunnies` means only once. On top of that, when you write `numberOfBunnies` only once, you have only one chance (instead of two chances) to type the variable name incorrectly. With simple expressions like `numberOfBunnies++`, these advantages hardly make a difference. But with more complicated expressions, such as `inventoryItems[(quantityReceived--*itemsPerBox+17)]++`, the efficiency and accuracy that you gain by using `++` and `--` are significant.

STATEMENTS AND EXPRESSIONS

You can describe the pre- and postincrement and pre- and postdecrement operators in two ways: the way everyone understands them and the right way. The way that I explain the concept in most of this section (in terms of time, with *before* and *after*) is the way that everyone understands it. Unfortunately, the way everyone understands the concept isn't really the right way. When you see ++ or --, you can think in terms of time sequence. But occasionally a programmer uses ++ or -- in a convoluted way, and the notions of *before* and *after* break down. So if you're ever in a tight spot, think about these operators in terms of statements and expressions.

First, remember that a statement tells the computer to do something, and an expression has a value. (I discuss statements in Chapter 3, and I describe expressions elsewhere in this chapter.) Which category does `numberOfBunnies++` belong to? The surprising answer is both. The Java code `numberOfBunnies++` is both a statement and an expression.

Assume that, before the computer executes the code `out.println(numberOfBunnies++)`, the value of `numberOfBunnies` is 28.

- As a statement, `numberOfBunnies++` tells the computer to add 1 to `numberOfBunnies`.
- As an expression, the value of `numberOfBunnies++` is 28, not 29.

So even though the computer adds 1 to `numberOfBunnies`, the code `out.println(numberOfBunnies++)` really means `out.println(28)`.

Now, almost everything you just read about `numberOfBunnies++` is true about `++numberOfBunnies`. The only difference is that as an expression, `++numberOfBunnies` behaves in a more intuitive way.

- As a statement, `++numberOfBunnies` tells the computer to add 1 to `numberOfBunnies`.
- As an expression, the value of `++numberOfBunnies` is 29.

So, with `out.println(++numberOfBunnies)`, the computer adds 1 to the variable `numberOfBunnies`, and the code `out.println(++numberOfBunnies)` really means `out.println(29)`.

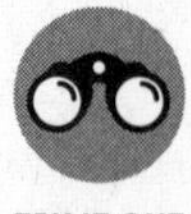

TRY IT OUT

Before you run the following code, try to predict what the code's output will be. Then run the code to find out whether your prediction is correct:

```
public class Main {

  public static void main(String[] args) {
    int i = 10;
    System.out.println(i++);
    System.out.println(--i);
    --i;
    i--;
    System.out.println(i);
    System.out.println(++i);
    System.out.println(i--);
    System.out.println(i);
    i++;
    i = i++ + ++i;
    System.out.println(i);
    i = i++ + i++;
    System.out.println(i);
  }
}
```

Type the boldface text, one line after another, into JShell, and see how JShell responds.

```
jshell> int i = 8
jshell> i++
jshell> i
jshell> i
jshell> i++
jshell> i
jshell> ++i
jshell> i
```

Assignment operators

If you read the preceding section, which is about operators that add 1, you may be wondering whether you can manipulate these operators to add 2 or add 5 or add 1000000. Can you write `numberOfBunnies++++` and still call yourself a Java programmer? Well, you can't. If you try it, an error message appears when you try to compile your code.

What can you do? As luck would have it, Java has plenty of assignment operators you can use. With an *assignment operator*, you can add, subtract, multiply, or divide by anything you want. You can do other cool operations, too. Listing 4-8 has a smorgasbord of assignment operators (the things with equal signs). Figure 4-17 shows the output from running Listing 4-8.

LISTING 4-8: Assignment Operators

```
public class UseAssignmentOperators {

    public static void main(String args[]) {
        int numberOfBunnies = 27;
        int numberExtra = 53;

        numberOfBunnies += 1;
        System.out.println(numberOfBunnies);

        numberOfBunnies += 5;
        System.out.println(numberOfBunnies);

        numberOfBunnies += numberExtra;
        System.out.println(numberOfBunnies);

        numberOfBunnies *= 2;
        System.out.println(numberOfBunnies);

        System.out.println(numberOfBunnies -= 7);

        System.out.println(numberOfBunnies = 100);
    }
}
```

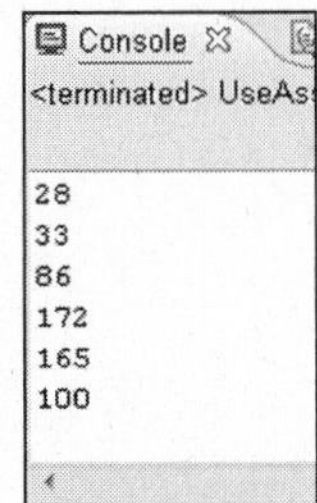

FIGURE 4-17: A run of the code in Listing 4-8.

Listing 4-8 shows how versatile Java's assignment operators are. With the assignment operators, you can add, subtract, multiply, or divide a variable by any number. Notice how `+= 5` adds 5 to `numberOfBunnies`, and how `*= 2` multiplies `numberOfBunnies` by 2. You can even use another expression's value (in Listing 4-8, `numberExtra`) as the number to be applied.

The last two lines in Listing 4-8 demonstrate a special feature of Java's assignment operators. You can use an assignment operator as part of a larger Java statement. In the next-to-last line of Listing 4-8, the operator subtracts 7 from numberOfBunnies, decreasing the value of numberOfBunnies from 172 to 165. Then the whole assignment business is stuffed into a call to System.out.println, so 165 prints onscreen.

Lo and behold, the last line of Listing 4-8 shows how you can do the same thing with Java's plain old equal sign. The thing that I call an assignment statement near the start of this chapter is really one of the assignment operators that I describe in this section. Therefore, whenever you assign a value to something, you can make that assignment be part of a larger statement.

TECHNICAL STUFF

Each use of an assignment operator does double duty as a statement and an expression. In all cases, the expression's value equals whatever value you assign. For example, before executing the code System.out.println(numberOfBunnies -= 7), the value of numberOfBunnies is 172. As a statement, numberOfBunnies -= 7 tells the computer to subtract 7 from numberOfBunnies (so the value of numberOfBunnies goes from 172 to 165). As an expression, the value of numberOfBunnies -= 7 is 165. So the code System.out.println(numberOfBunnies -= 7) really means System.out.println(165). The number 165 displays on the computer screen.

For a richer explanation of this kind of thing, see the sidebar "Statements and expressions," earlier in this chapter.

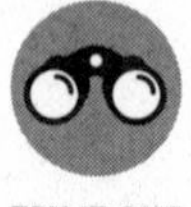

TRY IT OUT

Before you run the following code, try to predict what the code's output will be. Then run the code to find out whether your prediction is correct:

```
public class Main {

  public static void main(String[] args) {
    int i = 10;

    i += 2;
    i -= 5;
    i *= 6;

    System.out.println(i);
    System.out.println(i += 3);
    System.out.println(i /= 2);
  }
}
```

» Forming logical conditions

» Putting statements inside one another

» Choosing among many alternatives

Chapter 5

Controlling Program Flow with Decision-Making Statements

The TV show *Dennis the Menace* aired on CBS from 1959 to 1963. I remember one episode in which Mr. Wilson was having trouble making an important decision. I think it was something about changing jobs or moving to a new town. Anyway, I can still see that shot of Mr. Wilson sitting in his yard, sipping lemonade, and staring into nowhere for the whole afternoon. Of course, the annoying character Dennis was constantly interrupting Mr. Wilson's peace and quiet. That's what made this situation funny.

What impressed me about this episode (the reason I remember it clearly even now) was Mr. Wilson's dogged intent in making the decision. This guy wasn't going about his everyday business, roaming around the neighborhood while thoughts about the decision wandered in and out of his mind. He was sitting quietly in his yard, making marks carefully and logically on his mental balance sheet. How many people actually make decisions this way?

At that time, I was still pretty young. I'd never faced the responsibility of making a big decision that affected my family and me. But I wondered what such a decision-making process would be like. Would it help to sit there like a stump for hours on end? Would I make my decisions by the careful weighing and tallying of options? Or would I shoot in the dark, take risks, and act on impulse? Only time would tell.

Making Decisions (Java if Statements)

When you're writing computer programs, you're constantly hitting forks in roads. Did the user correctly type the password? If yes, let the user work; if no, kick the bum out. So the Java programming language needs a way of making a program branch in one of two directions. Fortunately, the language has a way: It's called an `if` statement.

Guess the number

Listing 5-1 illustrates the use of an `if` statement. Two runs of the program in Listing 5-1 are shown in Figure 5-1.

LISTING 5-1: A Guessing Game

```
import static java.lang.System.out;
import java.util.Scanner;
import java.util.Random;

public class GuessingGame {

    public static void main(String args[]) {
        Scanner keyboard = new Scanner(System.in);

        out.print("Enter an int from 1 to 10: ");

        int inputNumber = keyboard.nextInt();
        int randomNumber = new Random().nextInt(10) + 1;

        if (inputNumber == randomNumber) {
            out.println("**********");
            out.println("*You win.*");
            out.println("**********");
        } else {
            out.println("You lose.");
            out.print("The random number was ");
            out.println(randomNumber + ".");
        }
```

```
        out.println("Thank you for playing.");

        keyboard.close();
    }
}
```

```
Enter an int from 1 to 10: 2
**********
*You win.*
**********
Thank you for playing.


Enter an int from 1 to 10: 4
You lose.
The random number was 10.
Thank you for playing.
```

FIGURE 5-1: Two runs of the guessing game.

The program in Listing 5-1 plays a guessing game with the user. The program gets a number (a guess) from the user and then generates a random number between 1 and 10. If the number that the user entered is the same as the random number, the user wins. Otherwise, the user loses and the program tells the user what the random number was.

She controlled keystrokes from the keyboard

Taken together, the lines

```
import java.util.Scanner;

        Scanner keyboard = new Scanner(System.in);

        int inputNumber = keyboard.nextInt();
```

in Listing 5-1 get whatever number the user types on the computer's keyboard. The last of the three lines puts this number into a variable named *inputNumber*. If these lines look complicated, don't worry: You can copy these lines almost word for word whenever you want to read from the keyboard. Include the first two lines (the `import` and `Scanner` lines) just once in your program. Later in your program, wherever the user types an `int` value, include a line with a call to `nextInt` (as in the last of the preceding three lines of code).

Of all the names in these three lines of code, the only two names that I coined myself are *inputNumber* and *keyboard*. All the other names are part of Java. So, if I want to be creative, I can write the lines this way:

```
import java.util.Scanner;

        Scanner readingThingie = new Scanner(System.in);

        int valueTypedIn = readingThingie.nextInt();
```

I can also beef up my program's import declarations, as I do later on in Listings 5-2 and 5-3. Other than that, I have very little leeway.

As you read on in this book, you'll start recognizing the patterns behind these three lines of code, so I don't clutter up this section with all the details. For now, you can just copy these three lines and keep the following in mind:

» **When you import `java.util.Scanner`, you don't use the word *static*.**

  But importing `Scanner` is different from importing `System.out`. When you import `java.lang.System.out`, you use the word `static`. (Refer to Listing 5-1.) The difference creeps into the code because `Scanner` is the name of a class, and `System.out` isn't the name of a class.

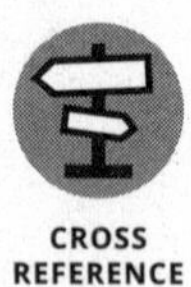

  For a quick look at the use of the word *static* in import declarations, see the sidebar in Chapter 4 about import declarations: the ugly truth. For a more complete story about the word, see Chapter 10.

» **Typically (on a desktop or laptop computer), the name *System.in* stands for the keyboard.**

  To get characters from some place other than the keyboard, you can type something other than `System.in` inside the parentheses.

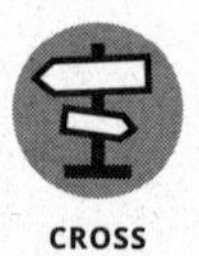

  What else can you put inside the `new Scanner(...)` parentheses? For some ideas, see Chapter 8.

  In Listing 5-1, I make the arbitrary decision to give one of my variables the name `keyboard`. The name `keyboard` reminds you, the reader, that this variable refers to a bunch of plastic buttons in front of your computer. Naming something `keyboard` doesn't tell Java anything about plastic buttons or about user input. On the other hand, the name `System.in` always tells Java about those plastic buttons. The code `Scanner keyboard = new Scanner(System.in)` in Listing 5-1 connects the name `keyboard` with the plastic buttons that we all know and love.

» **When you expect the user to type an `int` value (a whole number of some kind), use `nextInt()`.**

If you expect the user to type a `double` value (a number containing a decimal point), use `nextDouble()`. If you expect the user to type **true** or **false**, use `nextBoolean()`. If you expect the user to type a word like *Barry*, *Java*, or *Hello*, use `next()`.

WARNING

Decimal points vary from one country to another. In the United States, *10.5* (with a period) represents ten-and-a-half, but in France, *10,5* (with a comma) represents ten-and-a-half. In the Persian language, a decimal point looks like a slash (but it sits a bit lower than the digit characters). Your computer's operating system stores information about the country you live in, and Java reads that information to decide what ten-and-a-half looks like. If you run a program containing a `nextDouble()` method call, and Java responds with an `InputMismatchException`, check your input. You might have input 10.5 when your country's conventions require 10,5 (or another way of representing ten-and-a-half). For more information, see the "Where on Earth do you live?" sidebar in Chapter 8.

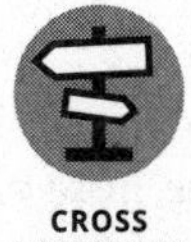

CROSS REFERENCE

For an example in which the user types a word, see Listing 5-3, later in this chapter. For an example in which the user types a single character, see Listing 6-4, in Chapter 6. For an example in which a program reads an entire line of text (all in one big gulp), see Chapter 8.

» **You can get several values from the keyboard, one after another.**

To do this, use the `keyboard.nextInt()` code several times.

To see a program that reads more than one value from the keyboard, go to Listing 5-4, later in this chapter.

» Whenever you use Java's `Scanner`, you should call the `close` method after your last `nextInt` call (or your last `nextDouble` call, or your last `next`*`Whatever`* call).

In Listing 5-1, the `main` method's last statement is

```
keyboard.close();
```

This statement does some housekeeping to disconnect the Java program from the computer keyboard. (The amount of required housekeeping is more than you might think!) If I omit this statement from Listing 5-1, nothing terrible happens. Java's Virtual Machine usually cleans up after itself very nicely. But using `close()` to explicitly detach from the keyboard is good practice, and some IDEs display warnings if you omit the `keyboard.close()` statement. In this book's example, I always remember to close my `Scanner` variables.

TECHNICAL STUFF

In Chapter 13, I show you a more reliable way to incorporate the `keyboard.close()` statement in your Java program.

When your program calls `System.out.println`, your program uses the computer's screen. So why don't you call a `close` method after all your `System.out.println` calls? The answer is subtle. In Listing 5-1, your own code connects to the keyboard by calling `new Scanner(System.in)`. So, later in the program, your code cleans up after itself by calling the `close` method. But with `System.out.println`, your own code doesn't create a connection to the screen. (The `out` variable refers to a `PrintStream`, but you don't call `new PrintStream()` to prepare for calling `System.out.println`.) Instead, the Java Virtual Machine connects to the screen on your behalf. The Java Virtual Machine's code (which you never have to see) contains a call to `new PrintStream()` in preparation for your calling `System.out.println`. So, because it's a well-behaved piece of code, the Java Virtual Machine eventually calls `out.close()` without any effort on your part.

Creating randomness

Achieving real randomness is surprisingly difficult. Mathematician Persi Diaconis says that if you flip a coin several times, always starting with the head side up, you're likely to toss heads more often than tails. If you toss several more times, always starting with the tail side up, you'll likely toss tails more often than heads. In other words, coin tossing isn't really fair.*

Computers aren't much better than coins and human thumbs. A computer mimics the generation of random sequences, but in the end the computer just does what it's told and does all of this in a purely deterministic fashion. So in Listing 5-1, when the computer executes

```
import java.util.Random;

        int randomNumber = new Random().nextInt(10) + 1;
```

the computer appears to give a randomly generated number — a whole number between 1 and 10. But it's all a fake. The computer only follows instructions. It's not really random, but without bending a computer over backward, it's the best that anyone can do.

*Diaconis, Persi. "The Search for Randomness." American Association for the Advancement of Science annual meeting. Seattle. 14 Feb. 2004.

Once again, I ask you to take this code on blind faith. Don't worry about what new Random().nextInt means until you have more experience with Java. Just copy this code into your own programs and have fun with it. And if the numbers from 1 to 10 aren't in your flight plans, don't fret. To roll an imaginary die, write the statement

```
int rollEmBaby = new Random().nextInt(6) + 1;
```

With the execution of this statement, the variable rollEmBaby gets a value from 1 to 6.

The if statement

At the core of Listing 5-1 is a Java if statement. This if statement represents a fork in the road. (See Figure 5-2.) The computer follows one of two prongs — the prong that prints You win or the prong that prints You lose. The computer decides which prong to take by testing the truth or falsehood of a *condition*. In Listing 5-1, the condition being tested is

```
inputNumber == randomNumber
```

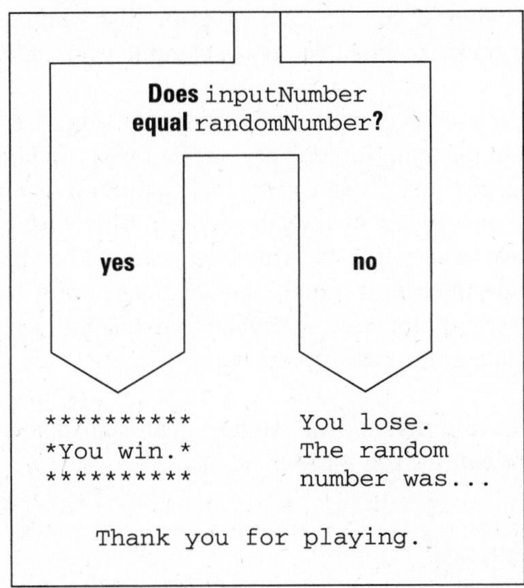

FIGURE 5-2: An if statement is like a fork in the road.

Does the value of inputNumber equal the value of randomNumber? When the condition is true, the computer does the stuff between the condition and the word *else*. When the condition turns out to be false, the computer does the stuff after the word *else*. Either way, the computer goes on to execute the last `println` call, which displays `Thank you for playing`.

REMEMBER

The condition in an `if` statement must be enclosed in parentheses. However, a line like `if (inputNumber == randomNumber)` is not a complete statement (just as "If I had a hammer" isn't a complete sentence). So this line `if (inputNumber == randomNumber)` shouldn't end with a semicolon.

TECHNICAL STUFF

Sometimes, when I'm writing about a condition that's being tested, I slip into using the word *expression* instead of *condition*. That's okay because every condition is an expression. An expression is something that has a value and, sure enough, every condition has a value. The condition's value is either `true` or `false`. (For revealing information about expressions and values like `true` and `false`, see Chapter 4.)

The double equal sign

In Listing 5-1, in the `if` statement's condition, notice the use of the double equal sign. Comparing two numbers to see whether they're the same isn't the same as setting something equal to something else. That's why the symbol to compare for equality isn't the same as the symbol that's used in an assignment or an initialization. In an `if` statement's condition, you can't replace the double equal sign with a single equal sign. If you do, your program just won't work. (You almost always get an error message when you try to compile your code.)

On the other hand, if you never make the mistake of using a single equal sign in a condition, you're not normal. Not long ago, while I was teaching an introductory Java course, I promised that I'd swallow my laser pointer if no one made the single equal sign mistake during any of the lab sessions. This wasn't an idle promise. I knew I'd never have to keep it. As it turned out, even if I had ignored the first ten times anybody made the single equal sign mistake during those lab sessions, I would still be laser-pointer-free. Everybody mistakenly uses the single equal sign several times in a programming career.

TIP

The trick is not to avoid making the single-equal-sign mistake; the trick is to catch the mistake whenever you make it.

Brace yourself

The `if` statement in Listing 5-1 has two halves: a top half and a bottom half. I have names for these two parts of an `if` statement. I call them the *if part* (the top half) and the *else part* (the bottom half).

The `if` part in Listing 5-1 seems to have more than one statement in it. I make this happen by enclosing the three statements of the `if` part in a pair of curly braces. When I do this, I form a block. A *block* is a bunch of statements scrunched together by a pair of curly braces.

With this block, three calls to `println` are tucked away safely inside the `if` part. With the curly braces, the rows of asterisks and the words `You win` display only when the user's guess is correct.

This business with blocks and curly braces applies to the else part as well. In Listing 5-1, whenever `inputNumber` doesn't equal `randomNumber`, the computer executes three `print`/`println` calls. To convince the computer that all three of these calls are inside the `else` clause, I put these calls into a block. That is, I enclose these three calls in a pair of curly braces.

TECHNICAL STUFF

Strictly speaking, Listing 5-1 has only one statement between the `if` and the `else` statements and only one statement after the `else` statement. The trick is that when you place a bunch of statements inside curly braces, you get a block; and a block behaves, in all respects, like a single statement. In fact, the official Java documentation lists blocks as one of the many kinds of statements. So, in Listing 5-1, the block that prints `You win` and asterisks is a single statement that has, within it, three smaller statements.

Indenting if statements in your code

Notice how, in Listing 5-1, the `print` and `println` calls inside the `if` statement are indented. (This includes both the `You win` and `You lose` statements. The `print` and `println` calls that come after the word `else` are still part of the `if` statement.) Strictly speaking, you don't have to indent the statements that are inside an `if` statement. For all the compiler cares, you can write your whole program on a single line or place all your statements in an artful, misshapen zigzag. The problem is that neither you nor anyone else can make sense of your code if you don't indent your statements in some logical fashion. In Listing 5-1, the indenting of the `print` and `println` statements helps your eye (and brain) see quickly that these statements are subordinate to the overall `if/else` flow.

In a small program, unindented or poorly indented code is barely tolerable. But in a complicated program, indentation that doesn't follow a neat, logical pattern is a big, ugly nightmare.

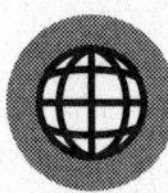

Many Java IDEs have tools to indent your code automatically. In fact, code indentation is one of my favorite IDE features. So don't walk — run — to a computer, and visit this book's website (`www.allmycode.com/JavaForDummies`) for more information on what Java IDEs can offer.

WARNING

When you write if statements, you may be tempted to chuck out the window all the rules about curly braces and simply rely on indentation. This works in other programming languages, such as Python and Haskell, but it doesn't work in Java. If you indent three statements after the word else and forget to enclose those statements in curly braces, the computer thinks that the else part includes only the first of the three statements. What's worse, the indentation misleads you into believing that the else part includes all three statements. This makes it more difficult for you to figure out why your code isn't behaving the way you think it should. Watch those braces!

Elseless in Ifrica

Okay, so the title of this section is contrived. Big deal! The idea is that you can create an if statement without the else part. Take, for instance, the code in Listing 5-1, shown earlier. Maybe you'd rather not rub it in whenever the user loses the game. The modified code in Listing 5-2 shows you how to do this (and Figure 5-3 shows you the result).

LISTING 5-2: A Kinder, Gentler Guessing Game

```
import static java.lang.System.in;
import static java.lang.System.out;
import java.util.Scanner;
import java.util.Random;

public class DontTellThemTheyLost {

    public static void main(String args[]) {
        Scanner keyboard = new Scanner(in);

        out.print("Enter an int from 1 to 10: ");

        int inputNumber = keyboard.nextInt();
        int randomNumber = new Random().nextInt(10) + 1;

        if (inputNumber == randomNumber) {
            out.println("*You win.*");
        }

        out.println("That was a very good guess :-)");
        out.print("The random number was ");
        out.println(randomNumber + ".");
        out.println("Thank you for playing.");

        keyboard.close();
    }
}
```

The `if` statement in Listing 5-2 has no `else` part. When `inputNumber` is the same as `randomNumber`, the computer prints `You win`. When `inputNumber` is different from `randomNumber`, the computer doesn't print `You win`.

Listing 5-2 illustrates another new idea. With an `import` declaration for `System.in`, I can reduce `new Scanner(System.in)` to the shorter `new Scanner(in)`. Adding this `import` declaration is hardly worth the effort. In fact, I do more typing with the `import` declaration than without it. Nevertheless, the code in Listing 5-2 demonstrates that it's possible to import `System.in`.

```
Enter an int from 1 to 10: 4
*You win.*
That was a very good guess :-)
The random number was 4.
Thank you for playing.


Enter an int from 1 to 10: 4
That was a very good guess :-)
The random number was 6.
Thank you for playing.
```

FIGURE 5-3: Two runs of the game in Listing 5-2.

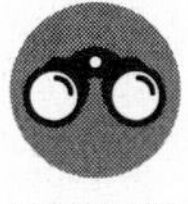

TRY IT OUT

In Chapter 4, Listing 4-5 tells you whether you can or cannot fit ten people on an elevator. A run of the listing's code looks something like this:

```
True or False?
You can fit all ten of the
Brickenchicker dectuplets
on the elevator:

false
```

Use what you know about Java's `if` statements to make the program's output more natural. Depending on the value of the program's `elevatorWeightLimit` variable, the output should be either

```
You can fit all ten of the
Brickenchicker dectuplets
on the elevator.
```

or

```
You can't fit all ten of the
Brickenchicker dectuplets
on the elevator.
```

Using Blocks in JShell

Chapter 4 introduces Java 9's interactive JShell environment. You type a statement, and JShell responds immediately by executing the statement. That's fine for simple statements, but what happens when you have a statement inside of a block?

In JShell, you can start typing a statement with one or more blocks. JShell doesn't respond until you finish typing the entire statement — blocks and all. To see how it works, look over this conversation that I had recently with JShell:

```
jshell> import static java.lang.System.out

jshell> import java.util.Random

jshell> int randomNumber = new Random().nextInt(10) + 1
randomNumber ==> 4

jshell> int inputNumber = 4
inputNumber ==> 4

jshell> if (inputNumber == randomNumber) {
   ...>     out.println("*You win.*");
   ...> }
*You win.*

jshell>
```

In this dialogue, I've set the text that I type in bold. JShell's responses aren't set in bold.

When I type `if (inputNumber == randomNumber) {` and press Enter, JShell doesn't do much. JShell only displays a `...>` prompt, which indicates that whatever lines I've typed don't form a complete statement. I have to respond by typing the rest of the `if` statement.

When I finish the `if` statement with a close curly brace, JShell finally acknowledges that I've typed an entire statement. JShell executes the statement and (in this example) displays `*You win.*`.

Notice the semicolon at the end of the `out.println` line:

» When you type a statement that's not inside of a block, JShell lets you omit the semicolon at the end of the statement.

» When you type a statement that's inside of a block, JShell (like the plain old Java in Listing 5-2) doesn't let you omit the semicolon.

TIP

When you type a block in JShell, you always have the option of typing the entire block on one line, with no line breaks, like so:

```
if (inputNumber == randomNumber) { out.println("*You win.*"); }
```

Forming Conditions with Comparisons and Logical Operators

The Java programming language has plenty of little squiggles and doodads for your various condition-forming needs. This section tells you all about them.

Comparing numbers; comparing characters

Table 5-1 shows you the operators that you can use to compare one value with another.

TABLE 5-1 Comparison Operators

Operator Symbol	Meaning	Example
`==`	is equal to	`numberOfCows == 5`
`!=`	is not equal to	`buttonClicked != panicButton`
`<`	is less than	`numberOfCows < 5`
`>`	is greater than	`myInitial > 'B'`
`<=`	is less than or equal to	`numberOfCows <= 5`
`>=`	is greater than or equal to	`myInitial >= 'B'`

You can use all of Java's comparison operators to compare numbers and characters. When you compare numbers, things go pretty much the way you think they should go. But when you compare characters, things are a little strange. Comparing uppercase letters with one another is no problem. Because the letter *B* comes alphabetically before *H*, the condition `'B' < 'H'` is true. Comparing lowercase letters with one another is also okay. What's strange is that when you compare an uppercase letter with a lowercase letter, the uppercase letter is always smaller. So, even though `'Z' < 'A'` is `false`, `'Z' < 'a'` is `true`.

TECHNICAL STUFF

Under the hood, the letters *A* through *Z* are stored with numeric codes 65 through 90. The letters *a* through *z* are stored with codes 97 through 122. That's why each uppercase letter is smaller than each lowercase letter.

WARNING

Be careful when you compare two numbers for equality (with ==) or inequality (with !=). After you do some calculations and obtain two `double` values or two `float` values, the values that you have are seldom dead-on equal to one another. (The problem comes from those pesky digits beyond the decimal point.) For instance, the Fahrenheit equivalent of 21 degrees Celsius is 69.8, and when you calculate `9.0 / 5 * 21 + 32` by hand, you get 69.8. But the condition `9.0 / 5 * 21 + 32 == 69.8` turns out to be false. That's because, when the computer calculates `9.0 / 5 * 21 + 32`, it gets 69.80000000000001, not 69.8.

Comparing objects

When you start working with objects, you find that you can use == and != to compare objects with one another. For instance, a button you see on the computer screen is an object. You can ask whether the thing that was just mouse-clicked is a particular button on your screen. You do this with Java's equality operator:

```
if (e.getSource() == bCopy) {
    clipboard.setText(which.getText());
```

CROSS REFERENCE

To find out more about responding to button clicks, read Chapter 16.

The big gotcha with Java's comparison scheme comes when you compare two strings. (For a word or two about Java's `String` type, see the section about reference types in Chapter 4.) When you compare two strings with one another, you don't want to use the double equal sign. Using the double equal sign would ask, "Is this string stored in exactly the same place in memory as that other string?" Usually, that's not what you want to ask. Instead, you usually want to ask, "Does this string have the same characters in it as that other string?" To ask the second question (the more appropriate question), Java's `String` type has a method named `equals`. (Like everything else in the known universe, this `equals` method is defined in the Java API, short for application programming interface.) The `equals` method compares two strings to see whether they have the same characters in them. For an example using Java's `equals` method, see Listing 5-3. (Figure 5-4 shows a run of the program in Listing 5-3.)

```
What's the password? swordfish
You typed >>swordfish<<

The word you typed is not
stored in the same place as
the real password, but that's
no big deal.

The word you typed has the
same characters as the real
password. You can use our
precious system.
```

FIGURE 5-4: The results of using == and using Java's `equals` method.

LISTING 5-3: Checking a Password

```
import static java.lang.System.*;
import java.util.Scanner;

public class CheckPassword {

    public static void main(String args[]) {

        out.print("What's the password?");

        Scanner keyboard = new Scanner(in);
        String password = keyboard.next();

        out.println("You typed >>" + password + "<<");
        out.println();

        if (password == "swordfish") {
            out.println("The word you typed is stored");
            out.println("in the same place as the real");
            out.println("password. You must be a");
            out.println("hacker.");
        } else {
            out.println("The word you typed is not");
            out.println("stored in the same place as");
            out.println("the real password, but that's");
            out.println("no big deal.");
        }
        out.println();

        if (password.equals("swordfish")) {
            out.println("The word you typed has the");
            out.println("same characters as the real");
```

(continued)

LISTING 5-3: (continued)

```
            out.println("password. You can use our");
            out.println("precious system.");
        } else {
            out.println("The word you typed doesn't");
            out.println("have the same characters as");
            out.println("the real password. You can't");
            out.println("use our precious system.");
        }

        keyboard.close();
    }
}
```

In Listing 5-3, the call `keyboard.next()` grabs whatever word the user types on the computer keyboard. The code shoves this word into the variable named *password.* Then the program's `if` statements use two different techniques to compare `password` with `"swordfish"`.

The more appropriate of the two techniques uses Java's `equals` method. The `equals` method looks funny because when you call it, you put a dot after one string and put the other string in parentheses. But that's the way you have to do it.

In calling Java's `equals` method, it doesn't matter which string gets the dot and which gets the parentheses. For instance, in Listing 5-3, you could have written

```
if ("swordfish".equals(password))
```

The method would work just as well.

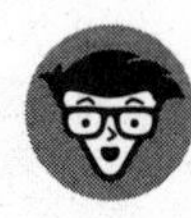

TECHNICAL STUFF

A call to Java's `equals` method looks imbalanced, but it's not. There's a reason behind the apparent imbalance between the dot and the parentheses. The idea is that you have two objects: the `password` object and the `"swordfish"` object. Each of these two objects is of type `String`. (However, `password` is a variable of type `String`, and `"swordfish"` is a `String` literal.) When you write `password.equals("swordfish")`, you're calling an `equals` method that belongs to the `password` object. When you call that method, you're feeding `"swordfish"` to the method as the method's parameter (pun intended).

CROSS REFERENCE

You can read more about methods belonging to objects in Chapter 7.

When comparing strings with one another, use the `equals` method — not the double equal sign.

Importing everything in one fell swoop

The first line of Listing 5-3 illustrates a lazy way of importing both `System.out` and `System.in`. To import everything that `System` has to offer, you use the asterisk wildcard character (`*`). In fact, importing `java.lang.System.*` is like having about 30 separate import declarations, including `System.in`, `System.out`, `System.err`, `System.nanoTime`, and many other `System` things.

The use of an asterisk in an `import` declaration is generally considered bad programming practice, so I don't do it often in this book's examples. But for larger programs — programs that use dozens of names from the Java API — the lazy asterisk trick is handy.

TECHNICAL STUFF

You can't toss an asterisk anywhere you want inside an `import` declaration. For example, you can't import everything starting with `java` by writing `import java.*`. You can substitute an asterisk only for the name of a class or for the name of something static that's tucked away inside a class. For more information about asterisks in `import` declarations, see Chapter 9. For information about `static` things, see Chapter 10.

Java's logical operators

Mr. Spock would be pleased: Java has all the operators that you need for mixing and matching logical tests. The operators are shown in Table 5-2.

TABLE 5-2 Logical Operators

<table>
<tr><th>Operator Symbol</th><th>What It Means</th><th>Example</th></tr>
<tr><td>&&</td><td>and</td><td><code>5 < x && x < 10</code></td></tr>
<tr><td>||</td><td>or</td><td><code>x < 5 || 10 < x</code></td></tr>
<tr><td>!</td><td>not</td><td><code>!password.equals("swordfish")</code></td></tr>
</table>

You can use these operators to form all kinds of elaborate conditions. Listing 5-4 has an example.

LISTING 5-4: Checking Username and Password

```
import javax.swing.JOptionPane;

public class Authenticator {

    public static void main(String args[]) {

        String username = JOptionPane.showInputDialog("Username:");
        String password = JOptionPane.showInputDialog("Password:");

        if (
            username != null && password != null &&
            (
              (username.equals("bburd") && password.equals("swordfish")) ||
              (username.equals("hritter") && password.equals("preakston"))
            )
          )
        {
            JOptionPane.showMessageDialog(null, "You're in.");
        } else {
            JOptionPane.showMessageDialog(null, "You're suspicious.");
        }
    }
}
```

Several runs of the program of Listing 5-4 are shown in Figure 5-5. When the username is *bburd* and the password is *swordfish* or when the username is *hritter* and the password is *preakston*, the user gets a nice message. Otherwise, the user is a bum who gets the nasty message that he or she deserves.

Confession: Figure 5-5 is a fake! To help you read the usernames and passwords, I added an extra statement to Listing 5-4. The extra statement (`UIManager.put("TextField.font", new Font("Dialog", Font.BOLD, 14))`) enlarges each text field's font size. Yes, I modified the code before creating the figure. Shame on me!

Listing 5-4 illustrates a new way to get user input; namely, to show the user an input dialog box. The statement

```
String password = JOptionPane.showInputDialog("Password:");
```

in Listing 5-4 performs more or less the same task as the statement

```
String password = keyboard.next();
```

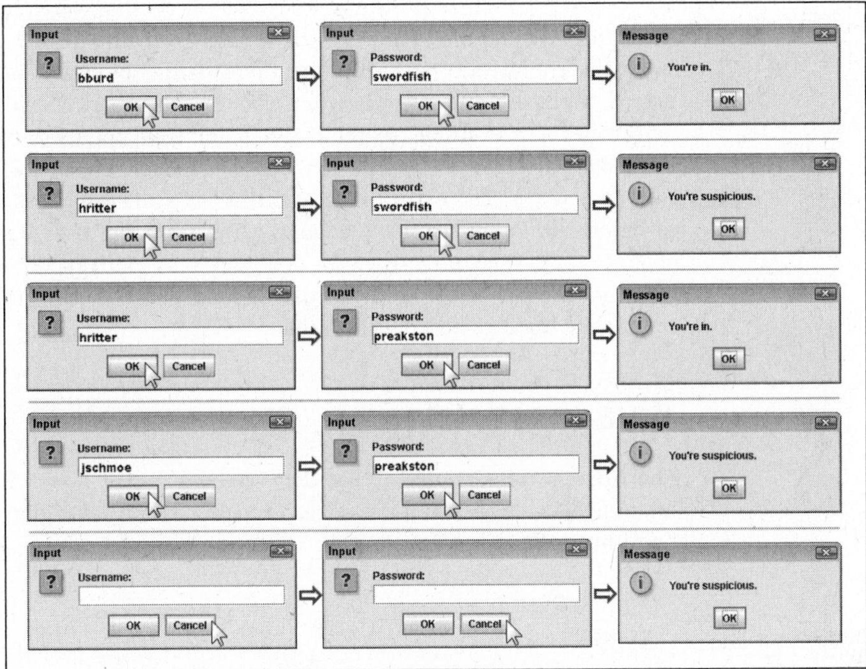

FIGURE 5-5: Several runs of the code from Listing 5-4.

from Listing 5-3. The big difference is, while `keyboard.next()` displays dull-looking text in a console, `JOptionPane.showInputDialog("Username:")` displays a fancy dialog box containing a text field and buttons. (Compare Figures 5-4 and 5-5.) When the user clicks OK, the computer takes whatever text is in the text field and hands that text over to a variable. In fact, Listing 5-4 uses `JOptionPane.showInputDialog` twice — once to get a value for the username variable and a second time to get a value for the password variable.

Near the end of Listing 5-4, I use a slight variation on the `JOptionPane` business,

```
JOptionPane.showMessageDialog(null, "You're in.");
```

With `showMessageDialog`, I show a very simple dialog box — a box with no text field. (Again, see Figure 5-5.)

Like thousands of other names, the name `JOptionPane` is defined in Java's API. (To be more specific, `JOptionPane` is defined inside something called `javax.swing`, which in turn is defined inside Java's API.) So, to use the name `JOptionPane` throughout Listing 5-4, I import `javax.swing.JOptionPane` at the top of the listing.

TIP

In Listing 5-4, JOptionPane.showInputDialog works nicely because the user's input (username and password) are mere strings of characters. If you want the user to input a number (an int or a double, for example), you have to do some extra work. For example, to get an int value from the user, type something like int numberOfCows = Integer.parseInt(JOptionPane.showInputDialog("How many cows?")). The extra Integer.parseInt stuff forces your text field's input to be an int value. To get a double value from the user, type something like double fractionOfHolsteins = Double.parseDouble(JOptionPane.showInputDialog("Holsteins:")). The extra Double.parseDouble business forces your text field's input to be a double value.

Vive les nuls!

The French translations of *For Dummies* books are books *Pour les Nuls.* So a "dummy" in English is a "nul" in French.* But in Java, the word null means "nothing." When you see

```
if (
     username != null
```

in Listing 5-4, you can imagine that you see

```
if (
     username isn't nothing
```

or

```
if (
     username has any value at all
```

To find out how username can have no value, see the last row in Figure 5-5. When you click Cancel in the first dialog box, the computer hands null to your program. So, in Listing 5-4, the variable username becomes null. The comparisons username != null checks to make sure that you haven't clicked Cancel in the program's first dialog box. The comparison password != null performs the same kind of check for the program's second dialog box. When you see the if statement in Listing 5-4, you can imagine that you see the following:

*In Russian, a "dummy" is a "чайник" which, when interpreted literally, means a "teapot." So in Russian, this book is "Java For Teapots." I've never been called a "teapot," and I'm not sure how I'd react if I were.

```
if (
      you didn't press Cancel in the username dialog and
      you didn't press Cancel in the password dialog and
      (
        (you typed bburd in the username dialog and
         you typed swordfish in the password dialog) or
        (you typed hritter in the username dialog and
         you typed preakston in the password dialog)
      )
   )
```

WARNING

In Listing 5-4, the comparisons `username != null` and `password != null` are not optional. If you forget to include these and click Cancel when the program runs, you get a nasty `NullPointerException` message, and the program comes crashing down before your eyes. The word `null` represents nothing, and in Java, you can't compare nothing to a string like `"bburd"` or `"swordfish"`. In Listing 5-4, the purpose of the comparison `username != null` is to prevent Java from moving on to check `username.equals("bburd")` whenever you happen to click Cancel. Without this preliminary `username != null` test, you're courting trouble.

TECHNICAL STUFF

The last couple of `null`s in Listing 5-4 are different from the others. In the code `JOptionPane.showMessageDialog (null, "You're in.")`, the word `null` stands for "no other dialog box." In particular, the call `showMessageDialog` tells Java to pop up a new dialog box, and the word `null` indicates that the new dialog box doesn't grow out of any existing dialog box. One way or another, Java insists that you say something about the origin of the newly popped dialog box. (For some reason, Java doesn't insist that you specify the origin of the `showInputDialog` box. Go figure!) Anyway, in Listing 5-4, having a `showMessageDialog` box pop up from nowhere is quite useful.

(Conditions in parentheses)

Keep an eye on those parentheses! When you're combining conditions with logical operators, it's better to waste typing effort and add unneeded parentheses than to goof up your result by using too few parentheses. Take, for example, the expression

```
2 < 5 || 100 < 6 && 27 < 1
```

By misreading this expression, you might conclude that the expression is false. That is, you could wrongly read the expression as meaning `(`*`something-or-other`*`) && 27 < 1`. Because `27 < 1` is false, you would conclude that the whole expression is false. The fact is that, in Java, any `&&` operator is evaluated before any || operator. So the expression really asks whether `2 < 5 || (something-or-other)`. Because `2 < 5` is true, the whole expression is true.

To change the expression's value from `true` to `false`, you can put the expression's first two comparisons in parentheses, like this:

```
(2 < 5 || 100 < 6) && 27 < 1
```

TIP

Java's || operator is *inclusive*. This means that you get a `true` value whenever the thing on the left side is true, the thing on the right side is true, or both things are true. For instance, the expression `2 < 10 || 20 < 30` is true.

WARNING

In Java, you can't combine comparisons the way you do in ordinary English. In English, you may say, "We'll have between three and ten people at the dinner table." But in Java, you get an error message if you write `3 <= people <= 10`. To do this comparison, you need something like `3 <= people && people <= 10`.

In Listing 5-4, the `if` statement's condition has more than a dozen parentheses. What happens if you omit two of them?

```
if (
    username != null && password != null &&
    // open parenthesis omitted
        (username.equals("bburd") && password.equals("swordfish")) ||
        (username.equals("hritter") && password.equals("preakston"))
    // close parenthesis omitted
   )
```

Java tries to interpret your wishes by grouping everything before the "or" (the || operator):

```
if (
    username != null && password != null &&
    (username.equals("bburd") && password.equals("swordfish"))

    ||

    (username.equals("hritter") && password.equals("preakston"))
   )
```

When the user clicks Cancel and username is `null`, Java says, "Okay! The stuff before the || operator is false, but maybe the stuff after the || operator is true. I'll check the stuff after the || operator to find out whether it's true." (Java often talks to itself. The psychiatrists are monitoring this situation.)

Anyway, when Java finally checks `username.equals("hritter")`, your program aborts with an ugly `NullPointerException` message. You've made Java angry by trying to apply `.equals` to a `null` username. (Psychiatrists have recommended anger management sessions for Java, but Java's insurance plan refuses to pay for the sessions.)

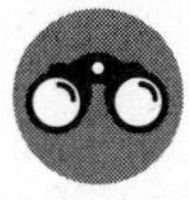

TRY IT OUT

Make some changes to the code in Listing 5-4:

- Add a third username/password combination to the list of acceptable logins.
- Modify the `if` statement's condition so that an all-uppercase entry for either username is acceptable. In other words, the input `BBURD` yields the same result as `bburd` and the input `HRITTER` yields the same result as `hritter`.
- In Listing 5-4, change

  ```
  username != null && password != null
  ```

  to

  ```
  !(username == null || password == null)
  ```

  Does the program still work? Why, or why not?
- In Listing 5-4, change

  ```
  username != null && password != null
  ```

  to

  ```
  !(username == null && password == null)
  ```

  This is almost the same as the previous experiment. The only difference is the use of `&&` instead of `||` between the two `== null` tests.

  Does the program still work? Why, or why not?

Building a Nest

Have you seen those cute Russian matryoshka nesting dolls? Open one, and another one is inside. Open the second, and a third one is inside it. You can do the same thing with Java's `if` statements. (Talk about fun!) Listing 5-5 shows you how.

LISTING 5-5: Nested if Statements

```
import static java.lang.System.out;
import java.util.Scanner;

public class Authenticator2 {

    public static void main(String args[]) {
        Scanner keyboard = new Scanner(System.in);

        out.print("Username: ");
        String username = keyboard.next();

        if (username.equals("bburd")) {
            out.print("Password: ");
            String password = keyboard.next();

            if (password.equals("swordfish")) {
                out.println("You're in.");
            } else {
                out.println("Incorrect password");
            }

        } else {
            out.println("Unknown user");
        }

        keyboard.close();
    }
}
```

Figure 5-6 shows several runs of the code in Listing 5-5. The main idea is that to log on, you have to pass two tests. (In other words, two conditions must be true.) The first condition tests for a valid username; the second condition tests for the correct password. If you pass the first test (the username test), you march right into another `if` statement that performs a second test (the password test). If you fail the first test, you never make it to the second test. Figure 5-7 shows the overall plan.

WARNING

The code in Listing 5-5 does a good job with nested `if` statements, but it does a terrible job with real-world user authentication. First, never show a password in plain view (without asterisks to masquerade the password). Second, don't handle passwords without encrypting them. Third, don't tell the malicious user which of the two words (the username or the password) was entered incorrectly. Fourth . . . well, I could go on and on. The code in Listing 5-5 just isn't meant to illustrate good username/password practices.

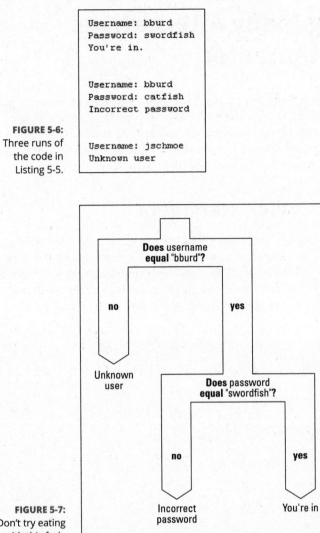

```
Username: bburd
Password: swordfish
You're in.


Username: bburd
Password: catfish
Incorrect password


Username: jschmoe
Unknown user
```

FIGURE 5-6: Three runs of the code in Listing 5-5.

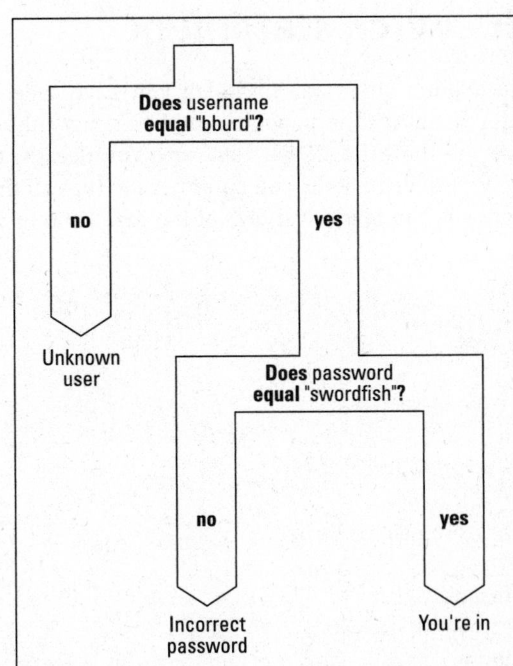

FIGURE 5-7: Don't try eating with this fork.

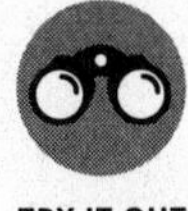

TRY IT OUT

Modify the program in Listing 5-4 so that, if the user clicks Cancel for either the username or the password, the program replies with a `Not enough information` message.

Choosing among Many Alternatives (Java switch Statements)

I'm the first to admit that I hate making decisions. If things go wrong, I would rather have the problem be someone else's fault. Writing the previous sections (on making decisions with Java's `if` statement) knocked the stuffing right out of me. That's why my mind boggles as I begin this section on choosing among many alternatives. What a relief it is to have that confession out of the way!

Your basic switch statement

Now, it's time to explore situations in which you have a decision with many branches. Take, for instance, the popular campfire song "Al's All Wet." (For a review of the lyrics, see the "Al's All Wet" sidebar.) You're eager to write code that prints this song's lyrics. Fortunately, you don't have to type all the words over and over again. Instead, you can take advantage of the repetition in the lyrics.

"AL'S ALL WET"

Sung to the tune of "Gentille Alouette":

> Al's all wet. Oh, why is Al all wet? Oh,
>
> Al's all wet 'cause he's standing in the rain.
>
> Why is Al out in the rain?
>
> That's because he has no brain.
>
> Has no brain, has no brain,
>
> In the rain, in the rain.
>
> Ohhhhhhhh ...
>
> Al's all wet. Oh, why is Al all wet? Oh,

Al's all wet 'cause he's standing in the rain.

Why is Al out in the rain?

That's because he is a pain.

He's a pain, he's a pain,

Has no brain, has no brain,

In the rain, in the rain.

Ohhhhhhhh ...

Al's all wet. Oh, why is Al all wet? Oh,

Al's all wet 'cause he's standing in the rain.

Why is Al out in the rain?

'Cause this is the last refrain.

Last refrain, last refrain,

He's a pain, he's a pain,

Has no brain, has no brain,

In the rain, in the rain.

Ohhhhhhhh ...

Al's all wet. Oh, why is Al all wet? Oh,

Al's all wet 'cause he's standing in the rain.

—Harriet Ritter and Barry Burd

A complete program to display the "Al's All Wet" lyrics won't come until Chapter 6. In the meantime, assume that you have a variable named verse. The value of verse is 1, 2, 3, or 4, depending on which verse of "Al's All Wet" you're trying to print. You could have a big, clumsy bunch of if statements that checks each possible verse number:

```
if (verse == 1) {
    out.println("That's because he has no brain.");
}
if (verse == 2) {
    out.println("That's because he is a pain.");
}
if (verse == 3) {
    out.println("'Cause this is the last refrain.");
}
```

But that approach seems wasteful. Why not create a statement that checks the value of verse just once and then takes an action based on the value it finds? Fortunately, just such a statement exists. It's called a *switch* statement. Listing 5-6 has an example of a switch statement.

LISTING 5-6: A switch Statement

```
import static java.lang.System.out;
import java.util.Scanner;

public class JustSwitchIt {

    public static void main(String args[]) {
        Scanner keyboard = new Scanner(System.in);
        out.print("Which verse? ");
        int verse = keyboard.nextInt();

        switch (verse) {
        case 1:
            out.println("That's because he has no brain.");
            break;
        case 2:
            out.println("That's because he is a pain.");
            break;
        case 3:
            out.println("'Cause this is the last refrain.");
            break;
```

```
        default:
            out.println("No such verse. Please try again.");
            break;
        }

        out.println("Ohhhhhhhh . . . .");

        keyboard.close();
    }
}
```

Figure 5-8 shows two runs of the program in Listing 5-6. (Figure 5-9 illustrates the program's overall idea.) First, the user types a number, like the number 2. Then execution of the program reaches the top of the `switch` statement. The computer checks the value of the `verse` variable. When the computer determines that the `verse` variable's value is `2`, the computer checks each case of the `switch` statement. The value `2` doesn't match the topmost case, so the computer proceeds to the middle of the three cases. The value posted for the middle case (the number 2) matches the value of the `verse` variable, so the computer executes the statements that come immediately after case 2. These two statements are

```
out.println("That's because he is a pain.");
break;
```

```
Which verse? 2
That's because he is a pain.
Ohhhhhhhh. . . .

Which verse? 6
No such verse. Please try again.
Ohhhhhhhh. . . .
```

FIGURE 5-8: Running the code of Listing 5-6 two times.

The first of the two statements displays the line `That's because he is a pain.` on the screen. The second statement is called a `break` statement. (What a surprise!) When the computer encounters a `break` statement, the computer jumps out of whatever `switch` statement it's in. So, in Listing 5-6, the computer skips right past the case that would display `'Cause this is the last refrain.` In fact, the computer jumps out of the entire `switch` statement and goes straight to the statement just after the end of the `switch` statement. The computer displays `Ohhhhhhhh . . .` because that's what the statement after the `switch` statement tells the computer to do.

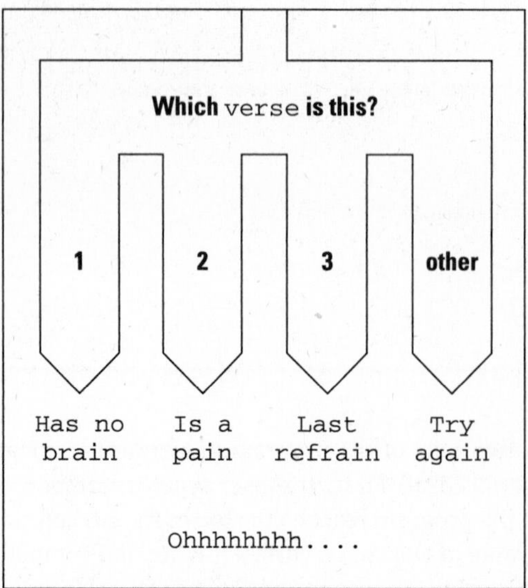

FIGURE 5-9: The big fork in the code of Listing 5-6.

If the pesky user asks for verse 6, the computer bypasses cases 1, 2, and 3. The computer goes straight to the default. In the default, the computer displays `No such verse. Please try again`, and then breaks out of the `switch` statement. After the computer is out of the `switch` statement, the computer displays `Ohhhhhhhh . . .`

TIP

You don't really need to put a `break` at the very end of a `switch` statement. In Listing 5-6, the last `break` (the `break` that's part of the default) is just for the sake of overall tidiness.

To break or not to break

In every Java programmer's life, a time comes when he or she forgets to use `break` statements. At first, the resulting output is confusing, but then the programmer remembers fall-through. The term *fall-through* describes what happens when you end a case without a `break` statement. What happens is that execution of the code falls right through to the next case in line. Execution keeps falling through until you eventually reach a `break` statement or the end of the entire `switch` statement.

Usually, when you're using a `switch` statement, you don't want fall-through, so you pepper `break` statements throughout the `switch` statements. But, occasionally, fall-through is just the thing you need. Take, for instance, the "Al's All Wet" song. (The classy lyrics are shown in the sidebar bearing the song's name.) Each verse of "Al's All Wet" adds new lines in addition to the lines from previous verses. This situation (accumulating lines from one verse to another) cries out for a `switch` statement with fall-through. Listing 5-7 demonstrates the idea.

LISTING 5-7: A switch Statement with Fall-Through

```
import static java.lang.System.out;
import java.util.Scanner;

public class FallingForYou {

    public static void main(String args[]) {
        Scanner keyboard = new Scanner(System.in);
        out.print("Which verse? ");
        int verse = keyboard.nextInt();

        switch (verse) {
        case 3:
            out.print("Last refrain, ");
            out.println("last refrain,");
        case 2:
            out.print("He's a pain, ");
            out.println("he's a pain,");
        case 1:
            out.print("Has no brain, ");
            out.println("has no brain,");
        }

        out.println("In the rain, in the rain.");
        out.println("Ohhhhhhhh...");
        out.println();

        keyboard.close();
    }
}
```

Figure 5-10 shows several runs of the program in Listing 5-7. Because the switch has no `break` statements in it, fall-through happens all over the place. For instance, when the user selects verse 2, the computer executes the two statements in case 2:

```
out.print("He's a pain, ");
out.println("he's a pain,");
```

Then the computer marches right on to execute the two statements in case 1:

```
out.print("Has no brain, ");
out.println("has no brain,");
```

That's good because the song's second verse has all these lines in it.

```
Which verse? 1
Has no brain, has no brain,
In the rain, in the rain.
Ohhhhhhhh...


Which verse? 2
He's a pain, he's a pain,
Has no brain, has no brain,
In the rain, in the rain.
Ohhhhhhhh...


Which verse? 3
Last refrain, last refrain,
He's a pain, he's a pain,
Has no brain, has no brain,
In the rain, in the rain.
Ohhhhhhhh...


Which verse? 6
In the rain, in the rain.
Ohhhhhhhh...
```

FIGURE 5-10: Running the code of Listing 5-7 four times.

Notice what happens when the user asks for verse 6. The `switch` statement in Listing 5-7 has no case 6 and no default, so none of the actions inside the `switch` statement is executed. Even so, with statements that print `In the rain, in the rain` and `Ohhhhhhhh ...` right after the `switch` statement, the computer displays something when the user asks for verse 6.

Strings in a switch statement

In Listings 5-6 and 5-7, shown earlier, the variable `verse` (an `int` value) steers the `switch` statement to one case or another. An `int` value inside a `switch` statement works in any version of Java, old or new. (For that matter, `char` values and a few other kinds of values have worked in Java's `switch` statements ever since Java was a brand-new language.)

Starting with Java 7, you can set it up so that the case to be executed in a `switch` statement depends on the value of a particular string. Listing 5-8 illustrates the use of strings in `switch` statements. Figure 5-11 shows a run of the code in Listing 5-8.

LISTING 5-8: A switch Statement with a String

```
import static java.lang.System.out;
import java.util.Scanner;

public class SwitchIt7 {

    public static void main(String args[]) {
       Scanner keyboard = new Scanner(System.in);
       out.print("Which verse (one, two or three)? ");
       String verse = keyboard.next();

       switch (verse) {
       case "one":
          out.println("That's because he has no brain.");
          break;
       case "two":
          out.println("That's because he is a pain.");
          break;
       case "three":
          out.println("'Cause this is the last refrain.");
          break;
       default:
          out.println("No such verse. Please try again.");
          break;
       }

       out.println("Ohhhhhhhh... .");

       keyboard.close();
    }
}
```

```
Which verse (one, two or three)? two
That's because he is a pain.
Ohhhhhhhh. . . .
```

FIGURE 5-11: Running the code of Listing 5-8.

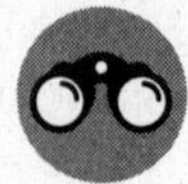

TRY IT OUT

Get some practice with `if` statements and `switch` statements!

- Write a program that inputs the name of a month and outputs the number of days in that month. In this first version of the program, assume that February always has 28 days.
- Make your code even better! Have the user input a month name, but also have the user input yes or no in response to the question `Is it a leap year?`

» **Counting as you loop**

» **Repeating relentlessly (until the user gives you a clear answer)**

Chapter 6

Controlling Program Flow with Loops

In 1966, the company that brings you Head & Shoulders shampoo made history. On the back of the bottle, the directions for using the shampoo read, "LATHER-RINSE-REPEAT." Never before had a complete set of directions (for doing anything, let alone shampooing your hair) been summarized so succinctly. People in the direction-writing business hailed this as a monumental achievement. Directions like these stood in stark contrast to others of the time. (For instance, the first sentence on a can of bug spray read, "Turn this can so that it points away from your face." Duh!)

Aside from their brevity, the thing that made the Head & Shoulders directions so cool was that, with three simple words, it managed to capture a notion that's at the heart of all instruction-giving — the notion of repetition. That last word, *REPEAT*, took an otherwise bland instructional drone and turned it into a sophisticated recipe for action.

The fundamental idea is that when you're following directions, you don't just follow one instruction after another. Instead, you take turns in the road. You make decisions ("If HAIR IS DRY, then USE CONDITIONER") and you go into loops ("LATHER-RINSE, and then LATHER-RINSE again."). In computer programming, you use decision-making and looping all the time. This chapter explores looping in Java.

Repeating Instructions Over and Over Again (Java while Statements)

Here's a guessing game for you. The computer generates a random number from 1 to 10. The computer asks you to guess the number. If you guess incorrectly, the game continues. As soon as you guess correctly, the game is over. Listing 6-1 shows the program to play the game, and Figure 6-1 shows a round of play.

LISTING 6-1: A Repeating Guessing Game

```
import static java.lang.System.out;
import java.util.Scanner;
import java.util.Random;

public class GuessAgain {

    public static void main(String args[]) {
        Scanner keyboard = new Scanner(System.in);

        int numGuesses = 0;
        int randomNumber = new Random().nextInt(10) + 1;

        out.println("       ************         ");
        out.println("Welcome to the Guessing Game");
        out.println("       ************         ");
        out.println();

        out.print("Enter an int from 1 to 10: ");
        int inputNumber = keyboard.nextInt();
        numGuesses++;

        while (inputNumber != randomNumber) {
            out.println();
            out.println("Try again...");
            out.print("Enter an int from 1 to 10: ");
            inputNumber = keyboard.nextInt();
            numGuesses++;
        }
```

```
            out.print("You win after ");
            out.println(numGuesses + " guesses.");

            keyboard.close();
        }
    }
```

```
        ************
Welcome to the Guessing Game
        ************

Enter an int from 1 to 10: 2

Try again...
Enter an int from 1 to 10: 5

Try again...
Enter an int from 1 to 10: 8

Try again...
Enter an int from 1 to 10: 3
You win after 4 guesses.
```

FIGURE 6-1: Play until you drop.

In Figure 6-1, the user makes four guesses. Each time around, the computer checks to see whether the guess is correct. An incorrect guess generates a request to try again. For a correct guess, the user gets a rousing `You win`, along with a tally of the number of guesses he or she made. The computer repeats several statements, checking each time through to see whether the user's guess is the same as a certain randomly generated number. Each time the user makes a guess, the computer adds 1 to its tally of guesses. When the user makes the correct guess, the computer displays that tally. Figure 6-2 illustrates the flow of action.

When you look over Listing 6-1, you see the code that does all this work. At the core of the code is a thing called a *while statement* (also known as a *while loop*). Rephrased in English, the `while` statement says:

```
while the inputNumber is not equal to the randomNumber
keep doing all the stuff in curly braces: {

}
```

The stuff in curly braces (the stuff that repeats) is the code that prints `Try again` and `Enter an int ...`, gets a value from the keyboard, and adds 1 to the count of the user's guesses.

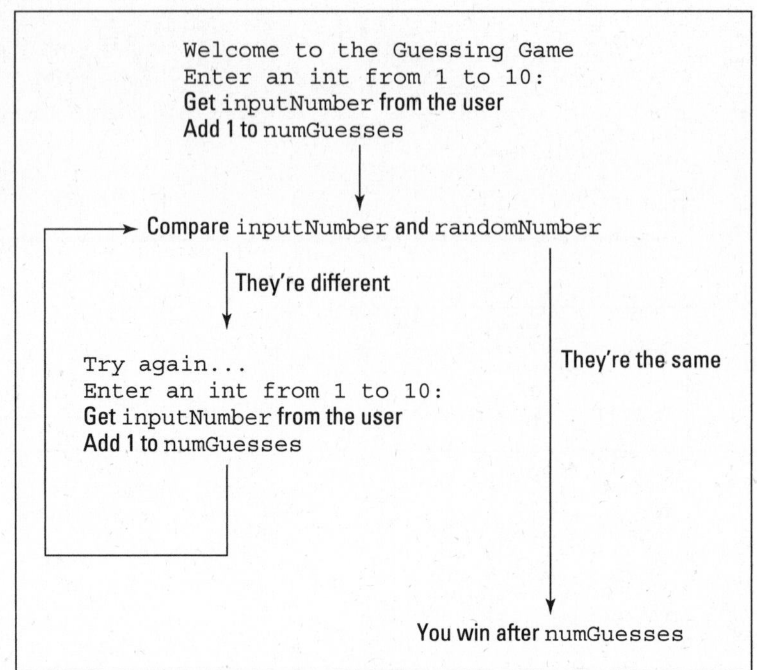
Welcome to the Guessing Game
Enter an int from 1 to 10:
Get inputNumber from the user
Add 1 to numGuesses
Compare inputNumber and randomNumber
They're different
Try again...
Enter an int from 1 to 10:
Get inputNumber from the user
Add 1 to numGuesses
They're the same
You win after numGuesses

FIGURE 6-2: Around and around you go.

TIP

When you're dealing with counters, like `numGuesses` in Listing 6-1, you may easily become confused and be off by 1 in either direction. You can avoid this headache by making sure that the ++ statements stay close to the statements whose events you're counting. For example, in Listing 6-1, the variable `numGuesses` starts with a value of `0`. That's because, when the program starts running, the user hasn't made any guesses. Later in the program, right after each call to `keyboard.nextInt`, is a `numGuesses++` statement. That's how you do it — you increment the counter as soon as the user enters another guess.

The statements in curly braces are repeated as long as `inputNumber != randomNumber` is true. Each repetition of the statements in the loop is called an iteration of the loop. In Figure 6-1, the loop undergoes three iterations. (If you don't believe that Figure 6-1 has exactly three iterations, count the number of `Try again` printings in the program's output. A `Try again` appears for each incorrect guess.)

When, at long last, the user enters the correct guess, the computer goes back to the top of the `while` statement, checks the condition in parentheses, and finds itself in double double-negative land. The not equal (`!=`) relationship between `inputNumber` and `randomNumber` no longer holds. In other words, the `while` statement's condition, `inputNumber != randomNumber`, is false. Because the `while` statement's condition is false, the computer jumps past the `while` loop and goes on to the statements just below the `while` loop. In these two statements, the computer prints `You win` after four guesses.

REMEMBER

With code of the kind shown in Listing 6-1, the computer never jumps out in mid-loop. When the computer finds that `inputNumber` isn't equal to `randomNumber`, the computer marches on and executes all five statements inside the loop's curly braces. The computer performs the test again (to see whether `inputNumber` is still not equal to `randomNumber`) only after it fully executes all five statements in the loop.

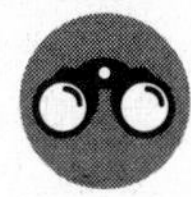

TRY IT OUT

I have two things for you to try:

- Modify the program in Listing 6-1 so that the randomly generated number is a number from 1 and 100. To make life bearable for the game player, have the program give a hint whenever the player guesses incorrectly. Hints such as `Try a higher number` or `Try a lower number` are very helpful.
- Write a program in which the user types `int` values, one after another. The program stops looping when the user types a number that isn't positive (for example, the number 0 or the number –17). After all the looping, the program displays the largest number that the user typed. For example, if the user types the numbers

  ```
  7
  25
  3
  9
  0
  ```

  the program displays the number 25.

Repeating a Certain Number of Times (Java for Statements)

"Write *I will not talk in class* on the blackboard 100 times."

What your teacher really meant was this:

```
Set the count to 0.
As long as the count is less than 100,
    Write 'I will not talk in class' on the blackboard,
    Add 1 to the count.
```

Fortunately, you didn't know about loops and counters at the time. If you pointed out all this stuff to your teacher, you'd have gotten into a lot more trouble than you were already in.

One way or another, life is filled with examples of counting loops. And computer programming mirrors life — or is it the other way around? When you tell a computer what to do, you're often telling the computer to print three lines, process ten accounts, dial a million phone numbers, or whatever. Because counting loops is so common in programming, the people who create programming languages have developed statements just for loops of this kind. In Java, the statement that repeats something a certain number of times is called a *for statement.* Listings 6-2 and 6-3 illustrate the use of the for statement. Listing 6-2 has a rock-bottom simple example, and Listing 6-3 has a more exotic example. Take your pick.

LISTING 6-2: The World's Most Boring for Loop

```
import static java.lang.System.out;

public class Yawn {

    public static void main(String args[]) {

        for (int count = 1; count <= 10; count++) {
            out.print("The value of count is ");
            out.print(count);
            out.println(".");
        }

        out.println("Done!");
    }
}
```

Figure 6-3 shows you what you get when you run the program of Listing 6-2. (You get exactly what you deserve.) The for statement in Listing 6-2 starts by setting the count variable to 1. Then the statement tests to make sure that count is less than or equal to 10 (which it certainly is). Then the for statement dives ahead and executes the printing statements between the curly braces. (At this early stage of the game, the computer prints The value of count is 1.) Finally, the for statement does that last thing inside its parentheses — it adds 1 to the value of count.

With count now equal to 2, the for statement checks again to make sure that count is less than or equal to 10. (Yes, 2 is smaller than 10.) Because the test turns out okay, the for statement marches back into the curly braced statements and prints The value of count is 2 on the screen. Finally, the for statement does that last thing inside its parentheses — it adds 1 to the value of count, increasing the value of count to 3.

```
The value of count is 1.
The value of count is 2.
The value of count is 3.
The value of count is 4.
The value of count is 5.
The value of count is 6.
The value of count is 7.
The value of count is 8.
The value of count is 9.
The value of count is 10.
Done!
```

FIGURE 6-3: Counting to ten.

And so on. This whole thing repeats until, after ten iterations, the value of `count` finally reaches 11. When this happens, the check for `count` being less than or equal to ten fails, and the loop's execution ends. The computer jumps to whatever statement comes immediately after the `for` statement. In Listing 6-2, the computer prints `Done!` as its output. Figure 6-4 illustrates the whole process.

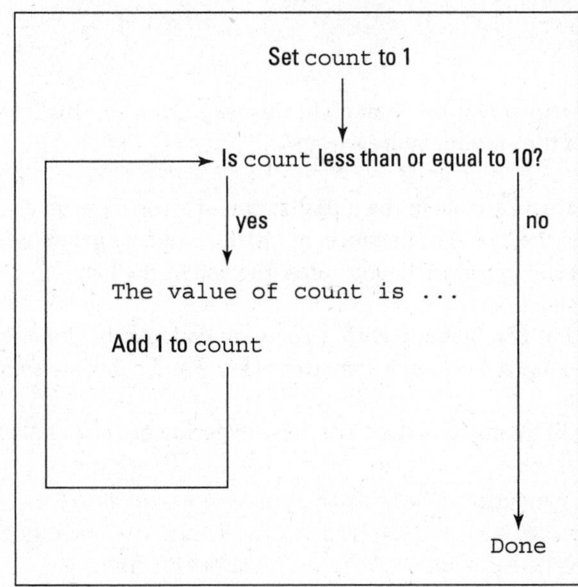

FIGURE 6-4: The action of the `for` loop in Listing 6-2.

The anatomy of a for statement

After the word *for*, you always put three things in parentheses. The first of these three is called an *initialization*, the second is an *expression*, and the third is an *update*:

```
for ( initialization ; expression ; update )
```

Each of the three items in parentheses plays its own distinct role:

- **The initialization** is executed once, when the run of your program first reaches the `for` statement.
- **The expression** is evaluated several times (before each iteration).
- **The update** is also evaluated several times (at the end of each iteration).

If it helps, think of the loop as though its text is shifted all around:

```
int count = 1
for count <= 10 {
    out.print("The value of count is ");
    out.print(count);
    out.println(".");
    count++;
}
```

You can't write a real `for` statement this way. Even so, this is the order in which the parts of the statement are executed.

If you declare a variable in the initialization of a `for` loop, you can't use that variable outside the loop. For instance, in Listing 6-2, you get an error message if you try putting `out.println(count)` after the end of the loop.

Anything that can be done with a `for` loop can also be done with a `while` loop. Choosing to use a `for` loop is a matter of style and convenience, not necessity.

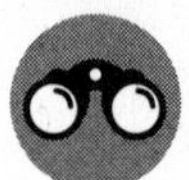

Would you like some practice? Try these experiments and challenges:

- A `for` statement's initialization may have several parts. A `for` statement's update may also have several parts. To find out how, enter the following lines in Java's JShell, or add the lines to a small Java program:

  ```
  import static java.lang.System.out
  for (int i = 0, j = 10; i < j; i++, j--) {out.println(i + " " + j);}
  ```

- What's the output of the following code?

  ```
  int total = 0;
  for (int i = 0; i < 10; i++) {
    total += i;
  }
  System.out.println(total);
  ```

In this code, the variable `total` is called an *accumulator* because it accumulates (adds up) a bunch of values inside the loop.

- In mathematics, the exclamation point (!) means *factorial* — the number you get when you multiply all the positive `int` values up to and including a certain number. For example, 3! is 1 × 2 × 3, which is 6. And 5! is 1 × 2 × 3 × 4 × 5, which is 120.

  Write a program in which the user types a positive `int` value (call it *n*), and Java displays the value of *n*! as its output.

- Without running the following code, try to predict what the code's output will be:

```
for (int row = 0; row < 5; row++) {
  for (int column = 0; column < 5; column++) {
    System.out.print("*");
  }
  System.out.println();
}
```

  After making your prediction, run the code to find out whether your prediction is correct.

- The code in this experiment is a slight variation on the code in the previous experiment. First, try to predict what the code will output. Then run the code to find out whether your prediction is correct:

```
for (int row = 0; row < 5; row++) {
  for (int column = 0; column <= row; column++) {
    System.out.print("*");
  }
  System.out.println();
}
```

- Write a program that uses loops to display three copies of the following pattern, one after another:

```
*
**
***
****
*****
```

The world premiere of "Al's All Wet"

Listing 6-2 is very nice, but the program in that listing doesn't do anything interesting. For a more eye-catching example, see Listing 6-3. In Listing 6-3, I make good on a promise I make in Chapter 5. The program in Listing 6-3 prints all the lyrics of the hit single "Al's All Wet." (You can find the lyrics in Chapter 5.)

LISTING 6-3: The Unabridged "Al's All Wet" Song

```
import static java.lang.System.out;

public class AlsAllWet {

   public static void main(String args[]) {

      for (int verse = 1; verse <= 3; verse++) {
        out.print("Al's all wet. ");
        out.println("Oh, why is Al all wet? Oh,");
        out.print("Al's all wet 'cause ");
        out.println("he's standing in the rain.");
        out.println("Why is Al out in the rain?");

        switch (verse) {
        case 1:
          out.println("That's because he has no brain.");
          break;
        case 2:
          out.println("That's because he is a pain.");
          break;
        case 3:
          out.println("'Cause this is the last refrain.");
          break;
        }

        switch (verse) {
        case 3:
          out.println("Last refrain, last refrain,");
        case 2:
          out.println("He's a pain, he's a pain,");
        case 1:
          out.println("Has no brain, has no brain,");
        }

        out.println("In the rain, in the rain.");
        out.println("Ohhhhhhhh...");
        out.println();
      }
```

```
        out.print("Al's all wet. ");
        out.println("Oh, why is Al all wet? Oh,");
        out.print("Al's all wet 'cause ");
        out.println("he's standing in the rain.");
    }
}
```

Listing 6-3 is nice because it combines many of the ideas from Chapters 5 and 6. In Listing 6-3, two switch statements are nested inside a for loop. One of the switch statements uses break statements; the other switch statement uses fall-through. As the value of the for loop's counter variable (verse) goes from 1 to 2 and then to 3, all the cases in the switch statements are executed. When the program is near the end of its run and execution has dropped out of the for loop, the program's last four statements print the song's final verse.

TECHNICAL STUFF

When I boldly declare that a for statement is for counting, I'm stretching the truth just a bit. Java's for statement is very versatile. You can use a for statement in situations that have nothing to do with counting. For instance, a statement with no update part, such as for (i = 0; i < 10;), just keeps on going. The looping ends when some action inside the loop assigns a big number to the variable i. You can even create a for statement with nothing inside the parentheses. The loop for (; ;) runs forever, which is good if the loop controls a serious piece of machinery. Usually, when you write a for statement, you're counting how many times to repeat something. But, in truth, you can do just about any kind of repetition with a for statement.

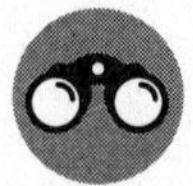

TRY IT OUT

Look! I have some experiments for you to try!

- Listing 6-3 uses break statements to jump out of a switch. But a break statement can also play a role inside a loop. To find out how it works, run a program containing the following code:

```
Scanner keyboard = new Scanner(System.in);
while (true) {
  System.out.print("Enter an int value: ");
  int i = keyboard.nextInt();
  if (i == 0) {
    break;
  }
  System.out.println(i);
}
System.out.println("Done!");
keyboard.close();
```

The loop's condition is always `true`. It's like starting a loop with the line

```
while (1 + 1 == 2)
```

If it weren't for the `break` statement, the loop would run forever. Fortunately, when you execute the `break` statement, Java jumps to the code immediately after the loop.

- In addition to its `break` statement, Java has a `continue` statement. When you execute a `continue` statement, Java skips to the end of its loop and begins the next iteration of that loop. To see it in action, run a program containing the following code:

```
Scanner keyboard = new Scanner(System.in);

while (true) {
  System.out.print("Enter an int value: ");
  int i = keyboard.nextInt();
  if (i > 10) {
    continue;
  }
  if (i == 0) {
    break;

  }
  System.out.println(i);
}

System.out.println("Done!");
keyboard.close();
```

Repeating until You Get What You Want (Java do Statements)

Fools rush in where angels fear to tread.

—ALEXANDER POPE

Today, I want to be young and foolish (or, at the very least, foolish). Look back at Figure 6-2 and notice how Java's `while` loop works. When execution enters a `while` loop, the computer checks to make sure that the loop's condition is true. If the condition isn't true, the statements inside the loop are never executed — not even once. In fact, you can easily cook up a `while` loop whose statements are never executed (although I can't think of a reason why you would ever want to do it):

```
int twoPlusTwo = 2 + 2;

while (twoPlusTwo == 5) {
    out.println("Are you kidding?");
    out.println("2 + 2 doesn't equal 5");
    out.print("Everyone knows that");
    out.println(" 2 + 2 equals 3");
}
```

In spite of this silly `twoPlusTwo` example, the `while` statement turns out to be the most versatile of Java's looping constructs. In particular, the `while` loop is good for situations in which you must look before you leap. For example, "While money is in my account, write a mortgage check every month." When you first encounter this statement, if your account has a zero balance, you don't want to write a mortgage check — not even one check.

But at times (not many), you want to leap before you look. Take, for instance, the situation in which you're asking the user for a response. Maybe the user's response makes sense, but maybe it doesn't. If it doesn't, you want to ask again. Maybe the user's finger slipped, or perhaps the user didn't understand the question.

Figure 6-5 shows some runs of a program to delete a file. Before deleting the file, the program asks the user whether making the deletion is okay. If the user answers *y* or *n*, the program proceeds according to the user's wishes. But if the user enters any other character (any digit, uppercase letter, punctuation symbol, or whatever), the program asks the user for another response.

```
Delete evidence? (y/n) n
Sorry, buddy. Just asking.


Delete evidence? (y/n) u
Delete evidence? (y/n) Y
Delete evidence? (y/n) L
Delete evidence? (y/n) 8
Delete evidence? (y/n) .
Delete evidence? (y/n) y
Okay, here goes...
The evidence has been deleted.
```

FIGURE 6-5: Two runs of the code in Listing 6-4.

To write this program, you need a loop — a loop that repeatedly asks the user whether the file should be deleted. The loop keeps asking until the user gives a meaningful response. Now, the thing to notice is that the loop doesn't need to check anything before asking the user the first time. Indeed, before the user gives the first response, the loop has nothing to check. The loop doesn't start with "as long as such-and-such is true, then get a response from the user." Instead, the loop just leaps ahead, gets a response from the user, and then checks the response to see whether it makes sense.

That's why the program in Listing 6-4 has a *do* loop (also known as a *do . . . while* loop). With a do loop, the program jumps right in, takes action, and then checks a condition to see whether the result of the action makes sense. If the result makes sense, execution of the loop is done. If not, the program goes back to the top of the loop for another go-round.

LISTING 6-4: To Delete or Not to Delete

```
import java.io.File;
import static java.lang.System.out;
import java.util.Scanner;

public class DeleteEvidence {

   public static void main(String args[]) {
      File evidence = new File("cookedBooks.txt");
      Scanner keyboard = new Scanner(System.in);
      char reply;

      do {
         out.print("Delete evidence? (y/n) ");
         reply = keyboard.findWithinHorizon(".",0).charAt(0);
      } while (reply != 'y' && reply != 'n');

      if (reply == 'y') {
         out.println("Okay, here goes...");
         evidence.delete();
         out.println("The evidence has been deleted.");
      } else {
         out.println("Sorry, buddy. Just asking.");
      }

      keyboard.close();
   }
}
```

Figure 6-5 shows two runs of the code in Listing 6-4. The program accepts lowercase letters *y* and *n*, but not the uppercase letters *Y* and *N*. To make the program accept uppercase letters, change the conditions in the code as follows:

```
do {
    out.print("Delete evidence? (y/n) ");
    reply = keyboard.findWithinHorizon(".", 0).charAt(0);
} while (reply != 'y' && reply != 'Y' && reply != 'n' && reply!='N');

if (reply == 'y' || reply == 'Y') {
```

Figure 6-6 shows the flow of control in the loop of Listing 6-4. With a do loop, the situation in the twoPlusTwo program (shown at the beginning of this section) can never happen. Because the do loop carries out its first action without testing a condition, every do loop is guaranteed to perform at least one iteration.

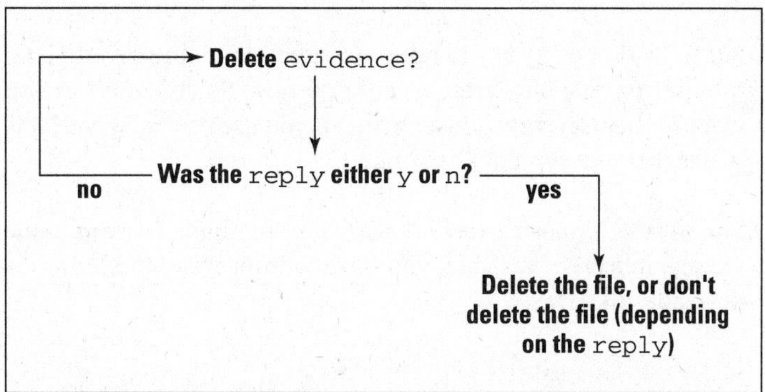

FIGURE 6-6: Here we go loop, do loop.

TIP

The location of Listing 6-4's cookedBooks.txt file on your computer's hard drive depends on several factors. If you create a cookedBooks.txt file in the wrong directory, the code in Listing 6-4 cannot delete your file. (More precisely, if cookedBooks.txt is in the wrong directory on your hard drive, the code in Listing 6-4 can't find the cookedBooks.txt file in preparation for deleting the file.) In most settings, you start testing Listing 6-4 by creating a project within your IDE. The new project lives in a folder on your hard drive, and the cookedBooks.txt file belongs directly inside that folder. For example, I have a project named 06-04. That project lives on my hard drive in a folder named 06-04. Inside that folder, I have a file named cookedBooks.txt. If you have trouble with this, add the following code to Listing 6-4 immediately after the new File statement:

```
try {
  out.println("Looking for " + evidence.getCanonicalPath());
} catch (java.io.IOException e) {
  e.printStackTrace();
}
```

When you run the code, Java tells you where, on your hard drive, the `cookedBooks.txt` file should be.

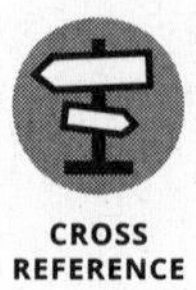

CROSS REFERENCE

For more information about files and their folders, see Chapter 8.

Reading a single character

Over in Listing 5-3 from Chapter 5, the user types a word on the keyboard. The `keyboard.next` method grabs the word and places the word into a `String` variable named *password.* Everything works nicely because a `String` variable can store many characters at once, and the `next` method can read many characters at once.

But in Listing 6-4, you're not interested in reading several characters. You expect the user to type one letter — either **y** or **n**. So you don't create a `String` variable to store the user's response. Instead, you create a `char` variable — a variable that stores just one symbol at a time.

The Java API doesn't have a `nextChar` method. To read something suitable for storage in a `char` variable, you have to improvise. In Listing 6-4, the improvisation looks like this:

```
keyboard.findWithinHorizon(".", 0).charAt(0)
```

You can use this code exactly as it appears in Listing 6-4 whenever you want to read a single character.

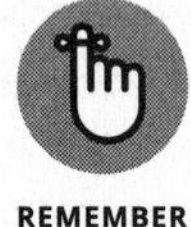

REMEMBER

A `String` variable can contain many characters or just one. But a `String` variable that contains only one character isn't the same as a `char` variable. No matter what you put in a `String` variable, `String` variables and `char` variables have to be treated differently.

File handling in Java

In Listing 6-4, the actual file-handling statements deserve some attention. These statements involve the use of classes, objects, and methods. Many of the meaty details about these things are in other chapters, like Chapters 7 and 9. Even so, I can't do any harm by touching on some highlights right here.

So, you can find a class in the Java language API named *java.io.File.* The statement

```
File evidence = new File("cookedBooks.txt");
```

creates a new object in the computer's memory. This object, formed from the java.io.File class, describes everything that the program needs to know about the disk file cookedBooks.txt. From this point on in Listing 6-4, the variable evidence refers to the disk file cookedBooks.txt.

The evidence object, as an instance of the java.io.File class, has a delete method. (What can I say? It's in the API documentation.) When you call evidence.delete, the computer gets rid of the file for you.

Of course, you can't get rid of something that doesn't already exist. When the computer executes

```
File evidence = new File("cookedBooks.txt");
```

Java doesn't check to make sure that you have a file named cookedBooks.txt. To force Java to do the checking, you have a few options. The simplest is to call the exists method. When you call evidence.exists(), the method looks in the folder where Java expects to find cookedBooks.txt. The call evidence.exists() returns true if Java finds cookedBooks.txt inside that folder. Otherwise, the call evidence.exists() returns false. Here's a souped-up version of Listing 6-4, with a call to exists included in the code:

```
import java.io.File;
import static java.lang.System.out;
import java.util.Scanner;

public class DeleteEvidence {

  public static void main(String args[]) {
    File evidence = new File("cookedBooks.txt");
    if (evidence.exists()) {
      Scanner keyboard = new Scanner(System.in);
      char reply;

      do {
        out.print("Delete evidence? (y/n) ");
        reply =
           keyboard.findWithinHorizon(".", 0).charAt(0);
      } while (reply != 'y' && reply != 'n');

      if (reply == 'y') {
        out.println("Okay, here goes...");
        evidence.delete();
        out.println("The evidence has been deleted.");
```

```
        } else {
          out.println("Sorry, buddy. Just asking.");
        }

        keyboard.close();
      }
    }
  }
```

Variable declarations and blocks

A bunch of statements surrounded by curly braces forms a block. If you declare a variable inside a block, you generally can't use that variable outside the block. For instance, in Listing 6-4, you get an error message if you make the following change:

```
do {
   out.print("Delete evidence? (y/n) ");
   char reply = keyboard.findWithinHorizon(".", 0).charAt(0);
} while (reply != 'y' && reply != 'n');

if (reply == 'y')
```

With the declaration `char reply` inside the loop's curly braces, no use of the name `reply` makes sense anywhere outside the braces. When you try to compile this code, you get three error messages — two for the `reply` words in `while (reply != 'y' && reply != 'n')` and a third for the `if` statement's `reply`.

So in Listing 6-4, your hands are tied. The program's first real use of the `reply` variable is inside the loop. But to make that variable available after the loop, you have to declare `reply` before the loop. In this situation, you're best off declaring the `reply` variable without initializing the variable. Very interesting!

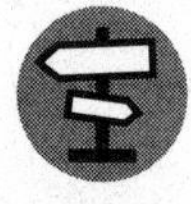

CROSS REFERENCE

To read more about variable initializations, see Chapter 4. To find out more about blocks, see Chapter 5.

All versions of Java have the three kinds of loops described in this chapter (`while` loops, `for` loops, and `do ... while` loops). But newer Java versions (namely, Java 5 and beyond) have yet another kind of loop, called an *enhanced for loop*. For a look at Java's `enhanced for` loop, see Chapter 11.

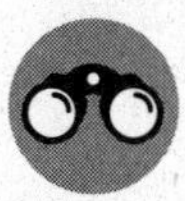

TRY IT OUT

Copy the code from Listing 6-1, but with the following change:

```
out.print("Enter an int from 1 to 10: ");
int inputNumber = keyboard.nextInt();
numGuesses++;

do {
    out.println();
    out.println("Try again...");
    out.print("Enter an int from 1 to 10: ");
    inputNumber = keyboard.nextInt();
    numGuesses++;
} while (inputNumber != randomNumber);

out.print("You win after ");
out.println(numGuesses + " guesses.");
```

The code in Listing 6-1 has a `while` loop, but this modified code has a `do` loop. Does this modified code work correctly? Why, or why not?

3 Working with the Big Picture: Object-Oriented Programming

IN THIS PART . . .

Find out what classes and objects are (without bending your brain out of shape).

Find out how object-oriented programming helps you reuse existing code (saving you time and money).

Be the emperor of your own virtual world by constructing brand-new objects.

» Passing values to and from methods

» Hiding details in your object-oriented code

Chapter 7

Thinking in Terms of Classes and Objects

As a computer book author, I've been told this over and over again: I shouldn't expect people to read sections and chapters in their logical order. People jump around, picking what they need and skipping what they don't feel like reading. With that in mind, I realize that you may have skipped Chapter 1. If that's the case, please don't feel guilty. You can compensate in just 60 seconds by reading the following information, culled from Chapter 1:

> *Because Java is an object-oriented programming language, your primary goal is to describe classes and objects. A class is the idea behind a certain kind of thing. An object is a concrete instance of a class. The programmer defines a class, and from the class definition, Java makes individual objects.*

Of course, you can certainly choose to skip over the 60-second summary paragraph. If that's the case, you may want to recoup some of your losses. You can do that by reading the following two-word summary of Chapter 1:

> *Classes; objects.*

Defining a Class (What It Means to Be an Account)

What distinguishes one bank account from another? If you ask a banker this question, you hear a long sales pitch. The banker describes interest rates, fees, penalties — the whole routine. Fortunately for you, I'm not interested in all that. Instead, I want to know how my account is different from your account. After all, my account is named *Barry Burd, trading as Burd Brain Consulting,* and your account is named *Jane Q. Reader, trading as Budding Java Expert.* My account has $24.02 in it. How about yours?

When you come right down to it, the differences between one account and another can be summarized as values of variables. Maybe there's a variable named `balance`. For me, the value of `balance` is `24.02`. For you, the value of `balance` is `55.63`. The question is, when writing a computer program to deal with accounts, how do I separate my `balance` variable from your `balance` variable?

The answer is to create two separate objects. Let one `balance` variable live inside one of the objects and let the other `balance` variable live inside the other object. While you're at it, put a `name` variable and an `address` variable in each of the objects. And there you have it: two objects, and each object represents an account. More precisely, each object is an instance of the `Account` class. (See Figure 7-1.)

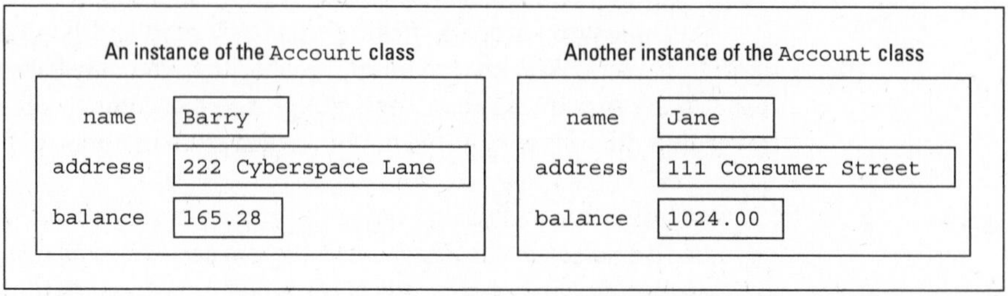

FIGURE 7-1: Two objects.

So far, so good. However, you still haven't solved the original problem. In your computer program, how do you refer to my `balance` variable, as opposed to your `balance` variable? Well, you have two objects sitting around, so maybe you have variables to refer to these two objects. Create one variable named *myAccount* and another variable named *yourAccount.* The `myAccount` variable refers to my object (my instance of the `Account` class) with all the stuff that's inside it. To refer to my balance, write

```
myAccount.balance
```

To refer to my name, write

```
myAccount.name
```

Then yourAccount.balance refers to the value in your object's balance variable, and yourAccount.name refers to the value of your object's name variable. To tell Java how much I have in my account, you can write

```
myAccount.balance = 24.02;
```

To display your name on the screen, you can write

```
out.println(yourAccount.name);
```

These ideas come together in Listings 7-1 and 7-2. Here's Listing 7-1:

LISTING 7-1: What It Means to Be an Account

```
public class Account {
    String name;
    String address;
    double balance;
}
```

The Account class in Listing 7-1 defines what it means to be an Account. In particular, Listing 7-1 tells you that each of the Account class's instances has three variables: name, address, and balance. This is consistent with the information in Figure 7-1. Java programmers have a special name for variables of this kind (variables that belong to instances of classes). Each of these variables — name, address, and balance — is called a *field.*

REMEMBER

A variable declared inside a class but not inside any particular method is a *field.* In Listing 7-1, the variables name, address, and balance are fields. Another name for a field is an *instance variable.*

If you've been grappling with the material in Chapters 4 through 6, the code for class Account (refer to Listing 7-1) may come as a big shock to you. Can you really define a complete Java class with only four lines of code (give or take a curly brace)? You certainly can. A class is a grouping of existing things. In the Account class of Listing 7-1, those existing things are two String values and a double value.

WARNING

The field declarations in Listing 7-1 have *default access*, which means that I didn't add a word before the type name `String`. The alternatives to default access are *public*, *protected*, and *private* access:

```
public String name;
protected String address;
private double balance;
```

Professional programmers shun the use of default access because default access doesn't shield a field from accidental misuse. But in my experience, you learn best when you learn about the simplest stuff first, and in Java, default access is the simplest stuff. In this book, I delay the discussion of private access until this chapter's section "Hiding Details with Accessor Methods." And I delay the discussion of protected access until Chapter 14. As you read this chapter's examples, please keep in mind that default access isn't the best thing to use in a Java program. And, if a professional programmer asks you where you learned to use default access, please lie and blame someone else's book.

Declaring variables and creating objects

A young fellow approaches me while I'm walking down the street. He tells me to print "You'll love Java!" so I print those words. If you must know, I print them with chalk on the sidewalk. But where I print the words doesn't matter. What matters is that some guy issues instructions, and I follow the instructions.

Later that day, an elderly woman sits next to me on a park bench. She says, "An account has a name, an address, and a balance." And I say, "That's fine, but what do you want me to do about it?" In response she just stares at me, so I don't do anything about her *account* pronouncement. I just sit there, she sits there, and we both do absolutely nothing.

Listing 7-1, shown earlier, is like the elderly woman. This listing defines what it means to be an `Account`, but the listing doesn't tell me to do anything with my account, or with anyone else's account. In order to do something, I need a second piece of code. I need another class — a class that contains a `main` method. Fortunately, while the woman and I sit quietly on the park bench, a young child comes by with Listing 7-2.

LISTING 7-2: Dealing with Account Objects

```
import static java.lang.System.out;

public class UseAccount {

    public static void main(String args[]) {
        Account myAccount;
        Account yourAccount;

        myAccount = new Account();
        yourAccount = new Account();

        myAccount.name = "Barry Burd";
        myAccount.address = "222 Cyberspace Lane";
        myAccount.balance = 24.02;

        yourAccount.name = "Jane Q. Public";
        yourAccount.address = "111 Consumer Street";
        yourAccount.balance = 55.63;

        out.print(myAccount.name);
        out.print(" (");
        out.print(myAccount.address);
        out.print(") has $");
        out.print(myAccount.balance);
        out.println();

        out.print(yourAccount.name);
        out.print(" (");
        out.print(yourAccount.address);
        out.print(") has $");
        out.print(yourAccount.balance);
    }
}
```

Taken together, the two classes — Account and UseAccount — form one complete program. The code in Listing 7-2 defines the UseAccount class, and the UseAccount class has a main method. This main method has variables of its own — yourAccount and myAccount.

In a way, the first two lines inside the main method of Listing 7-2 are misleading. Some people read Account yourAccount as if it's supposed to mean, "yourAccount is an Account," or "The variable yourAccount refers to an instance of the Account class." That's not really what this first line means. Instead, the line Account yourAccount means, "If and when I make the variable yourAccount refer to something, that something will be an instance of the Account class." So, what's the difference?

The difference is that simply declaring `Account yourAccount` doesn't make the `yourAccount` variable refer to an object. All the declaration does is reserve the variable name *yourAccount* so that the name can eventually refer to an instance of the `Account` class. The creation of an actual object doesn't come until later in the code, when Java executes `new Account()`.

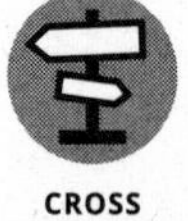

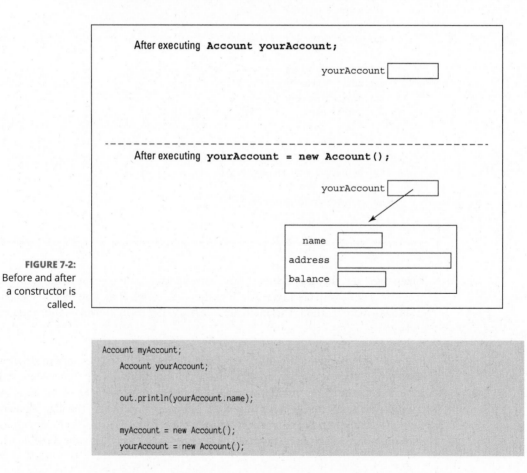
CROSS REFERENCE

Technically, when Java executes `new Account()`, you're creating an object by calling the `Account` class's *constructor*. I have more to say about that in Chapter 9.

When Java executes the assignment `yourAccount = new Account()`, Java creates a new object (a new instance of the `Account` class) and makes the variable `yourAccount` refer to that new object. (The equal sign makes the variable refer to the new object.) Figure 7-2 illustrates the situation.

To test the claim that I made in the last few paragraphs, I added an extra line to the code of Listing 7-2. I tried to print `yourAccount.name` after declaring `yourAccount` but before calling `new Account()`:

FIGURE 7-2: Before and after a constructor is called.

```
Account myAccount;
    Account yourAccount;

    out.println(yourAccount.name);

    myAccount = new Account();
    yourAccount = new Account();
```

When I tried to compile the new code, I got this error message: `variable yourAccount might not have been initialized`. That settles it. Before you do `new Account()`, you can't print the name variable of an object because an object doesn't exist.

REMEMBER

When a variable has a reference type, simply declaring the variable isn't enough. You don't get an object until you call a constructor and use the keyword `new`.

For information about reference types, see Chapter 4.

Initializing a variable

In Chapter 4, I announce that you can initialize a primitive type variable as part of the variable's declaration.

```
int weightOfAPerson = 150;
```

You can do the same thing with reference type variables, such as `myAccount` and `yourAccount` in Listing 7-2. You can combine the first four lines in the listing's main method into just two lines, like this:

```
Account myAccount = new Account();
Account yourAccount = new Account();
```

If you combine lines this way, you automatically avoid the `variable might not have been initialized` error that I describe in the preceding section. Sometimes you find a situation in which you can't initialize a variable. But when you can initialize, it's usually a plus.

Using an object's fields

After you've bitten off and chewed the `main` method's first four lines, the rest of the code in the earlier Listing 7-2 is sensible and straightforward. You have three lines that put values in the `myAccount` object's fields, three lines that put values in the `yourAccount` object's fields, and four lines that do some printing. Figure 7-3 shows the program's output.

FIGURE 7-3: Running the code in Listings 7-1 and 7-2.

```
Barry Burd (222 Cyberspace Lane) has $24.02
Jane Q. Public (111 Consumer Street) has $55.63
```

One program; several classes

Each program in Chapters 3 to 6 consists of a single class. That's great for a book's introductory chapters. But in real life, a typical program consists of hundreds or even thousands of classes. The program that spans Listings 7-1 and 7-2 consists of two classes. Sure, having two classes isn't like having thousands of classes, but it's a step in that direction.

In practice, most programmers put each class in a file of its own. When you create a program, such as the one in Listings 7-1 and 7-2, you create two files on your computer's hard drive. Therefore, when you download this section's example from the web, you get two separate files — `Account.java` and `UseAccount.java`.

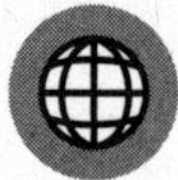

For information about running a program consisting of more than one `.java` file in Eclipse, NetBeans, and IntelliJ IDEA, visit this book's website (`www.allmycode.com/JavaForDummies`).

Public classes

The first line of Listing 7-1 is

```
public class Account {
```

The `Account` class is public. A public class is available for use by all other classes. For example, if you write an ATMController program in some remote corner of cyberspace, then your ATMController program can contain code, such as `myAccount.balance = 24.02`, making use of the `Account` class declared in Listing 7-1. (Of course, your code has to know where in cyberspace I've stored the code in Listing 7-1, but that's another story.)

Listing 7-2 contains the code `myAccount.balance = 24.02`. You might say to yourself, "The `Account` class has to be public because another class (the code in Listing 7-2) uses the `Account` class." Unfortunately, the real lowdown about public classes is a bit more complicated. In fact, when the planets align themselves correctly, one class can make use of another class's code, even though the other class isn't public. (I cover the proper aligning of planets in Chapter 14.)

The dirty secret in this chapter's code is that declaring certain classes to be public simply makes me feel good. Yes, programmers do certain things to feel good. In Listing 7-1, my esthetic sense of goodness comes from the fact that an `Account` class is useful to many other programmers. When I create a class that declares something useful and nameable — an `Account`, an `Engine`, a `Customer`, a `BrainWave`, a `Headache`, or a `SevenLayerCake` class — I declare the class to be public.

The UseAccount class in Listing 7-2 is also public. When a class contains a main method, Java programmers tend to make the class public without thinking too much about who uses the class. So even if no other class makes use of my main method, I declare the UseAccount class to be public. Most of the classes in this book contain main methods, so most of the classes in this book are public.

WARNING

When you declare a class to be public, you must declare the class in a file whose name is exactly the same as the name of the class (but with the .java extension added). For example, if you declare public class MyImportantCode, you must put the class's code in a file named MyImportantCode.java, with uppercase letters M, I, and C and all other letters lowercase. This file-naming rule has an important consequence: If your code declares two public classes, your code must consist of at least two .java files. In other words, you can't declare two public classes in one .java file.

For more news about the word *public* and other such words, see Chapter 14.

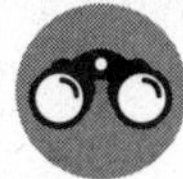

TRY IT OUT

In this section, I create an Account class. You can create classes too.

- An Organization has a name (such as *XYZ Company*), an annual revenue (such as $100,000.00), and a boolean value indicating whether the organization is or is not a profit-making organization. Companies that manufacture and sell products are generally profit-making organizations; groups that provide aid to victims of natural disasters are generally not profit-making organizations.

  Declare your own Organization class. Declare another class that creates organizations and displays information about those organizations.

- A product for sale in a food store has several characteristics: a type of food (peach slices), a weight (500 grams), a cost ($1.83), a number of servings (4), and a number of calories per serving (70).

  Declare a FoodProduct class. Declare another class that creates FoodProduct instances and displays information about those instances.

Defining a Method within a Class (Displaying an Account)

Imagine a table containing the information about two accounts. (If you have trouble imagining such a thing, just look at Table 7-1.)

TABLE 7-1

Without Object-Oriented Programming

Name	Address	Balance
Barry Burd	222 Cyberspace Lane	24.02
Jane Q. Public	111 Consumer Street	55.63

In Table 7-1, each account has three things — a name, an address, and a balance. That's how things were done before object-oriented programming came along. But object-oriented programming involved a big shift in thinking. With object-oriented programming, each account can have a name, an address, a balance, and a way of being displayed.

In object-oriented programming, each object has its own built-in functionality. An account knows how to display itself. A string can tell you whether it has the same characters inside it as another string has. A `PrintStream` instance, such as `System.out`, knows how to do `println`. In object-oriented programming, each object has its own methods. These methods are little subprograms that you can call to have an object do things to (or for) itself.

And why is this a good idea? It's good because you're making pieces of data take responsibility for themselves. With object-oriented programming, all the functionality that's associated with an account is collected inside the code for the `Account` class. Everything you have to know about a string is located in the file `String.java`. Anything having to do with year numbers (whether they have two or four digits, for instance) is handled right inside the `Year` class. Therefore, if anybody has problems with your `Account` class or your `Year` class, he or she knows just where to look for all the code. That's great!

Imagine an enhanced account table. In this new table, each object has built-in functionality. Each account knows how to display itself on the screen. Each row of the table has its own copy of a `display` method. Of course, you don't need much imagination to picture this table. I just happen to have a table you can look at. It's Table 7-2.

TABLE 7-2

The Object-Oriented Way

Name	Address	Balance	Display
Barry Burd	222 Cyberspace Lane	24.02	`out.print ...`
Jane Q. Public	111 Consumer Street	55.63	`out.print ...`

An account that displays itself

In Table 7-2, each account object has four things — a name, an address, a balance, and a way of displaying itself on the screen. After you make the jump to object-oriented thinking, you'll never turn back. Listings 7-3 and 7-4 show programs that implement the ideas in Table 7-2.

LISTING 7-3: An Account Displays Itself

```
import static java.lang.System.out;

public class Account {
    String name;
    String address;
    double balance;

    public void display() {
        out.print(name);
        out.print(" (");
        out.print(address);
        out.print(") has $");
        out.print(balance);
    }
}
```

LISTING 7-4: Using the Improved Account Class

```
public class UseAccount {

    public static void main(String args[]) {
        Account myAccount = new Account();
        Account yourAccount = new Account();

        myAccount.name = "Barry Burd";
        myAccount.address = "222 Cyberspace Lane";
        myAccount.balance = 24.02;

        yourAccount.name = "Jane Q. Public";
        yourAccount.address = "111 Consumer Street";
        yourAccount.balance = 55.63;

        myAccount.display();
        System.out.println();
        yourAccount.display();
    }
}
```

A run of the code in Listings 7-3 and 7-4 looks just like a run for Listings 7-1 and 7-2. You can see the action earlier, in Figure 7-3.

In Listing 7-3, the `Account` class has four things in it: a name, an address, a balance, and a display method. These things match up with the four columns in Table 7-2. So each instance of the `Account` class has a name, an address, a balance, and a way of displaying itself. The way you call these things is nice and uniform. To refer to the name stored in `myAccount`, you write

```
myAccount.name
```

To get `myAccount` to display itself on the screen, you write

```
myAccount.display()
```

The only difference is the parentheses.

REMEMBER

When you call a method, you put parentheses after the method's name.

The display method's header

Look again at Listings 7-3 and 7-4. A call to the display method is inside the `UseAccount` class's `main` method, but the declaration of the `display` method is up in the `Account` class. The declaration has a header and a body. (See Chapter 3.) The header has three words and some parentheses:

- **The word *public* serves roughly the same purpose as the word *public* in Listing 7-1.** Roughly speaking, any code can contain a call to a public method, even if the calling code and the public method belong to two different classes. In this section's example, the decision to make the `display` method public is a matter of taste. Normally, when I create a method that's useful in a wide variety of applications, I declare the method to be public.
- **The word *void* tells Java that when the `display` method is called, the `display` method doesn't return anything to the place that called it.** To see a method that does return something to the place that called it, see the next section.
- **The word *display* is the method's name.** Every method must have a name. Otherwise, you don't have a way to call the method.
- **The parentheses contain all the things you're going to pass to the method when you call it.** When you call a method, you can pass information to that method on the fly. The `display` method in Listing 7-3 looks strange

because the parentheses in the method's header have nothing inside them. This nothingness indicates that no information is passed to the `display` method when you call it. For a meatier example, see the next section.

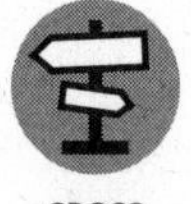
CROSS REFERENCE

Listing 7-3 contains the `display` method's declaration, and Listing 7-4 contains a call to the `display` method. Although Listings 7-3 and 7-4 contain different classes, both uses of `public` in Listing 7-3 are optional. To find out why, check out Chapter 14.

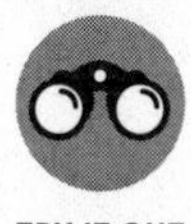
TRY IT OUT

In the previous section, you create `Organization` and `FoodProduct` classes. Add `display` methods to both of these classes and create separate classes that make use of these `display` methods.

Sending Values to and from Methods (Calculating Interest)

Think about sending someone to the supermarket to buy bread. When you do this, you say, "Go to the supermarket and buy some bread." (Try it at home. You'll have a fresh loaf of bread in no time at all!) Of course, some other time, you send that same person to the supermarket to buy bananas. You say, "Go to the supermarket and buy some bananas." And what's the point of all of this? Well, you have a method, and you have some on-the-fly information that you pass to the method when you call it. The method is named *goToTheSupermarketAndBuySome.* The on-the-fly information is either *bread* or *bananas,* depending on your culinary needs. In Java, the method calls would look like this:

```
goToTheSupermarketAndBuySome(bread);
goToTheSupermarketAndBuySome(bananas);
```

The things in parentheses are called *parameters* or *parameter lists.* With parameters, your methods become much more versatile. Instead of getting the same thing each time, you can send somebody to the supermarket to buy bread one time, bananas another time, and birdseed the third time. When you call your `goToTheSupermarketAndBuySome` method, you decide right there what you're going to ask your pal to buy.

And what happens when your friend returns from the supermarket? "Here's the bread you asked me to buy," says your friend. By carrying out your wishes, your friend returns something to you. You make a method call, and the method returns information (or a loaf of bread).

The thing returned to you is called the method's *return value.* The general type of thing that is returned to you is called the method's *return type.* These concepts are made more concrete in Listings 7-5 and 7-6.

LISTING 7-5: An Account That Calculates Its Own Interest

```
import static java.lang.System.out;

public class Account {
    String name;
    String address;
    double balance;

    public void display() {
        out.print(name);
        out.print(" (");
        out.print(address);
        out.print(") has $");
        out.print(balance);
    }

    public double getInterest(double percentageRate) {
        return balance * percentageRate / 100.00;
    }
}
```

LISTING 7-6: Calculating Interest

```
import static java.lang.System.out;

public class UseAccount {

    public static void main(String args[]) {
        Account myAccount = new Account();
        Account yourAccount = new Account();

        myAccount.name = "Barry Burd";
        myAccount.address = "222 Cyberspace Lane";
        myAccount.balance = 24.02;

        yourAccount.name = "Jane Q. Public";
        yourAccount.address = "111 Consumer Street";
        yourAccount.balance = 55.63;

        myAccount.display();
```

```
        out.print(" plus $");
        out.print(myAccount.getInterest(5.00));
        out.println(" interest ");

        yourAccount.display();

        double yourInterestRate = 7.00;
        out.print(" plus $");
        double yourInterestAmount = yourAccount.getInterest(yourInterestRate);
        out.print(yourInterestAmount);
        out.println(" interest ");
    }
}
```

Figure 7-4 shows the output of the code in Listings 7-5 and 7-6. In Listing 7-5, the Account class has a getInterest method. This getInterest method is called twice from the main method in Listing 7-6. The actual account balances and interest rates are different each time.

```
Barry Burd (222 Cyberspace Lane) has $24.02 plus $1.2009999999999998 interest
Jane Q. Public (111 Consumer Street) has $55.63 plus $3.8941000000000003 interest
```

FIGURE 7-4: Running the code in Listings 7-5 and 7-6.

- **In the first call, the balance is 24.02, and the interest rate is 5.00.** The first call, myAccount.getInterest(5.00), refers to the myAccount object and to the values stored in the myAccount object's fields. (See Figure 7-5.) When this call is made, the expression balance * percentageRate / 100.00 stands for 24.02 * 5.00 / 100.00.
- **In the second call, the balance is 55.63, and the interest rate is 7.00.** In the main method, just before this second call is made, the variable yourInterestRate is assigned the value 7.00. The call itself, yourAccount.getInterest(yourInterestRate), refers to the yourAccount object and to the values stored in the yourAccount object's fields. (Again, see Figure 7-5.) So, when the call is made, the expression balance * percentageRate / 100.00 stands for 55.63 * 7.00 / 100.00.

By the way, the main method in Listing 7-6 contains two calls to getInterest. One call has the literal 5.00 in its parameter list; the other call has the variable yourInterestRate in its parameter list. Why does one call use a literal and the other call use a variable? No reason. I just want to show you that you can do it either way.

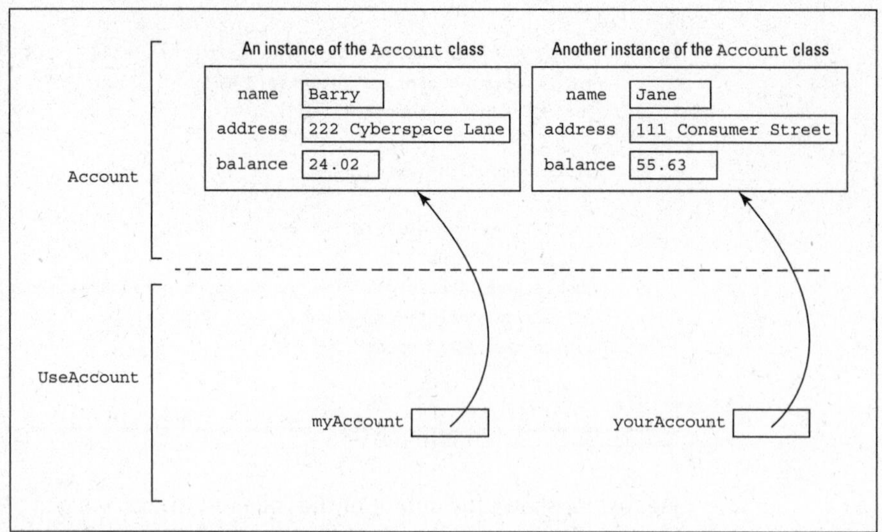

FIGURE 7-5: My account and your account.

Passing a value to a method

Take a look at the `getInterest` method's header. (As you read the explanation in the next few bullets, you can follow some of the ideas visually with the diagram in Figure 7-6.)

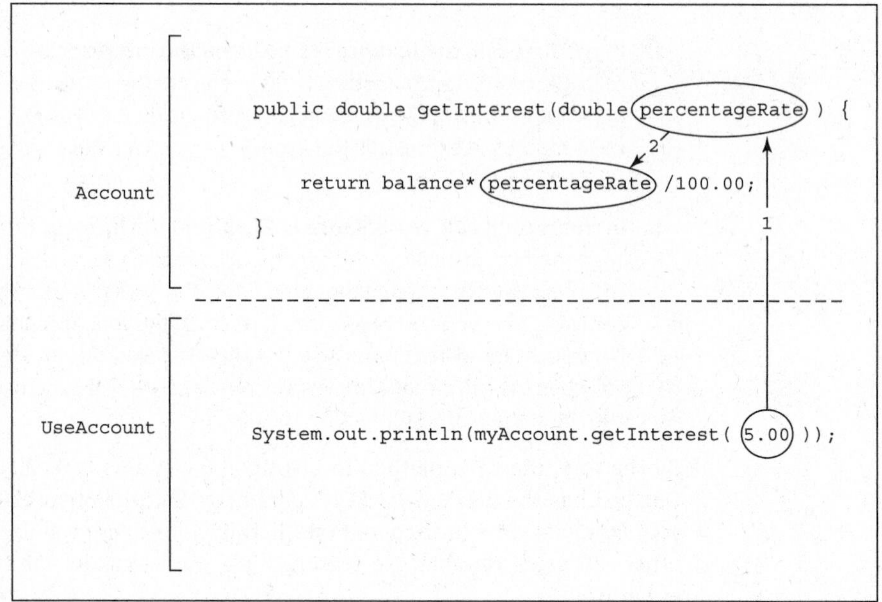

FIGURE 7-6: Passing a value to a method.

» **The word *double* tells Java that when the `getInterest` method is called, the `getInterest` method returns a double value back to the place that called it.** The statement in the `getInterest` method's body confirms this. The statement says `return balance * percentageRate / 100.00`, and the expression `balance * percentageRate / 100.00` has type `double`. (That's because all the things in the expression — `balance`, `percentageRate`, and `100.00` — have type `double`.)

When the `getInterest` method is called, the `return` statement calculates `balance * percentageRate / 100.00` and hands the calculation's result back to the code that called the method.

» **The word *getInterest* is the method's name.** That's the name you use to call the method when you're writing the code for the `UseAccount` class.

» **The parentheses contain all the things that you pass to the method when you call it.** When you call a method, you can pass information to that method on the fly. This information is the method's parameter list. The `getInterest` method's header says that the `getInterest` method takes one piece of information and that piece of information must be of type `double`:

```
public double getInterest(double  percentageRate)
```

Sure enough, if you look at the first call to `getInterest` (down in the `useAccount` class's main method), that call has the number `5.00` in it. And `5.00` is a `double` literal. When I call `getInterest`, I'm giving the method a value of type `double`.

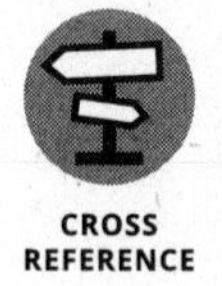
CROSS REFERENCE

If you don't remember what a literal is, see Chapter 4.

The same story holds true for the second call to `getInterest`. Down near the bottom of Listing 7-6, I call `getInterest` and feed the variable `yourInterestRate` to the method in its parameter list. Luckily for me, I declared `yourInterestRate` to be of type `double` just a few lines before that.

When you run the code in Listings 7-5 and 7-6, the flow of action isn't from top to bottom. The action goes from `main` to `getInterest`, and then back to `main`, and then back to `getInterest`, and, finally, back to `main` again. Figure 7-7 shows the whole business.

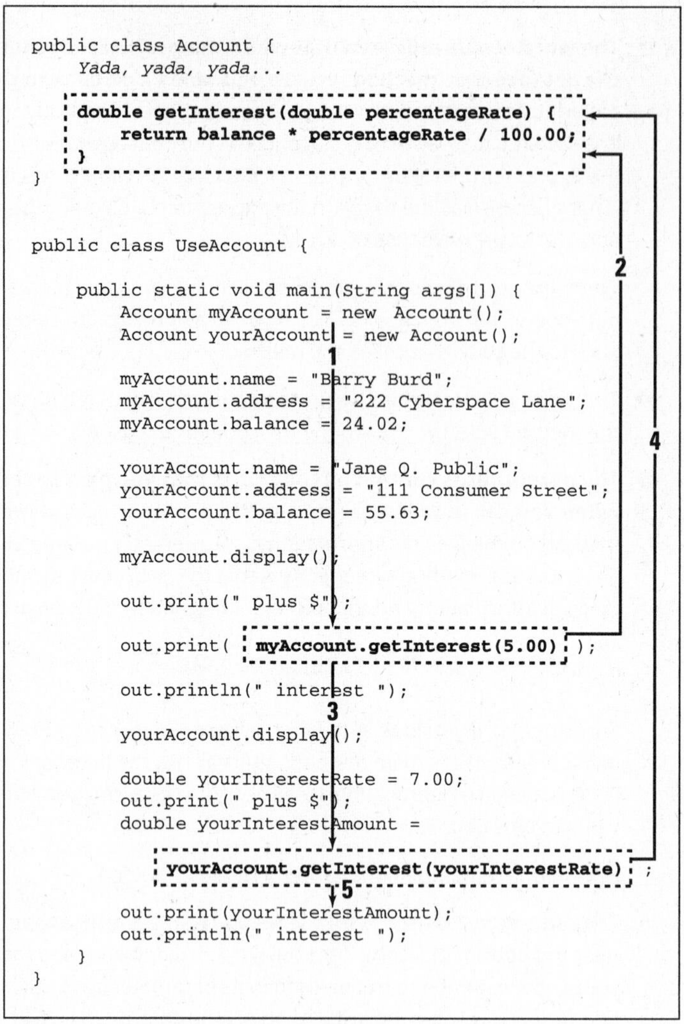

```
public class Account {
    Yada, yada, yada...

    double getInterest(double percentageRate) {
        return balance * percentageRate / 100.00;
    }
}


public class UseAccount {

    public static void main(String args[]) {
        Account myAccount = new  Account();
        Account yourAccount = new Account();

        myAccount.name = "Barry Burd";
        myAccount.address = "222 Cyberspace Lane";
        myAccount.balance = 24.02;

        yourAccount.name = "Jane Q. Public";
        yourAccount.address = "111 Consumer Street";
        yourAccount.balance = 55.63;

        myAccount.display();

        out.print(" plus $");

        out.print( myAccount.getInterest(5.00) );

        out.println(" interest ");

        yourAccount.display();

        double yourInterestRate = 7.00;
        out.print(" plus $");
        double yourInterestAmount =
            yourAccount.getInterest(yourInterestRate) ;
        out.print(yourInterestAmount);
        out.println(" interest ");
    }
}
```


FIGURE 7-7: The flow of control in Listings 7-5 and 7-6.

Returning a value from the getInterest method

When the `getInterest` method is called, the method executes the one statement that's in the method's body: a `return` statement. The `return` statement computes the value of `balance * percentageRate / 100.00`. If `balance` happens to be `24.02`, and `percentageRate` is `5.00`, the value of the expression is `1.201` — around $1.20. (Because the computer works exclusively with 0s and 1s, Java gets this number wrong by an ever-so-tiny amount. Java gets 1.2009999999999998. That's just something that humans have to live with.)

Anyway, after this value is calculated, Java executes the `return`, which sends the value back to the place in `main` where `getInterest` was called. At that point in the process, the entire method call — `myAccount.getInterest(5.00)` — takes on the value 1.2009999999999998. The call itself is inside a `println`:

```
out.println(myAccount.getInterest(5.00));
```

So the `println` ends up with the following meaning:

```
out.println(1.2009999999999998);
```

The whole process, in which a value is passed back to the method call, is illustrated in Figure 7-8.

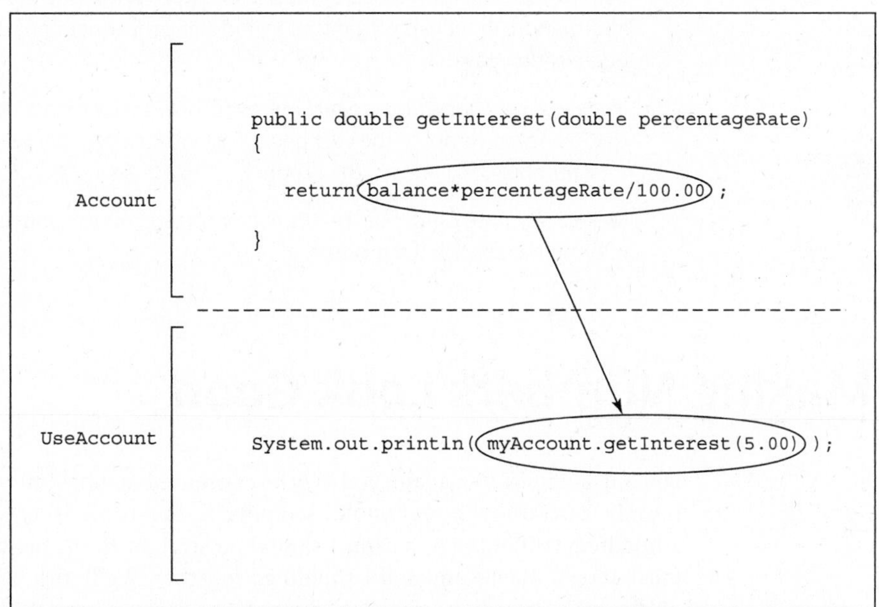

FIGURE 7-8: A method call is an expression with a value.

REMEMBER

If a method returns anything, a call to the method is an expression with a value. That value can be printed, assigned to a variable, added to something else, or whatever. Anything you can do with any other kind of value, you can do with a method call.

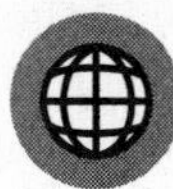

You might use the `Account` class in Listing 7-5 to solve a real problem. You'd call the `Account` class's `display` and `getInterest` methods in the course of an actual banking application. But the `UseAccount` class in Listing 7-6 is artificial. The `UseAccount` code creates some fake account data and then calls some `Account` class methods to convince you that the `Account` class's code works correctly. (You don't seriously think that a bank has depositors named "Jane Q. Public" and "Barry Burd," do you?) The `UseAccount` class in Listing 7-6 is a *test case* — a short-lived class whose sole purpose is to test another class's code. Like the code in Listing 7-6, each test case in this book is an ordinary class — a free-form class containing its own `main` method. Free-form classes are okay, but they're not optimal. Java developers have something better — a more disciplined way of writing test cases. The "better way" is called *JUnit*, and it's described on this book's website (`www.allmycode.com/JavaForDummies`).

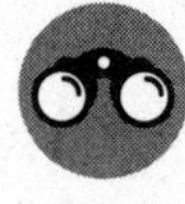

TRY IT OUT

- In previous sections, you create your own `Organization` class. Add a method to the class that computes the amount of tax the organization pays. A profit-making organization pays 10 percent of its revenue in tax, but a nonprofit organization pays only 2 percent of its revenue in tax.

  Make a separate class that creates two or three organizations and displays information about each organization, including the amount of tax the organization pays.

- In previous sections, you create your own `FoodProduct` class. Add methods to the class to compute the cost per 100 grams, the cost per serving, and the total number of calories in the product.

  Make a separate class that creates two or three products and displays information about each product.

Making Numbers Look Good

Looking at Figure 7-4 again, you may be concerned that the interest on my account is only $1.2009999999999998. Seemingly, the bank is cheating me out of 2 hundred-trillionths of a cent. I should go straight to the bank and demand my fair interest. Maybe you and I should go together. We'll kick up some fur at that old bank and bust this scam right open. If my guess is correct, this is part of a big salami scam. In a *salami scam*, someone shaves tiny amounts off millions of accounts. People don't notice their tiny little losses, but the person doing the shaving collects enough for a quick escape to Barbados (or for a whole truckload of salami).

Wait a minute! What about you? In Listing 7-6, you have `yourAccount`. And in Figure 7-4, your name is Jane Q. Public. Nothing is motivating you to come with me to the bank. Checking Figure 7-4 again, I see that you're way ahead of the game. According to my calculations, the program overpays you by 3 hundred-trillionths of a cent. Between the two of us, we're ahead by a hundred-trillionth of a cent. What gives?

Well, because computers use 0s (zeros) and 1s and don't have an infinite amount of space to do calculations, such inaccuracies as the ones shown in Figure 7-4 are normal. The quickest solution is to display the inaccurate numbers in a more sensible fashion. You can round the numbers and display only two digits beyond the decimal point, and some handy tools from Java's API (application programming interface) can help. Listing 7-7 shows the code, and Figure 7-9 displays the pleasant result.

LISTING 7-7: **Making Your Numbers Look Right**

```
import static java.lang.System.out;

public class UseAccount {

    public static void main(String args[]) {
        Account myAccount = new Account();
        Account yourAccount = new Account();

        myAccount.balance = 24.02;
        yourAccount.balance = 55.63;

        double myInterest = myAccount.getInterest(5.00);
        double yourInterest = yourAccount.getInterest(7.00);

        out.printf("$%4.2f\n", myInterest);
        out.printf("$%5.2f\n", myInterest);
        out.printf("$%.2f\n",  myInterest);
        out.printf("$%3.2f\n", myInterest);
        out.printf("$%.2f $%.2f", myInterest, yourInterest);
    }
}
```

FIGURE 7-9: Numbers that look like dollar amounts.

```
$1.20
$ 1.20
$1.20
$1.20
$1.20 $3.89
```

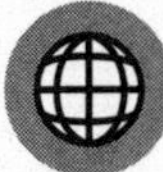

The inaccurate numbers in Figure 7-4 come from the computer's use of 0s and 1s. A mythical computer whose circuits were wired to use digits 0, 1, 2, 3, 4, 5, 6, 7, 8, and 9 wouldn't suffer from the same inaccuracies. So, to make things better, Java provides its own special way around the computer's inaccurate calculations. Java's API has a class named `BigDecimal` — a class that bypasses the computer's strange 0s and 1s and uses ordinary decimal digits to perform arithmetic calculations. For more information, visit this book's website (`www.allmycode.com/JavaForDummies`).

Listing 7-7 uses a handy method named `printf`. When you call `printf`, you always put at least two parameters inside the call's parentheses:

- **The first parameter is a *format string*.**

  The format string uses funny-looking codes to describe exactly how the other parameters are displayed.

- **All the other parameters (after the first) are values to be displayed.**

Look at the last `printf` call of Listing 7-7. The first parameter's format string has two placeholders for numbers. The first placeholder (`%.2f`) describes the display of `myInterest`. The second placeholder (another `%.2f`) describes the display of `yourInterest`. To find out exactly how these format strings work, see Figures 7-10 through 7-14.

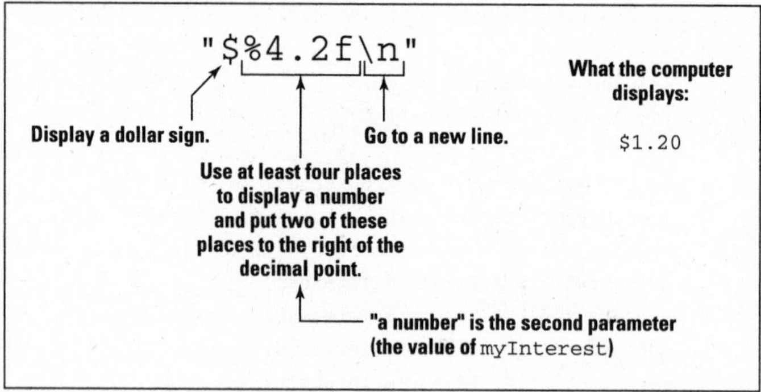

FIGURE 7-10: Using a format string.

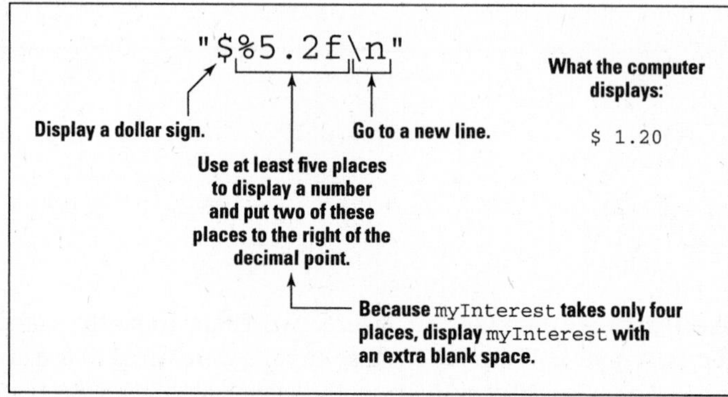

FIGURE 7-11: Adding extra places to display a value.

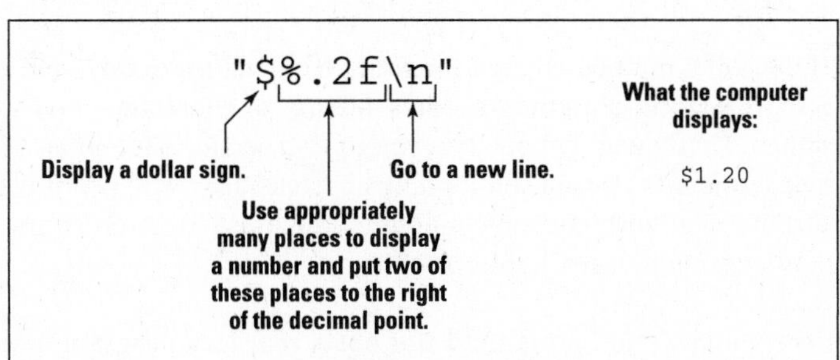

FIGURE 7-12: Displaying a value without specifying the exact number of places.

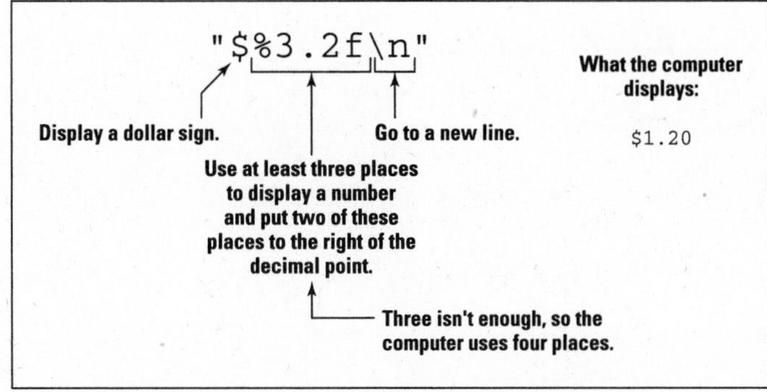

FIGURE 7-13: Specifying too few places to display a value.

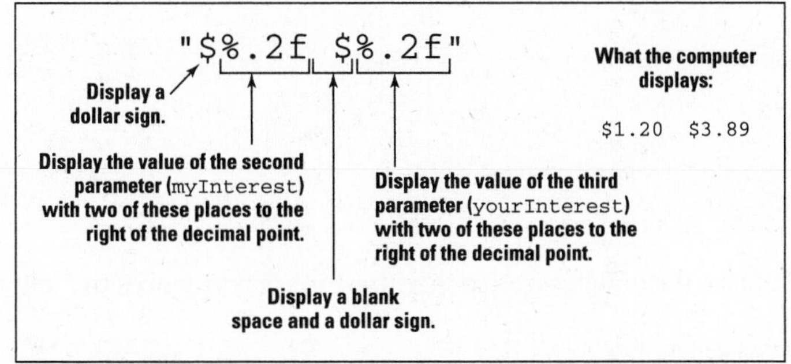

FIGURE 7-14: Displaying more than one value with a format string.

For more examples using the `printf` method and its format strings, see Chapters 8 and 9. For a complete list of options associated with the `printf` method's format string, see the `java.util.Formatter` page of Java's API documentation at `https://docs.oracle.com/javase/8/docs/api/java/util/Formatter.html`.

REMEMBER

The format string in a `printf` call doesn't change the way a number is stored internally for calculations. All the format string does is create a nice-looking bunch of digit characters that can be displayed on your screen.

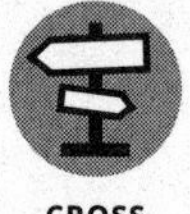

CROSS REFERENCE

The printf method is good for formatting values of any kind — ordinary numbers, hexadecimal numbers, dates, strings of characters, and some other strange values. That's why I show it to you in this section. But when you work with currency amounts, this section's printf tricks are fairly primitive. For some better ways to deal with currency amounts (such as the interest amounts in this section's example), see Chapter 11.

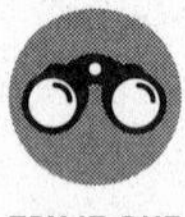

TRY IT OUT

Here's a Java "un-program." It's not a real Java program, because I've masked some of the characters in the code. I replaced these characters with underscores (_):

```
import static java.lang.System.out;

public class Main {

    public static void main(String[] args) {
        out.printf("%s%_%s", ">>", 7, "<<\n");
        out.printf("%s%___%s", ">>", 7, "<<\n");
        out.printf("%s%____%s", ">>", 7, "<<\n");
        out.printf("%s%____%s", ">>", 7, "<<\n");
        out.printf("%s%__%s", ">>", 7, "<<\n");
        out.printf("%s%__%s", ">>", -7, "<<\n");
        out.printf("%s%__%s", ">>", -7, "<<\n");
        out.printf("%s%_____%s", ">>", 7.0, "<<\n");
        out.printf("%s%_%s", ">>", "Hello", "<<\n");
        out.printf("%s%_%s", ">>", 'x', "<<\n");
        out.printf("%s%_%s", ">>", 'x', "<<\n");
    }
}
```

Replace the underscores so that this program produces the following output:

```
>>7<<
>>        7<<
>>7        <<
>>0000000007<<
>>+7<<
>>-7<<
>>(7)<<
>>   7.00000<<
>>HELLO<<
>>x<<
>>X<<
```

To do this, look for clues in the `java.util.Formatter` page of Java's API documentation at `https://docs.oracle.com/javase/8/docs/api/java/util/Formatter.html`.

Hiding Details with Accessor Methods

Put down this book and put on your hat. You've been such a loyal reader that I'm taking you out to lunch!

I have just one problem. I'm a bit short on cash. Would you mind if, on the way to lunch, we stopped at an automatic teller machine and picked up a few bucks? Also, we have to use your account. My account is a little low.

Fortunately, the teller machine is easy to use. Just step right up and enter your PIN. After you enter your PIN, the machine asks which of several variable names you want to use for your current balance. You have a choice of `balance324`, `myBal`, `currentBalance`, `b$`, `BALANCE`, `asj999`, or `conStanTinople`. Having selected a variable name, you're ready to select a memory location for the variable's value. You can select any number between 022FFF and 0555AA. (Those numbers are in hexadecimal format.) After you configure the teller machine's software, you can easily get your cash. You did bring a screwdriver, didn't you?

Good programming

When it comes to good computer programming practice, one word stands out above all others: *simplicity.* When you're writing complicated code, the last thing you want is to deal with somebody else's misnamed variables, convoluted solutions to problems, or clever, last-minute kludges. You want a clean interface that makes you solve your own problems and no one else's.

In the automatic teller machine scenario that I describe earlier, the big problem is that the machine's design forces you to worry about other people's concerns. When you should be thinking about getting money for lunch, you're thinking instead about variables and storage locations. Sure, someone has to work out the teller machine's engineering problems, but the banking customer isn't the person.

REMEMBER

This section is about safety, not security. Safe code keeps you from making accidental programming errors. Secure code (a completely different story) keeps malicious hackers from doing intentional damage.

So, everything connected with every aspect of a computer program has to be simple, right? Well, no. That's not right. Sometimes, to make things simple in the long run, you have to do lots of preparatory work up front. The people who built the automated teller machine worked hard to make sure that the machine is consumer-proof. The machine's interface, with its screen messages and buttons, makes the machine a very complicated, but carefully designed, device.

The point is that making things look simple takes some planning. In the case of object-oriented programming, one of the ways to make things look simple is to prevent code outside a class from directly using fields defined inside the class. Take a peek at the code in Listing 7-1. You're working at a company that has just spent $10 million for the code in the `Account` class. (That's more than a million-and-a-half per line!) Now your job is to write the `UseAccount` class. You would like to write

```
myAccount.name = "Barry Burd";
```

but doing so would be getting you too far inside the guts of the `Account` class. After all, people who use an automatic teller machine aren't allowed to program the machine's variables. They can't use the machine's keypad to type the statement

```
balanceOnAccount29872865457 = balanceOnAccount29872865457 + 1000000.00;
```

Instead, they push buttons that do the job in an orderly manner. That's how a programmer achieves safety and simplicity.

To keep things nice and orderly, you need to change the `Account` class from Listing 7-1 by outlawing such statements as the following:

```
myAccount.name = "Barry Burd";
```

and

```
out.print(yourAccount.balance);
```

Of course, this poses a problem. You're the person who's writing the code for the `UseAccount` class. If you can't write `myAccount.name` or `yourAccount.balance`, how will you accomplish anything at all? The answer lies in things called *accessor methods.* Listings 7-8 and 7-9 demonstrate these methods.

LISTING 7-8: Hide Those Fields

```
public class Account {
    private String name;
    private String address;
    private double balance;

    public void setName(String n) {
        name = n;
    }

    public String getName() {
        return name;
    }

    public void setAddress(String a) {
        address = a;
    }

    public String getAddress() {
        return address;
    }

    public void setBalance(double b) {
        balance = b;
    }

    public double getBalance() {
        return balance;
    }
}
```

LISTING 7-9: Calling Accessor Methods

```
import static java.lang.System.out;

public class UseAccount {

    public static void main(String args[]) {
        Account myAccount = new Account();
        Account yourAccount = new Account();

        myAccount.setName("Barry Burd");
        myAccount.setAddress("222 Cyberspace Lane");
        myAccount.setBalance(24.02);
```

(continued)

LISTING 7-9: *(continued)*

```
        yourAccount.setName("Jane Q. Public");
        yourAccount.setAddress("111 Consumer Street");
        yourAccount.setBalance(55.63);

        out.print(myAccount.getName());
        out.print(" (");
        out.print(myAccount.getAddress());
        out.print(") has $");
        out.print(myAccount.getBalance());
        out.println();

        out.print(yourAccount.getName());
        out.print(" (");
        out.print(yourAccount.getAddress());
        out.print(") has $");
        out.print(yourAccount.getBalance());
    }
}
```

A run of the code in Listings 7-8 and 7-9 looks no different from a run of Listings 7-1 and 7-2. Either program's run is shown earlier, in Figure 7-3. The big difference is that in Listing 7-8, the `Account` class enforces the carefully controlled use of its `name`, `address`, and `balance` fields.

Public lives and private dreams: Making a field inaccessible

Notice the addition of the word *private* in front of each of the `Account` class's field declarations. The word *private* is a Java keyword. When a field is declared private, no code outside of the class can make direct reference to that field. So if you put `myAccount.name = "Barry Burd"` in the `UseAccount` class of Listing 7-9, you get an error message such as `name has private access in Account`.

Instead of referencing `myAccount.name`, the `UseAccount` programmer must call method `myAccount.setName` or method `myAccount.getName`. These methods, `setName` and `getName`, are called *accessor* methods because they provide access to the `Account` class's `name` field. (Actually, the term *accessor method* isn't formally a part of the Java programming language. It's just the term that people use for methods that do this sort of thing.) To zoom in even more, `setName` is called a *setter* method, and `getName` is called a *getter* method. (I bet you won't forget that terminology!)

TIP

With many IDEs, you don't have to type your own accessor methods. First, you type a field declaration like `private String name`. Then, in your IDE's menu bar, you choose Source ⇨ Generate Getters and Setters, or choose Code ⇨ Insert Code ⇨ Setter or some mix of those commands. After you make all your choices, the IDE creates accessor methods and adds them to your code.

Notice that all the setter and getter methods in Listing 7-8 are declared to be public. This ensures that anyone from anywhere can call these two methods. The idea here is that manipulating the actual fields from outside the `Account` code is impossible, but you can easily reach the approved setter and getter methods for using those fields.

Think again about the automatic teller machine. Someone using the ATM can't type a command that directly changes the value in his or her account's `balance` field, but the procedure for depositing a million-dollar check is easy to follow. The people who build the teller machines know that if the check-depositing procedure is complicated, plenty of customers will mess it up royally. So that's the story — make impossible anything that people shouldn't do and make sure that the tasks people should be doing are easy.

TIP

Nothing about having setter and getter methods is sacred. You don't have to write any setter and getter methods that you're not going to use. For instance, in Listing 7-8, I can omit the declaration of method `getAddress`, and everything still works. The only problem if I do this is that anyone else who wants to use my `Account` class and retrieve the address of an existing account is up a creek.

TIP

When you create a method to set the value in a `balance` field, you don't have to name your method `setBalance`. You can name it `tunaFish` or whatever you like. The trouble is that the `set`*`Fieldname`* convention (with lowercase letters in `set` and an uppercase letter to start the *`Fieldname`* part) is an established stylistic convention in the world of Java programming. If you don't follow the convention, you confuse the kumquats out of other Java programmers. If your integrated development environment has drag-and-drop GUI design capability, you may temporarily lose that capability. (For a word about drag-and-drop GUI design, see Chapters 2 and 16.)

REMEMBER

When you call a setter method, you feed it a value of the type that's being set. That's why, in Listing 7-9, you call `yourAccount.setBalance(55.63)` with a parameter of type `double`. In contrast, when you call a getter method, you usually don't feed any values to the method. That's why, in Listing 7-9, you call `yourAccount.getBalance()` with an empty parameter list. Occasionally, you may want to get and set a value with a single statement. To add a dollar to your account's existing balance, you write `yourAccount.setBalance(yourAccount.getBalance() + 1.00)`.

Enforcing rules with accessor methods

Go back to Listing 7-8 and take a quick look at the setName method. Imagine putting the method's assignment statement inside an if statement.

```
public void setName(String n) {
    if (!n.equals("")) {
        name = n;
    }
}
```

Now, if the programmer in charge of the UseAccount class writes myAccount.setName(""), the call to setName doesn't have any effect. Furthermore, because the name field is private, the following statement is illegal in the UseAccount class:

```
myAccount.name = "";
```

Of course, a call such as myAccount.setName("Joe Schmoe") still works because "Joe Schmoe" doesn't equal the empty string "".

That's cool. With a private field and an accessor method, you can prevent someone from assigning the empty string to an account's name field. With more elaborate if statements, you can enforce any rules you want.

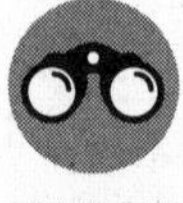
TRY IT OUT

In previous sections, you create your own Organization and FoodProduct classes. In those classes, replace the default access fields with private fields. Create getter and setter methods for those fields. In the setter methods, add code to ensure that the String values aren't empty and that numeric values aren't negative.

Barry's Own GUI Class

You may be getting tired of the bland, text-based programs that litter this book's pages. You may want something a bit flashier — something with text fields and buttons. Well, I've got some examples for you!

I've created a class that I call DummiesFrame. When you import my DummiesFrame class, you can create a simple graphical user interface (GUI) application with very little effort.

Listing 7-10 uses my DummiesFrame class, and Figures 7-15 to 7-17 show you the results.

LISTING 7-10: **Your First DummiesFrame Example**

```
import com.allmycode.dummiesframe.DummiesFrame;

public class GuessingGame {

    public static void main(String[] args) {
        DummiesFrame frame = new DummiesFrame("Greet Me!");
        frame.addRow("Your first name");
        frame.go();
    }

    public static String calculate(String firstName) {
        return "Hello, " + firstName + "!";
    }
}
```

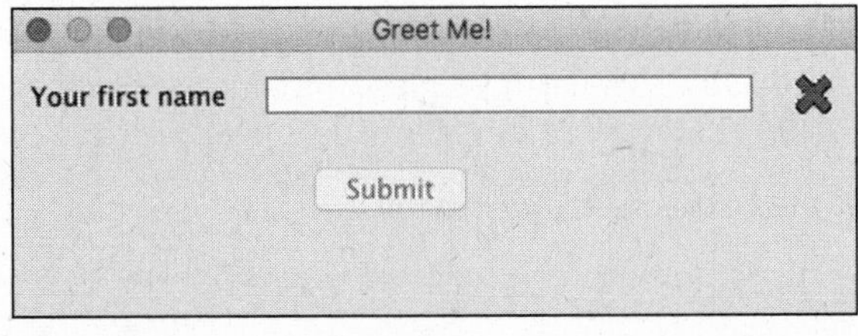

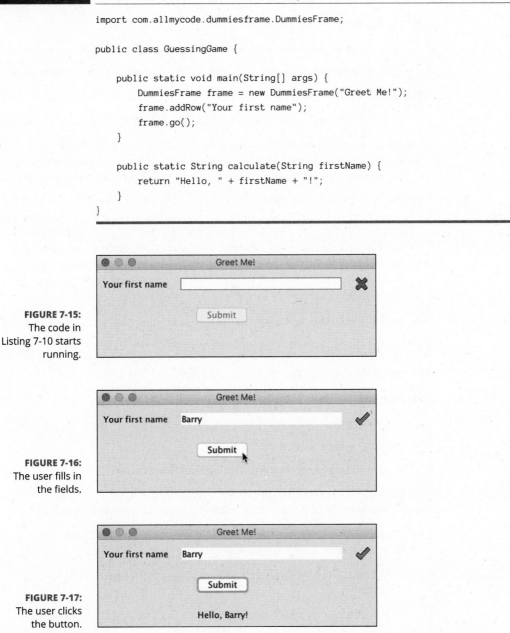

FIGURE 7-15: The code in Listing 7-10 starts running.

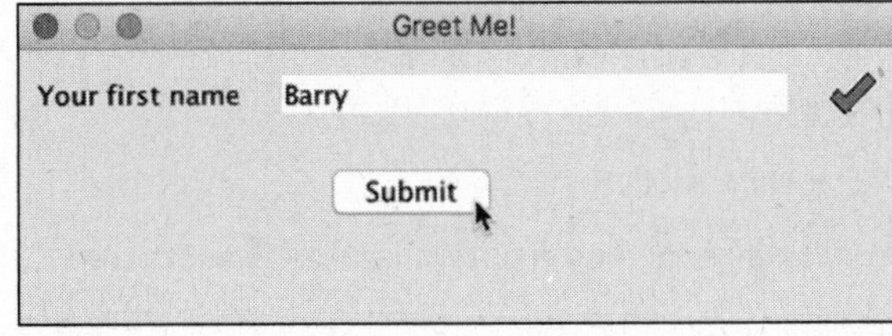

FIGURE 7-16: The user fills in the fields.

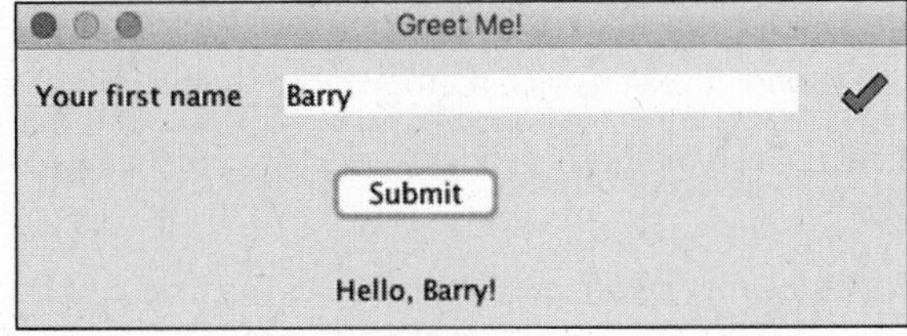

FIGURE 7-17: The user clicks the button.

Here's a blow-by-blow description of the lines in Listing 7-10:

- The first line

  ```
  import com.allmycode.dummiesframe.DummiesFrame;
  ```

  makes the name `DummiesFrame` available to the rest of the code in the listing.

- Inside the `main` method, the statement

  ```
  DummiesFrame frame = new DummiesFrame("Greet Me!");
  ```

  creates an instance of my `DummiesFrame` class and makes the variable name `frame` refer to that instance. A `DummiesFrame` object appears as a window on the user's screen. In this example, the text on the window's title bar is *Greet Me!*

- The next statement is a call to the `frame` object's `addRow` method:

  ```
  frame.addRow("Your first name");
  ```

  This call puts a row on the face of the application's window. The row consists of a label (whose text is *Your first name*), an empty text field, and a red X mark indicating that the user hasn't yet typed anything useful into the field. (Refer to Figure 7-15.)

- A call to the `frame` object's `go` method

  ```
  frame.go();
  ```

  makes the app's window appear on the screen.

- The header of the `calculate` method

  ```
  public static String calculate(String firstName) {
  ```

  tells Java two important things:

  - The `calculate` method returns a value of type `String`.
  - Java should expect the user to type a `String` value in the text field, and whatever the user types will become the `firstName` parameter's value.

  To use my `DummiesFrame` class, your code must have a method named `calculate`, and the `calculate` method must obey certain rules:

  - The `calculate` method's header must start with the words `public static`.
  - The method may return any Java type: `String`, `int`, `double`, or whatever. (That's actually not a rule; it's an opportunity!)
  - The `calculate` method must have the same number of parameters as there are rows in the application's window.

Listing 7-10 has only one addRow method call, so the window in Figure 7-10 has only one row (not including the *Submit* button), and so the `calculate` method has only one parameter.

When the user starts typing text into the window's text field, the red X mark turns into a green check mark. (Refer to Figure 7-16.) The green check mark indicates that the user has typed a value of the expected type (in this example, a `String` value) into the text field.

» When the user clicks the button, Java executes the `calculate` method. The expression in the method's `return` statement

```
return "Hello, " + firstName + "!";
```

tells Java what to display at the bottom of the window. (Refer to Figure 7-17.) In this example, the user types *Barry* in the one and only text field, so the value of `firstName` is `"Barry"`, and the calculate method returns the string `"Hello, Barry!"` (Ah! The perks of being a *For Dummies* author!)

Using my `DummiesFrame` class, you can build a simple GUI application with only ten lines of code.

REMEMBER

The `DummiesFrame` class isn't built into the Java API so, in order to run the code in Listing 7-10, my `DummiesFrame.java` file must be part of your project. When you download the code from this book's website (`www.allmycode.com/JavaForDummies`), you get a folder named `07-10` containing both the Listing 7-10 code and my `DummiesFrame.java` code. But if you create your own project containing the Listing 7-10, you have to add my `DummiesFrame.java` file manually. The way you do this depends on which IDE you use. One way or another, my `DummiesFrame` class is in a package named `com.allmycode.dummiesframe`, so the `DummiesFrame.java` file must be in a directory named `dummiesframe`, which is inside another directory named `allmycode`, which is inside yet another directory named `com`. For more about packages, see Chapters 9 and 14.

TECHNICAL STUFF

To keep things simple, I include the `DummiesFrame.java` file in the `07-10` folder that you download from this book's website. But, really, is that the best way to add my own code to your project? In Chapter 1, I describe files with the `.class` extension, and the role that those files play in the running of a Java program. Instead of handing you my `DummiesFrame.java` file, I should be putting only a `DummiesFrame.class` file in the download. And, on some other occasion, if I have to give you hundreds of `.class` files, I should bundle them all into one big archive file. Java has a name for a big file that encodes many smaller `.class` files. It's called a JAR file and it has the `.jar` extension. In a real-life application, if you're preparing your code for other people to use as part of their own applications, a JAR file is definitely the way to go.

My `DummiesFrame` class isn't exclusively for greetings and salutations. Listing 7-11 uses `DummiesFrame` to do arithmetic.

LISTING 7-11: A Really Simple Calculator

```
import com.allmycode.dummiesframe.DummiesFrame;

public class Addition {

    public static void main(String[] args) {
        DummiesFrame frame = new DummiesFrame("Adding Machine");
        frame.addRow("First number");
        frame.addRow("Second number");
        frame.setButtonText("Sum");
        frame.go();
    }

    public static int calculate(int firstNumber, int secondNumber) {
        return firstNumber + secondNumber;
    }
}
```

The window in Figure 7-18 has two rows because Listing 7-11 has two `addRow` calls and the listing's `calculate` method has two parameters. In addition, Listing 7-11 calls the `frame` object's `setButtonText` method. So, in Figure 7-18, the text on the face of the button isn't the default word *Submit.*

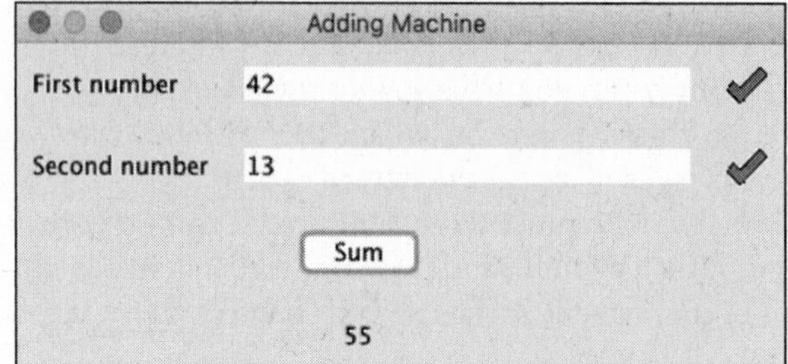

FIGURE 7-18: Look! The code in Listing 7-11 actually works!

Listing 7-12 contains a GUI version of the Guessing Game application from Chapter 5, and Figure 7-19 shows the game in action.

LISTING 7-12: I'm Thinking of a Number

```
import java.util.Random;
import com.allmycode.dummiesframe.DummiesFrame;

public class GuessingGame {
```

```
    public static void main(String[] args) {
        DummiesFrame frame = new DummiesFrame("Guessing Game");
        frame.addRow("Enter an int from 1 to 10");
        frame.setButtonText("Submit your guess");
        frame.go();
    }

    public static String calculate(int inputNumber) {
        Random random = new Random();
        int randomNumber = random.nextInt(10) + 1;

        if (inputNumber == randomNumber) {
            return "You win.";
        } else {
            return "You lose. The random number was " + randomNumber + ".";
        }
    }
}
```

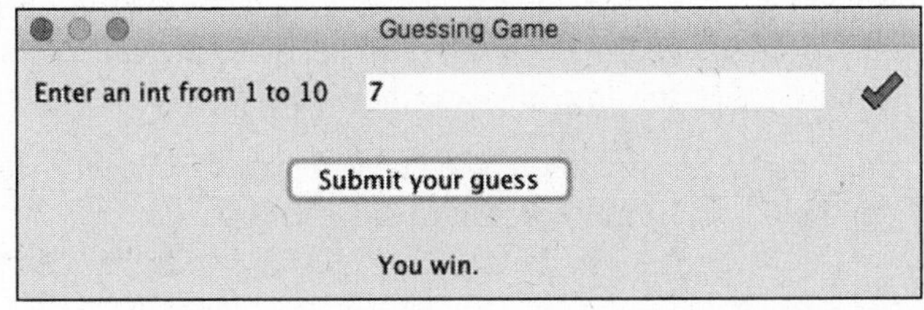

FIGURE 7-19: I win!

In Listing 7-13, I use this chapter's `Account` class alongside the `DummiesFrame` class. I could get the same results without creating an `Account` instance, but I want to show you how classes can cooperate to form a complete program. A run of the code is in Figure 7-20.

LISTING 7-13: Using the Account Class

```
import com.allmycode.dummiesframe.DummiesFrame;

public class UseAccount {

    public static void main(String args[]) {
        DummiesFrame frame = new DummiesFrame("Display an Account");
        frame.addRow("Full name");
        frame.addRow("Address");
        frame.addRow("Balance");
        frame.setButtonText("Display");
```

(continued)

LISTING 7-13: *(continued)*

```
        frame.go();
    }

    public static String calculate(String name, String address,
                                              double balance) {
        Account myAccount = new Account();

        myAccount.setName(name);
        myAccount.setAddress(address);
        myAccount.setBalance(balance);
        return myAccount.getName() + " (" + myAccount.getAddress() +
                ") has $" + myAccount.getBalance();
    }
}
```

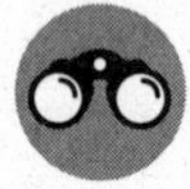

TRY IT OUT

Use the `DummiesFrame` class to create two GUI programs.

- A window has text fields for an organization's name, annual revenue, and status (profit-making or not profit-making). When the user clicks a button, the window displays the amount of tax the organization pays.

  A profit-making organization pays 10 percent of its revenue in tax; a nonprofit organization pays 2 percent of its revenue in tax.

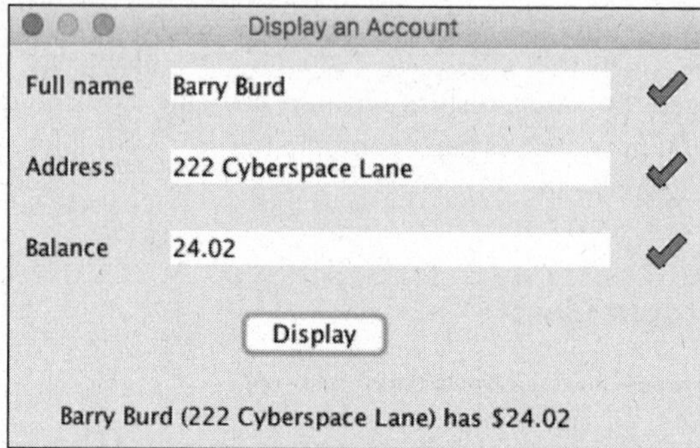

FIGURE 7-20: I'm rich.

- A window has text fields for a product's type of food, weight, cost, number of servings, and number of calories per serving. When the user clicks a button, the window displays the cost per 100 grams, the cost per serving, and the total number of calories in the product.

IN THIS CHAPTER

» Adding new life to old code

» Tweaking your code

» Making changes without spending a fortune

Chapter 8
Saving Time and Money: Reusing Existing Code

Once upon a time, there was a beautiful princess. When the princess turned 25 (the optimal age for strength, good looks, and fine moral character), her kind, old father brought her a gift in a lovely golden box. Anxious to know what was in the box, the princess ripped off the golden wrapping paper.

When the box was finally opened, the princess was thrilled. To her surprise, her father had given her what she had always wanted: a computer program that always ran correctly. The program did everything the princess wanted, and did it all exactly the way she wanted it to be done. The princess was happy, and so was her father.

Even as time marched on, the computer program never failed. For years on end, the princess changed her needs, expected more out of life, made increasing demands, expanded her career, reached for more and more fulfillment, juggled the desires of her husband and her kids, stretched the budget, and sought peace within her soul. Through all of this, the program remained her steady, faithful companion.

As the princess grew old, the program became old along with her. One evening, as she sat by the fireside, she posed a daunting question to the program: "How do you do it?" she asked. "How do you manage to keep giving the right answers, time after time, year after year?"

"Clean living," replied the program. "I swim 20 apps each day, I take C++ to Word off viruses, I avoid hogarithmic algorithms, I link Java in moderation, I say GNU to bugs, I don't smoke to back up, and I never byte off more than I can queue."

Needless to say, the princess was stunned.

Defining a Class (What It Means to Be an Employee)

Wouldn't it be nice if every piece of software did just what you wanted it to do? In an ideal world, you could buy a program, make it work right away, plug it seamlessly into new situations, and update it easily whenever your needs change. Unfortunately, software of this kind doesn't exist. (*Nothing* of this kind exists.) The truth is that no matter what you want to do, you can find software that does some of it, but not all of it.

This is one of the reasons why object-oriented programming has been successful. For years, companies were buying prewritten code, only to discover that the code didn't do what they wanted it to do. So, what did the companies do about it? They started messing with the code. Their programmers dug deep into the program files, changed variable names, moved subprograms around, reworked formulas, and generally made the code worse. The reality was that if a program didn't already do what you wanted it to do (even if it did something ever so close to what you wanted), you could never improve the situation by mucking around inside the code. The best option was always to chuck the whole program (expensive as that was) and start all over again. What a sad state of affairs!

With object-oriented programming, a big change has come about. At its heart, an object-oriented program is made to be modified. With correctly written software, you can take advantage of features that are already built-in, add new features of your own, and override features that don't suit your needs. And the best part is that the changes you make are clean. No clawing and digging into other people's brittle program code. Instead, you make nice, orderly additions and modifications without touching the existing code's internal logic. It's the ideal solution.

The last word on employees

When you write an object-oriented program, you start by thinking about the data. You're writing about accounts. So what's an account? You're writing code to handle button clicks. So what's a button? You're writing a program to send payroll checks to employees. What's an employee?

In this chapter's first example, an employee is someone with a name and a job title. Sure, employees have other characteristics, but for now I stick to the basics. The code in Listing 8-1 defines what it means to be an employee.

LISTING 8-1: What Is an Employee?

```
import static java.lang.System.out;

public class Employee {
    private String name;
    private String jobTitle;

    public void setName(String nameIn) {
        name = nameIn;
    }

    public String getName() {
        return name;
    }

    public void setJobTitle(String jobTitleIn) {
        jobTitle = jobTitleIn;
    }

    public String getJobTitle() {
        return jobTitle;
    }

    public void cutCheck(double amountPaid) {
        out.printf("Pay to the order of %s ", name);
        out.printf("(%s) ***$", jobTitle);
        out.printf("%,.2f\n", amountPaid);
    }
}
```

According to Listing 8-1, each employee has seven features. Two of these features are fairly simple: Each employee has a name and a job title. (In Listing 8-1, the `Employee` class has a `name` field and a `jobTitle` field.)

And what else does an employee have? Each employee has four methods to handle the values of the employee's name and job title. These methods are `setName`, `getName`, `setJobTitle`, and `getJobTitle`. I explain methods like these (*accessor* methods) in Chapter 7.

On top of all of that, each employee has a cutCheck method. The idea is that the method that writes payroll checks has to belong to one class or another. Because most of the information in the payroll check is customized for a particular employee, you may as well put the cutCheck method inside the Employee class.

For details about the printf calls in the cutCheck method, see the section "Cutting a check," later in this chapter.

Putting your class to good use

The Employee class in Listing 8-1 has no main method, so there's no starting point for executing code. To fix this deficiency, the programmer writes a separate program with a main method and uses that program to create Employee instances. Listing 8-2 shows a class with a main method — one that puts the code in Listing 8-1 to the test.

LISTING 8-2: Writing Payroll Checks

```
import java.util.Scanner;
import java.io.File;
import java.io.IOException;

public class DoPayroll {

    public static void main(String args[]) throws IOException {
        Scanner diskScanner = new Scanner(new File("EmployeeInfo.txt"));

        for (int empNum = 1; empNum <= 3; empNum++) {
            payOneEmployee(diskScanner);
        }
        diskScanner.close();
    }

    static void payOneEmployee(Scanner aScanner) {
        Employee anEmployee = new Employee();

        anEmployee.setName(aScanner.nextLine());
        anEmployee.setJobTitle(aScanner.nextLine());
        anEmployee.cutCheck(aScanner.nextDouble());
        aScanner.nextLine();
    }
}
```

WHERE ON EARTH DO YOU LIVE?

Grouping separators vary from one country to another. This makes a big difference when you try to read `double` values using Java's `Scanner` class. To see what I mean, have a serious look at the following JShell session.

```
jshell> import java.util.Scanner

jshell> import java.util.Locale

jshell> Scanner keyboard = new Scanner(System.in)
keyboard ==> java.util.Scanner[delimiters=\p{javaWhitespace}+] ... \E]
    [infinity string=\Q8\E]

jshell> keyboard.nextDouble()
1000.00
$4 ==> 1000.0

jshell> Locale.setDefault(Locale.FRANCE)

jshell> keyboard = new Scanner(System.in)
keyboard ==> java.util.Scanner[delimiters=\p{javaWhitespace}+] ... \E]
    [infinity string=\Q8\E]

jshell> keyboard.nextDouble()
1000,00
$7 ==> 1000.0

jshell> keyboard.nextDouble()
1000.00
|  java.util.InputMismatchException thrown:
|        at Scanner.throwFor (Scanner.java:860)
|        at Scanner.next (Scanner.java:1497)
|        at Scanner.nextDouble (Scanner.java:2467)
|        at (#8:1)

jshell>
```

I conducted this session on a computer in the United States. The country of origin is relevant because, in response to the first `keyboard.nextDouble()` call, I type `1000.00` (with a period before the last two zeros) and Java accepts this as meaning "one thousand."

But then, in the JShell session, I call `Locale.setDefault(Locale.FRANCE)`, which tells Java to behave as if my computer is in France. When I create another `Scanner` instance

(continued)

(continued)

and call `keyboard.nextDouble()` again, Java accepts `1000,00` (with a comma before the last two zeros) as an expression meaning *mille* (French for "one thousand"). What's more, Java no longer accepts the period in `1000.00`. When I type `1000.00` (with a period) I get an `InputMismatchException`.

By default, your computer's `Scanner` instance wants you to input `double` numbers the way you normally type them in your country. If you type numbers according to another country's convention, you get an `InputMismatchException`. So, when you run the code in Listing 8-2, the numbers in your `EmployeeInfo.txt` file must use your country's format.

This brings me to the running of the code in Listing 8-2. The `EmployeeInfo.txt` file that you download from this book's website starts with the following three lines:

Barry Burd

CEO

5000.00

That last number `5000.00` has a period in it, so if your country prefers a comma in place of my United States period, you get an `InputMismatchException`. In response to this, you have two choices:

- In the downloaded `EmployeeInfo.txt` file, change the periods to commas.
- In the code of Listing 8-2, add the statement `Locale.setDefault(Locale.US)` before the `diskScanner` declaration.

And finally, if you want your output to look like your own country's numbers, you can do it with Java's `Formatter` class. Add something like this to your code:

```
out.print(
    new java.util.Formatter().format(java.util.Locale.FRANCE, "%,.2f", 1000.00));
```

For all the details, see the API (Application Programming Interface) documentation for Java's `Formatter` class (`https://docs.oracle.com/javase/8/docs/api/java/util/Formatter.html` and `Locale` class (`https://docs.oracle.com/javase/8/docs/api/java/util/Locale.html`).

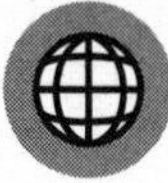

To run the code in Listing 8-2, your hard drive must contain a file named `EmployeeInfo.txt`. Fortunately, the stuff that you download from this book's website (`www.allmycode.com/JavaForDummies`) comes with an `EmployeeInfo.txt` file. You can import the downloaded material into any of the three most popular Java IDEs (Eclipse, NetBeans, or IntelliJ IDEA). If you import into Eclipse, you get a project named `08-01`. That project typically lives on your hard drive in a folder named `/Users/`*`your-user-name`*`/workspace/08-01`. Directly inside that folder, you have a file named `EmployeeInfo.txt`.

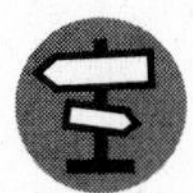

CROSS REFERENCE

For more words of wisdom about files on your hard drive, see the "Working with Disk Files (a Brief Detour)" section in this chapter.

The `DoPayroll` class in Listing 8-2 has two methods. One of the methods, `main`, calls the other method, `payOneEmployee`, three times. Each time around, the `payOneEmployee` method gets stuff from the `EmployeeInfo.txt` file and feeds this stuff to the `Employee` class's methods.

Here's how the variable name *anEmployee* is reused and recycled:

- » The first time that `payOneEmployee` is called, the statement `anEmployee = new Employee()` makes `anEmployee` refer to a new object.
- » The second time that `payOneEmployee` is called, the computer executes the same statement again. This second execution creates a new incarnation of the `anEmployee` variable that refers to a brand-new object.
- » The third time around, all the same stuff happens again. A new `anEmployee` variable ends up referring to a third object.

The whole story is pictured in Figure 8-1.

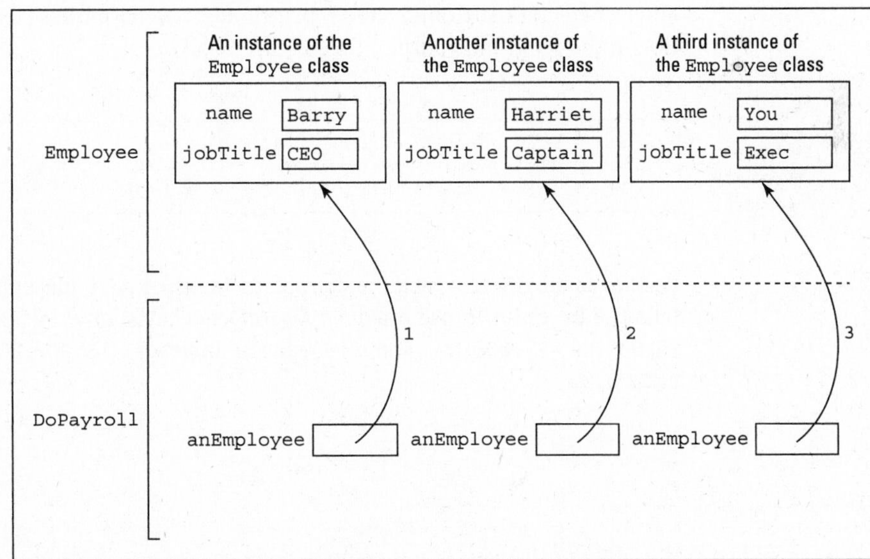

FIGURE 8-1: Three calls to the `payOneEmployee` method.

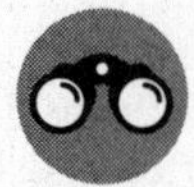

TRY IT OUT

There are always interesting things for you to try:

- A `PlaceToLive` has an address, a number of bedrooms, and an area (in square feet or square meters). Write the `PlaceToLive` class's code. Write code for a separate class named `DisplayThePlaces`. Your `DisplayThePlaces` class creates a few `PlaceToLive` instances by assigning values to their `address`, `numberOfBedrooms`, and `area` fields. The `DisplayThePlaces` class also reads (from the keyboard) the cost of living in each place. For each place, your code displays the cost per square foot (or square meter) and the cost per bedroom.
- Use your new `PlaceToLive` class and my `DummiesFrame` class (from Chapter 7) to create a GUI application. The GUI application takes information about a place to live and displays the place's cost per square foot (or meter) and the cost per bedroom.

Cutting a check

Listing 8-1 has three `printf` calls. Each `printf` call has a format string (like `"(%s) ***$"`) and a variable (like `jobTitle`). Each format string has a placeholder (like `%s`) that determines where and how the variable's value is displayed.

For example, in the second `printf` call, the format string has a `%s` placeholder. This `%s` holds a place for the `jobTitle` variable's value. According to Java's rules, the notation `%s` always holds a place for a string and, sure enough, the variable `jobTitle` is declared to be of type `String` in Listing 8-1. Parentheses and some other characters surround the `%s` placeholder, so parentheses surround each job title in the program's output. (See Figure 8-2.)

```
Pay to the order of Barry Burd (CEO) ***$5,000.00
Pay to the order of Harriet Ritter (Captain) ***$7,000.00
Pay to the order of Your Name Here (Honorary Exec of the Day) ***$10,000.00
```

FIGURE 8-2: Everybody gets paid.

Back in Listing 8-1, notice the comma inside the `%,.2f` placeholder. The comma tells the program to use *grouping separators*. That's why, in Figure 8-2, you see `$5,000.00`, `$7,000.00`, and `$10,000.00` instead of `$5000.00`, `$7000.00`, and `$10000.00`.

Working with Disk Files (a Brief Detour)

In previous chapters, programs read characters from the computer's keyboard. But the code in Listing 8-2 reads characters from a specific file. The file (named `EmployeeInfo.txt`) lives on your computer's hard drive.

This `EmployeeInfo.txt` file is like a word processing document. The file can contain letters, digits, and other characters. But unlike a word processing document, the `EmployeeInfo.txt` file contains no formatting — no italics, no bold, no font sizes, nothing of that kind.

The `EmployeeInfo.txt` file contains only ordinary characters — the kinds of keystrokes that you type while you play a guessing game from Chapters 5 and 6. Of course, getting guesses from a user's keyboard and reading employee data from a disk file aren't exactly the same. In a guessing game, the program displays prompts, such as `Enter an int from 1 to 10`. The game program conducts a back-and-forth dialogue with the person sitting at the keyboard. In contrast, Listing 8-2 has no dialogue. This `DoPayroll` program reads characters from a hard drive and doesn't prompt or interact with anyone.

Most of this chapter is about code reuse. But Listing 8-2 stumbles upon an important idea — an idea that's not directly related to code reuse. Unlike the examples in previous chapters, Listing 8-2 reads data from a stored disk file. So, in the following sections, I take a short side trip to explore disk files.

Storing data in a file

The code in Listing 8-2 doesn't run unless you have some employee data sitting in a file. Listing 8-2 says that this file is `EmployeeInfo.txt`. So, before running the code of Listing 8-2, I created a small `EmployeeInfo.txt` file. The file is shown in Figure 8-3; refer to Figure 8-2 for the resulting output.

```
Barry Burd
CEO
5000.00
Harriet Ritter
Captain
7000.00
Your Name Here
Honorary Exec of the Day
10000.00
```

FIGURE 8-3: An `EmployeeInfo.txt` file.

When you visit this book's website (`www.allmycode.com/JavaForDummies`) and you download the book's code listings, you get a copy of the `EmployeeInfo.txt` file.

WARNING

To keep Listing 8-2 simple, I insist that, when you type the characters in Figure 8-3, you finish up by typing `10000.00` and then pressing Enter. (Look again at Figure 8-3 and notice how the cursor is at the start of a brand-new line.) If you forget to finish by pressing Enter, the code in Listing 8-2 will crash when you try to run it.

WARNING

Grouping separators vary from one country to another. The file shown in Figure 8-3 works on a computer configured in the United States where *5000.00* means "five thousand." But the file doesn't work on a computer that's configured in what I call a "comma country" — a country where *5000,00* means "five thousand." If you live in a comma country, be sure to read this chapter's "Where on Earth do you live?" sidebar.

This book's website (`www.allmycode.com/JavaForDummies`) has tips for readers who need to create data files. This includes instructions for Windows, Linux, and Macintosh environments.

Copying and pasting code

In almost any computer programming language, reading data from a file can be tricky. You add extra lines of code to tell the computer what to do. Sometimes you can copy and paste these lines from other peoples' code. For example, you can follow the pattern in Listing 8-2:

```
/*
 * The pattern in Listing 8-2
 */
import java.util.Scanner;
import java.io.File;
import java.io.IOException;

class SomeClassName {

    public static void main(String args[]) throws IOException {

        Scanner scannerName = new Scanner(new File("SomeFileName"));

        //Some code goes here

        scannerName.nextInt();
        scannerName.nextDouble();
        scannerName.next();
        scannerName.nextLine();
```

```
        //Some code goes here

        scannerName.close();
    }
}
```

You want to read data from a file. You start by imagining that you're reading from the keyboard. Put the usual Scanner and next codes into your program. Then add some extra items from the Listing 8-2 pattern:

- Add two new import declarations — one for java.io.File and another for java.io.IOException.
- Type **throws IOException** in your method's header.
- Type **new File(" ")** in your call to new Scanner.
- Take a file that's already on your hard drive. Type that filename inside the quotation marks.
- Take the word that you use for the name of your scanner. Reuse that word in calls to next, nextInt, nextDouble, and so on.
- Take the word that you use for the name of your scanner. Reuse that word in a call to close.

Occasionally, copying and pasting code can get you into trouble. Maybe you're writing a program that doesn't fit the simple Listing 8-2 pattern. You need to tweak the pattern a bit. But to tweak the pattern, you need to understand some of the ideas behind the pattern.

That's how the next section comes to your rescue. It covers some of these ideas.

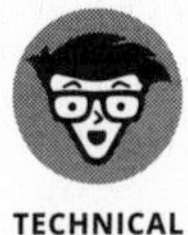

TECHNICAL STUFF

This paragraph is actually a confession. In almost every computer programming language, input from a disk file is a nasty business. There's no such thing as a simple INPUT command. You normally have to set up a connection between the code and the disk device, prepare for possible trouble reading from the device, do your reading, convert the characters you read into the type of value that you want and, finally, break your connection with the disk device. It's a big mess. That's why, in this book, I rely on Java's Scanner class. The Scanner class makes input relatively painless. But, I admit, professional Java programmers hardly ever use the Scanner class to do input. Instead, they use something called a BufferedReader or classes in the java.nio package. If you're not content with my use of the Scanner class and you want to see Listing 8-2 translated into a BufferedReader program, visit this book's website (www.allmycode.com/JavaForDummies).

Reading from a file

In previous chapters, programs read characters from the computer's keyboard. These programs use things like `Scanner`, `System.in`, and `nextDouble` — things defined in Java's API. The `DoPayroll` program in Listing 8-2 puts a new spin on this story. Rather than read characters from the keyboard, the program reads characters from the `EmployeeInfo.txt` file. The file lives on your computer's hard drive.

To read characters from a file, you use some of the same things that help you read characters from the keyboard. You use `Scanner`, `nextDouble`, and other goodies. But in addition to these goodies, you have a few extra hurdles to jump. Here's a list:

- **You need a new File object.** To be more precise, you need a new instance of the API's `File` class. You get this new instance with code like

  ```
  new File("EmployeeInfo.txt")
  ```

  The stuff in quotation marks is the name of a file — a file on your computer's hard drive. The file contains characters like those shown previously in Figure 8-3.

  At this point, the terminology makes mountains out of molehills. Sure, I use the phrases *new File object* and *new File instance,* but all you're doing is making `new File("EmployeeInfo.txt")` stand for a file on your hard drive. After you shove `new File("EmployeeInfo.txt")` into `new Scanner`,

  ```
  Scanner diskScanner = new Scanner(new File("EmployeeInfo.txt"));
  ```

  you can forget all about the `new File` business. From that point on in the code, `diskScanner` stands for the `EmployeeInfo.txt` filename on your computer's hard drive. (The name `diskScanner` stands for a file on your hard drive just as, in previous examples, the name `keyboard` stands for those buttons you press day in and day out.)

  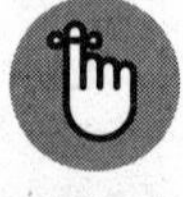

  Creating a `new File` object in Listing 8-2 is like creating a `new Employee` object later in the same listing. It's also like creating a `new Account` object in the examples of Chapter 7. The only difference is that the `Employee` and `Account` classes are defined in this book's examples. The `File` class is defined in Java's API.

  When you connect to a disk file with `new Scanner`, don't forget the `new File` part. If you write `new Scanner("EmployeeInfo.txt")` without `new File`, the compiler won't mind. (You don't get any warnings or error messages before you run the code.) But when you run the code, you don't get anything like the results that you expect to get.

» **You must refer to the File class by its full name: `java.io.File`.** You can do this with an import declaration like the one in Listing 8-2. Alternatively, you can clutter your code with a statement like

```
Scanner diskScanner = new Scanner(new java.io.File("EmployeeInfo.txt"));
```

» **You need a throws IOException clause.** Lots of things can go wrong when your program connects to `EmployeeInfo.txt`. For one thing, your hard drive may not have a file named `EmployeeInfo.txt`. For another, the file `EmployeeInfo.txt` may be in the wrong directory. To brace for this kind of calamity, the Java programming language takes certain precautions. The language insists that when a disk file is involved, you acknowledge the possible dangers of calling `new Scanner`.

You can acknowledge the hazards in several possible ways, but the simplest way is to use a `throws` clause. In Listing 8-2, the `main` method's header ends with the words *throws IOException.* By adding these two words, you appease the Java compiler. It's as if you're saying "I know that calling `new Scanner` can lead to problems. You don't have to remind me." And, sure enough, adding `throws IOException` to your `main` method keeps the compiler from complaining. (Without this `throws` clause, you get an `unreported exception` error message.)

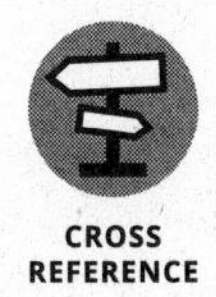
CROSS REFERENCE

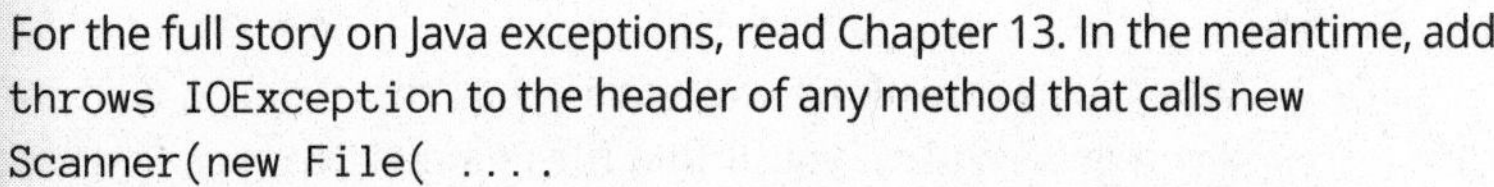
For the full story on Java exceptions, read Chapter 13. In the meantime, add `throws IOException` to the header of any method that calls `new Scanner(new File( ...`.

» **You must refer to the `IOException` class by its full name: `java.io.IOException`.**

You can do this with an `import` declaration like the one in Listing 8-2. Alternatively, you can enlarge the `main` method's `throws` clause:

```
public static void main(String args[])throws java.io.IOException {
```

» **You must pass the file scanner's name to the `payOneEmployee` method.**

In Listing 7-5 in Chapter 7, the `getInterest` method has a parameter named *percentageRate.* Whenever you call the `getInterest` method, you hand an extra, up-to-date piece of information to the method. (You hand a number — an interest rate — to the method. Figure 7-7 illustrates the idea.)

The same thing happens in Listing 8-2. The `payOneEmployee` method has a parameter named *aScanner.* Whenever you call the `payOneEmployee` method, you hand an extra, up-to-date piece of information to the method. (You hand a scanner — a reference to a disk file — to the method.)

You may wonder why the payOneEmployee method needs a parameter. After all, in Listing 8-2, the payOneEmployee method always reads data from the same file. Why bother informing this method, each time you call it, that the disk file is still the EmployeeInfo.txt file?

Well, there are plenty of ways to shuffle the code in Listing 8-2. Some ways don't involve a parameter. But the way that this example has arranged things, you have two separate methods: a main method and a payOneEmployee method. You create a scanner once inside the main method and then use the scanner three times — once inside each call to the payOneEmployee method.

Anything you define inside a method is like a private joke that's known only to the code inside that method. So the diskScanner that you define inside the main method isn't automatically known inside the payOneEmployee method. To make the payOneEmployee method aware of the disk file, you pass diskScanner from the main method to the payOneEmployee method.

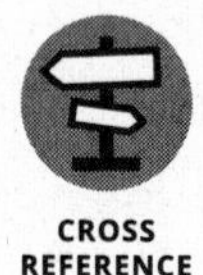
CROSS REFERENCE

To read more about things that you declare inside (and outside) of methods, see Chapter 10.

Who moved my file?

When you download the code from this book's website (www.allmycode.com/JavaForDummies), you'll find files named Employee.java and DoPayroll.java — the code in Listings 8-1 and 8-2. You'll also find a file named EmployeeInfo.txt. That's good because, if Java can't find the EmployeeInfo.txt file, the whole project doesn't run properly. Instead, you get a FileNotFoundException.

In general, when you get a FileNotFoundException, some file that your program needs isn't available to it. This is an easy mistake to make. It can be frustrating because, to you, a file such as EmployeeInfo.txt may look like it's available to your program. But remember: Computers are stupid. If you make a tiny mistake, the computer can't read between the lines for you. So, if your EmployeeInfo.txt file isn't in the right directory on your hard drive or the filename is spelled incorrectly, the computer chokes when it tries to run your code.

Sometimes you know darn well that an EmployeeInfo.txt (or *whatever.xyz*) file exists on your hard drive. But when you run your program, you still get a mean-looking FileNotFoundException. When this happens, the file is usually in the wrong directory on your hard drive. (Of course, it depends on your point of view. Maybe the file is in the right directory, but your Java program is looking for the file in the wrong directory.) To diagnose this problem, add the following code to Listing 8-2:

```
File employeeInfo = new File("EmployeeInfo.txt");
System.out.println("Looking for " + employeeInfo.getCanonicalPath());
```

When you run the code, Java tells you where, on your hard drive, the `EmployeeInfo.txt` file should be.

Adding directory names to your filenames

You can specify a file's exact location in your Java code. Code like `new File("C:\\Users\\bburd\\workspace\\08-01\\EmployeeInfo.txt")` looks really ugly, but it works.

In the preceding paragraph, did you notice the double backslashes in "`C:\\Users\\bburd\\workspace ...`"? If you're a Windows user, you'd be tempted to write `C:\Users\bburd\workspace ...` with single backslashes. But in Java, the single backslash has its own, special meaning. (For example, back in Listing 7-7, `\n` means to go to the next line.) So, in Java, to indicate a backslash inside a quoted string, you use a double backslash instead.

TECHNICAL STUFF

Macintosh and Linux users might find comfort in the fact that their path separator, `/`, has no special meaning in a Java string. On a Mac, the code `new File("/Users/bburd/workspace/08-01/EmployeeInfo.txt")` is as normal as breathing. (Well, it's almost that normal!) But Mac users and Linux wonks shouldn't claim superiority too quickly. Lines such as `new File("/Users/bburd/workspace ...` work in Windows as well. In Windows, you can use either a slash (`/`) or a backslash (`\`) as the path name separator. At the Windows command prompt, I can type `cd c:/users\bburd` to get to my home directory.

TIP

If you know where your Java program looks for files, you can worm your way from that place to the directory of your choice. Assume, for the moment, that the code in Listing 8-2 normally looks for the `EmployeeInfo.txt` file in a directory named `08-01`. As an experiment, go to the `08-01` directory and create a new subdirectory named *dataFiles*. Then move my `EmployeeInfo.txt` file to the new `dataFiles` directory. To read numbers and words from the file that you moved, modify Listing 8-2 with the code `new File("dataFiles\\EmployeeInfo.txt")` or `new File("dataFiles/EmployeeInfo.txt")`.

Reading a line at a time

In Listing 8-2, the `payOneEmployee` method illustrates some useful tricks for reading data. In particular, every scanner that you create has a `nextLine` method. (You might not use this `nextLine` method, but the method is available nonetheless.) When you call a scanner's `nextLine` method, the method grabs everything up to the end of the current line of text. In Listing 8-2, a call to `nextLine` can read a whole line from the `EmployeeInfo.txt` file. (In another program, a scanner's `nextLine` call may read everything the user types on the keyboard up to the pressing of the Enter key.)

Notice my careful choice of words: `nextLine` reads everything "up to the end of the current line." Unfortunately, what it means to read up to the end of the current line isn't always what you think it means. Intermingling `nextInt`, `nextDouble`, and `nextLine` calls can be messy. You have to watch what you're doing and check your program's output carefully.

To understand all of this, you need to be painfully aware of a data file's line breaks. Think of a line break as an extra character, stuck between one line of text and the next. Then imagine that calling `nextLine` means to read everything up to and including the next line break.

Now take a look at Figure 8-4:

- If one call to `nextLine` reads `Barry Burd[LineBreak]`, the subsequent call to `nextLine` reads `CEO[LineBreak]`.
- If one call to `nextDouble` reads the number 5000.00, the subsequent call to `nextLine` reads the `[LineBreak]` that comes immediately after the number 5000.00. (That's all the `nextLine` reads — a `[LineBreak]` and nothing more.)
- If a call to `nextLine` reads the `[LineBreak]` after the number 5000.00, the subsequent call to `nextLine` reads `Harriet Ritter[LineBreak]`.

So, after reading the number 5000.00, you need *two* calls to `nextLine` in order to scoop up the name *Harriet Ritter.* The mistake that I usually make is to forget the first of those two calls.

WARNING

Look again at the file in Figure 8-3. For this section's code to work correctly, you must have a line break after the last `10000.00`. If you don't, a final call to `nextLine` makes your program crash and burn. The error message reads `NoSuchElementException: No line found.`

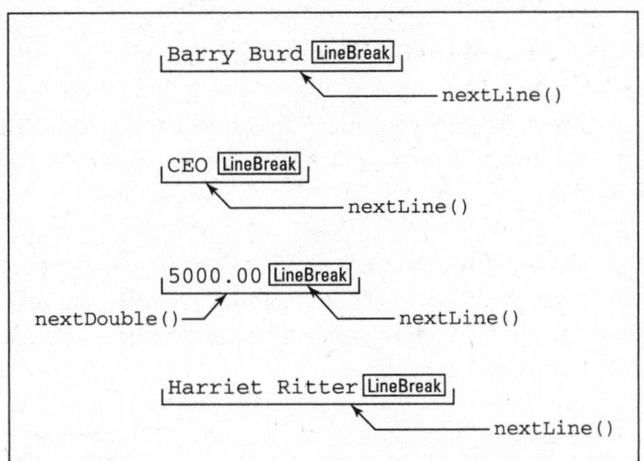

FIGURE 8-4: Calling next Double and nextLine.

TECHNICAL STUFF

I'm always surprised by the number of quirks that I find in each programming language's scanning methods. For example, the first `nextLine` that reads from the file in Figure 8-3 devours `Barry Burd[LineBreak]` from the file. But that `nextLine` call delivers `Barry Burd` (with no line break) to the running code. So `nextLine` looks for a line break, and then `nextLine` loses the line break. Yes, this is a subtle point. And no, this subtle point hardly ever causes problems for anyone.

TECHNICAL STUFF

If this business about `nextDouble` and `nextLine` confuses you, please don't put the blame on Java. Mixing input calls is delicate work in any computer programming language. And the really nasty thing is that each programming language approaches the problem a little differently. What you find out about `nextLine` in Java helps you understand the issues when you get to know C++ or Visual Basic, but it doesn't tell you all the details. Each language's details are unique to that language. (Yes, it's a big pain. But because all computer programmers become rich and famous, the pain eventually pays off.)

Closing the connection to a disk file

To the average computer user, a keyboard doesn't feel anything like a file stored on a computer's hard drive. But disk files and keyboard input have a lot in common. In fact, a basic principle of computer operating systems dictates that any differences between two kinds of input be, for the programmer, as blurry as possible. As a Java programmer, you should treat disk files and keyboard input almost the same way. That's why Listing 8-2 contains a `diskScanner.close()` call.

When you run a Java program, you normally execute the `main` method's statements, starting with the first statement in the method body and ending with the last statement in the method body. You take detours along the way, skipping past `else` parts and diving into method bodies, but basically you finish executing statements at the end of the `main` method. That's why, in Listing 8-2, the call to `close` is at the end of the `main` method's body. When you run the code in Listing 8-2, the last thing you do is disconnect from the disk file. And, fortunately, that disconnection takes place after you've executed all the `nextLine` and `nextDouble` calls.

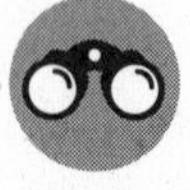

TRY IT OUT

Previously in this chapter, you create instances of your own `PlaceToLive` class and display information about those instances. Modify the text-based version of your code so that it gets each instance's characteristics (address, number of bedrooms, and area) from a disk file.

Defining Subclasses (What It Means to Be a Full-Time or Part-Time Employee)

This time last year, your company paid $10 million for a piece of software. That software came in the `Employee.class` file. People at Burd Brain Consulting (the company that created the software) don't want you to know about the innards of the software. (Otherwise, you may steal their ideas.) So you don't have the Java program file that the software came from. (In other words, you don't have `Employee.java`.) You can run the bytecode in the `Employee.class` file. You can also read the documentation in a web page named *Employee.html*. But you can't see the statements inside the `Employee.java` program, and you can't change any of the program's code.

Since this time last year, your company has grown. Unlike in the old days, your company now has two kinds of employees: full-time and part-time. Each full-time employee is on a fixed, weekly salary. (If the employee works nights and weekends, then in return for this monumental effort, the employee receives a hearty handshake.) In contrast, each part-time employee works for an hourly wage. Your company deducts an amount from each full-time employee's paycheck to pay for the company's benefits package. Part-time employees, however, don't get benefits.

The question is whether the software that your company bought last year can keep up with the company's growth. You invested in a great program to handle employees and their payroll, but the program doesn't differentiate between your full-time and part-time employees. You have several options:

- **Call your next-door neighbor, whose 12-year-old child knows more about computer programming than anyone in your company.** Get this uppity little brat to take the employee software apart, rewrite it, and hand it back to you with all the changes and additions your company requires.

On second thought, you can't do that. No matter how smart that kid is, the complexities of the employee software will probably confuse the kid. By the time you get the software back, it'll be filled with bugs and inconsistencies. Besides, you don't even have the `Employee.java` file to hand to the kid. All you have is the `Employee.class` file, which can't be read or modified with a text editor. (See Chapter 2.) Besides, your kid just beat up the neighbor's kid. You don't want to give your neighbor the satisfaction of seeing you beg for the whiz kid's help.

- **Scrap the $10 million employee software.** Get someone in your company to rewrite the software from scratch.

  In other words, say goodbye to your time and money.

- **Write a new front end for the employee software.** That is, build a piece of code that does some preliminary processing on full-time employees and then hands the preliminary results to your $10 million software. Do the same for part-time employees.

  This idea could be decent or spell disaster. Are you sure that the existing employee software has convenient *hooks* in it? (That is, does the employee software contain entry points that allow your front-end software to easily send preliminary data to the expensive employee software?) Remember: This plan treats the existing software as one big, monolithic lump, which can become cumbersome. Dividing the labor between your front-end code and the existing employee program is difficult. And if you add layer upon layer to existing black box code, you'll probably end up with a fairly inefficient system.

- **Call Burd Brain Consulting, the company that sold you the employee software.** Tell Dr. Burd that you want the next version of his software to differentiate between full-time and part-time employees.

  "No problem," says Dr. Burd. "It'll be ready by the start of the next fiscal quarter." That evening, Dr. Burd makes a discreet phone call to his next-door neighbor. . . .

- **Create two new Java classes named *FullTimeEmployee* and *PartTimeEmployee.*** Have each new class extend the existing functionality of the expensive `Employee` class, but have each new class define its own, specialized functionality for certain kinds of employees.

  Way to go! Figure 8-5 shows the structure that you want to create.

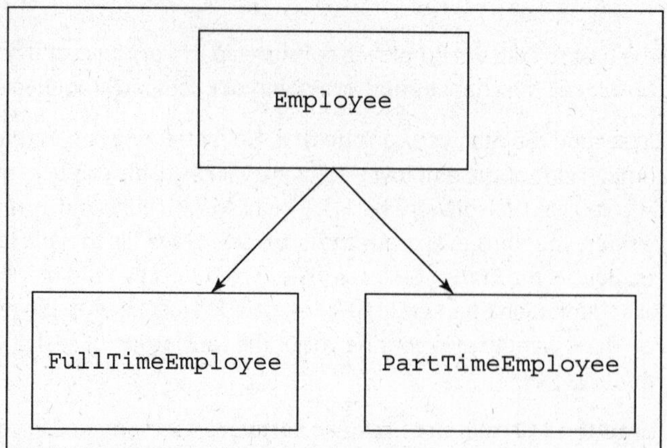

FIGURE 8-5: The Employee class family tree.

Creating a subclass

In Listing 8-1, I define an `Employee` class. I can use what I define in Listing 8-1 and extend the definition to create new, more specialized classes. So, in Listing 8-3, I define a new class: a `FullTimeEmployee` class.

LISTING 8-3: What Is a FullTimeEmployee?

```
public class FullTimeEmployee extends Employee {
    private double weeklySalary;
    private double benefitDeduction;

    public void setWeeklySalary(double weeklySalaryIn) {
        weeklySalary = weeklySalaryIn;
    }

    public double getWeeklySalary() {
        return weeklySalary;
    }

    public void setBenefitDeduction(double benefitDedIn) {
        benefitDeduction = benefitDedIn;
    }

    public double getBenefitDeduction() {
        return benefitDeduction;
    }

    public double findPaymentAmount() {
        return weeklySalary - benefitDeduction;
    }
}
```

Looking at Listing 8-3, you can see that each instance of the FullTimeEmployee class has two fields: weeklySalary and benefitDeduction. But are those the only fields that each FullTimeEmployee instance has? No, they're not. The first line of Listing 8-3 says that the FullTimeEmployee class extends the existing Employee class. This means that in addition to having a weeklySalary and a benefitDeduction, each FullTimeEmployee instance also has two other fields: name and jobTitle. These two fields come from the definition of the Employee class, which you can find in Listing 8-1.

In Listing 8-3, the magic word is *extends*. When one class extends an existing class, the extending class automatically inherits functionality that's defined in the existing class. So, the FullTimeEmployee class *inherits* the name and jobTitle fields. The FullTimeEmployee class also inherits all the methods that are declared in the Employee class: setName, getName, setJobTitle, getJobTitle, and cutCheck. The FullTimeEmployee class is a *subclass* of the Employee class. That means the Employee class is the *superclass* of the FullTimeEmployee class. You can also talk in terms of blood relatives: The FullTimeEmployee class is the *child* of the Employee class, and the Employee class is the *parent* of the FullTimeEmployee class.

It's almost (but not quite) as if the FullTimeEmployee class were defined by the code in Listing 8-4.

LISTING 8-4: Fake (But Informative) Code

```
import static java.lang.System.out;

public class FullTimeEmployee {
    private String name;
    private String jobTitle;
    private double weeklySalary;
    private double benefitDeduction;

    public void setName(String nameIn) {
        name = nameIn;
    }

    public String getName() {
        return name;
    }

    public void setJobTitle(String jobTitleIn) {
        jobTitle = jobTitleIn;
    }
```

(continued)

LISTING 8-4: *(continued)*

```
    public String getJobTitle() {
        return jobTitle;
    }

    public void setWeeklySalary(double weeklySalaryIn) {
        weeklySalary = weeklySalaryIn;
    }

    public double getWeeklySalary() {
        return weeklySalary;
    }

    public void setBenefitDeduction(double benefitDedIn) {
        benefitDeduction = benefitDedIn;
    }

    public double getBenefitDeduction() {
        return benefitDeduction;
    }

    public double findPaymentAmount() {
        return weeklySalary - benefitDeduction;
    }

    public void cutCheck(double amountPaid) {
        out.printf("Pay to the order of %s ", name);
        out.printf("(%s) ***$", jobTitle);
        out.printf("%,.2f\n", amountPaid);
    }
}
```

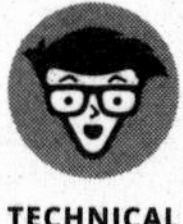

TECHNICAL STUFF

Why does the title for Listing 8-4 call that code fake? (Should the code feel insulted?) Well, the main difference between Listing 8-4 and the inheritance situation in Listings 8-1 and 8-3 is this: A child class can't directly reference the private fields of its parent class. To do anything with the parent class's private fields, the child class has to call the parent class's accessor methods. Back in Listing 8-3, calling `setName("Rufus")` would be legal, but the code `name="Rufus"` wouldn't be. If you believe everything you read in Listing 8-4, you'd think that code in the `FullTimeEmployee` class can do `name="Rufus"`. Well, it can't. (My, what a subtle point this is!)

REMEMBER

You don't need the `Employee.java` file on your hard drive to write code that extends the `Employee` class. All you need is the file `Employee.class`.

Creating subclasses is habit-forming

After you're accustomed to extending classes, you can get extend-happy. If you created a `FullTimeEmployee` class, you might as well create a `PartTimeEmployee` class, as shown in Listing 8-5.

LISTING 8-5: What Is a PartTimeEmployee?

```
public class PartTimeEmployee extends Employee {
    private double hourlyRate;

    public void setHourlyRate(double rateIn) {
        hourlyRate = rateIn;
    }

    public double getHourlyRate() {
        return hourlyRate;
    }

    public double findPaymentAmount(int hours) {
        return hourlyRate * hours;
    }
}
```

Unlike the `FullTimeEmployee` class, `PartTimeEmployee` has no salary or deduction. Instead `PartTimeEmployee` has an `hourlyRate` field. (Adding a `numberOfHoursWorked` field would also be a possibility. I chose not to do this, figuring that the number of hours a part-time employee works will change drastically from week to week.)

Using Subclasses

The preceding section tells a story about creating subclasses. It's a good story, but it's incomplete. Creating subclasses is fine, but you gain nothing from these subclasses unless you write code to use them. So in this section, you explore code that uses subclasses.

Now the time has come for you to classify yourself as either a type-F person, a type-P person, or a type-T person. (I'm this book's author, so I get to make up some personality types. I can even point to someone in public and say, "Look! He's a type-T person!")

» **A type-F person** wants to see the fundamentals. (The letter *F* stands for *fundamentals.*) "Show me a program that lays out the principles in their barest, most basic form," says the type-F person. A type-F person isn't worried about bells and whistles. The bells come later, and the whistles may never come. If you're a type-F person, you want to see a program that uses the `FullTimeEmployee` and `PartTimeEmployee` subclasses and then moves out of your way so that you can get some work done.

» **A type-P person** wants practical applications. (The letter *P* stands for *practical.*) Type-P people need to see ideas in context; otherwise, the ideas float away too quickly. "Show me a program that demonstrates the usefulness of the `FullTimeEmployee` and `PartTimeEmployee` subclasses," says the type-P person. "I have no use for your stinking abstractions. I want real-life examples, and I want them now!"

» **A type-T person** is inspired by something that I write about briefly in Chapter 7: The type-T person wants to *test* the code in the `FullTimeEmployee` and `PartTimeEmployee` subclasses. Testing the code means putting the code through its paces — checking the output's accuracy when the input is ordinary, when the input is unexpected, and even when the input is completely unrealistic. What's more, the type-T person wants to use a standard, easily recognizable outline for the testing code so that other programmers can quickly understand the test results. The type-T person creates JUnit tests that use the `FullTimeEmployee` and `PartTimeEmployee` subclasses.

Listing 8-6, which is for the type-F crowd, is lean and simple and makes good bedtime reading.

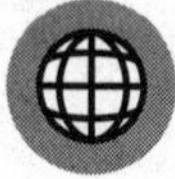

If you're a type-P or type-T person, please visit this book's website (`www.allmycode.com/JavaForDummies`). The site contains examples to satisfy type-P and type-T readers.

Listing 8-6 shows you a bare-bones program that uses the subclasses `FullTimeEmployee` and `PartTimeEmployee`. Figure 8-6 shows the program's output.

LISTING 8-6: Putting Subclasses to Good Use

```
public class DoPayrollTypeF {

  public static void main(String args[]) {

    FullTimeEmployee ftEmployee = new FullTimeEmployee();

    ftEmployee.setName("Barry Burd");
    ftEmployee.setJobTitle("CEO");
    ftEmployee.setWeeklySalary(5000.00);
```

```
        ftEmployee.setBenefitDeduction(500.00);
        ftEmployee.cutCheck(ftEmployee.findPaymentAmount());
        System.out.println();

        PartTimeEmployee ptEmployee = new PartTimeEmployee();

        ptEmployee.setName("Steve Surace");
        ptEmployee.setJobTitle("Driver");
        ptEmployee.setHourlyRate(7.53);
        ptEmployee.cutCheck(ptEmployee.findPaymentAmount(10));
    }
}
```

FIGURE 8-6: The output of the program in Listing 8-6.

```
Pay to the order of Barry Burd (CEO) ***$4,500.00

Pay to the order of Steve Surace (Driver) ***$75.30
```

To understand Listing 8-6, you need to keep an eye on three classes: `Employee`, `FullTimeEmployee`, and `PartTimeEmployee`. (For a look at the code that defines these classes, see Listings 8-1, 8-3, and 8-5.)

The first half of Listing 8-6 deals with a full-time employee. Notice how many methods are available for use with the `ftEmployee` variable? For instance, you can call `ftEmployee.setWeeklySalary` because `ftEmployee` has type `FullTimeEmployee`. You can also call `ftEmployee.setName` because the `FullTimeEmployee` class extends the `Employee` class.

Because `cutCheck` is declared in the `Employee` class, you can call `ftEmployee.cutCheck`. But you can also call `ftEmployee.findPaymentAmount` because a `findPaymentAmount` method is in the `FullTimeEmployee` class.

Making types match

Look again at the first half of Listing 8-6. Take special notice of that last statement — the one in which the full-time employee is actually cut a check. The statement forms a nice, long chain of values and their types. You can see this by reading the statement from the inside out:

» Method `ftEmployee.findPaymentAmount` is called with an empty parameter list. (Refer to Listing 8-6.) That's good because the `findPaymentAmount` method takes no parameters. (Refer to Listing 8-3.)

- The `findPaymentAmount` method returns a value of type `double`. (Again, refer to Listing 8-3.)
- The `double` value that `ftEmployee.findPaymentAmount` returns is passed to method `ftEmployee.cutCheck`. (Refer to Listing 8-6.) That's good because the `cutCheck` method takes one parameter of type `double`. (Refer to Listing 8-1.)

For a fanciful graphical illustration, see Figure 8-7.

REMEMBER

Always feed a method the value types that it wants in its parameter list.

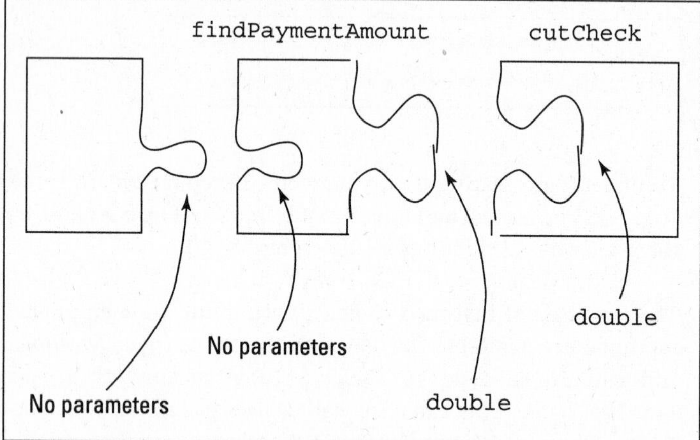

FIGURE 8-7: Matching parameters.

The second half of the story

In the second half of Listing 8-6, the code creates an object of type `PartTimeEmployee`. A variable of type `PartTimeEmployee` can do some of the same things a `FullTimeEmployee` variable can do. But the `PartTimeEmployee` class doesn't have the `setWeeklySalary` and `setBenefitDeduction` methods. Instead, the `PartTimeEmployee` class has the `setHourlyRate` method. (See Listing 8-5.) So in Listing 8-6 the next-to-last line is a call to the `setHourlyRate` method.

The last line of Listing 8-6 is by far the most interesting. On that line, the code hands the number `10` (the number of hours worked) to the `findPaymentAmount` method. Compare this with the earlier call to `findPaymentAmount` — the call for the full-time employee in the first half of Listing 8-6. Between the two subclasses, `FullTimeEmployee` and `PartTimeEmployee`, are two different findPaymentAmount methods. The two methods have two different kinds of parameter lists:

- The FullTimeEmployee class's findPaymentAmount method takes no parameters (refer to Listing 8-3).
- The PartTimeEmployee class's findPaymentAmount method takes one int parameter (refer to Listing 8-5).

This is par for the course. Finding the payment amount for a part-time employee isn't the same as finding the payment amount for a full-time employee. A part-time employee's pay changes each week, depending on the number of hours the employee works in a week. The full-time employee's pay stays the same each week. So the FullTimeEmployee and PartTimeEmployee classes both have findPaymentAmount methods, but each class's method works quite differently.

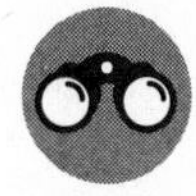
TRY IT OUT

Yes, I have some things for you to try:

- Previously in this chapter, you create instances of your own PlaceToLive class and display information about those instances. Create two subclasses of your PlaceToLive class: a House class and an Apartment class. Each House object has a mortgage cost (a monthly amount) and a property tax cost (a yearly amount). Each Apartment object has a rental cost (a monthly amount).

  A separate DisplayThePlaces class creates some houses and some apartments. For each house or apartment, your DisplayThePlaces class displays the total cost per square foot (or square meter) and the total cost per bedroom, both calculated monthly.

- In Chapter 7, you create an Organization class. Each instance of your Organization class has a name, an annual revenue amount, and a boolean value indicating whether the organization is or is not a profit-making organization.

  Create a new Organization_2.0 class. Each instance of this new class has only a name and an annual revenue amount. Create two subclasses: a ProfitMakingOrganization class and a NonProfitOrganization class. A profit-making organization pays 10 percent of its revenue in tax, but a nonprofit organization pays only 2 percent of its revenue in tax.

  Make a separate class that creates ProfitMakingOrganization instances and NonProfitOrganization instances while also displaying information about each instance, including the amount of tax the organization pays.

Overriding Existing Methods (Changing the Payments for Some Employees)

Wouldn't you know it! Some knucklehead in the human resources department offered double pay for overtime to one of your part-time employees. Now word is getting around, and some of the other part-timers want double pay for their overtime work. If this keeps up, you'll end up in the poorhouse, so you need to send out a memo to all the part-time employees, explaining why earning more money is not to their benefit.

In the meantime, you have two kinds of part-time employees — the ones who receive double pay for overtime hours and the ones who don't — so you need to modify your payroll software. What are your options?

- Well, you can dig right into the `PartTimeEmployee` class code, make a few changes, and hope for the best. (Not a good idea!)
- You can follow the previous section's advice and create a subclass of the existing `PartTimeEmployee` class. "But wait," you say. "The existing `PartTimeEmployee` class already has a `findPaymentAmount` method. Do I need some tricky way of bypassing this existing `findPaymentAmount` method for each double-pay-for-overtime employee?"

  At this point, you can thank your lucky stars that you're doing object-oriented programming in Java. With object-oriented programming, you can create a subclass that overrides the functionality of its parent class. Listing 8-7 has just such a subclass.

LISTING 8-7: Yet Another Subclass

```
public class PartTimeWithOver extends PartTimeEmployee {

    @Override
    public double findPaymentAmount(int hours) {

        if(hours <= 40) {
            return getHourlyRate() * hours;
        } else {
            return getHourlyRate() * 40 + getHourlyRate() * 2 * (hours - 40);
        }
    }
}
```

Figure 8-8 shows the relationship between the code in Listing 8-7 and other pieces of code in this chapter. In particular, PartTimeWithOver is a subclass of a subclass. In object-oriented programming, a chain of this kind is not the least bit unusual. In fact, as subclasses go, this chain is rather short.

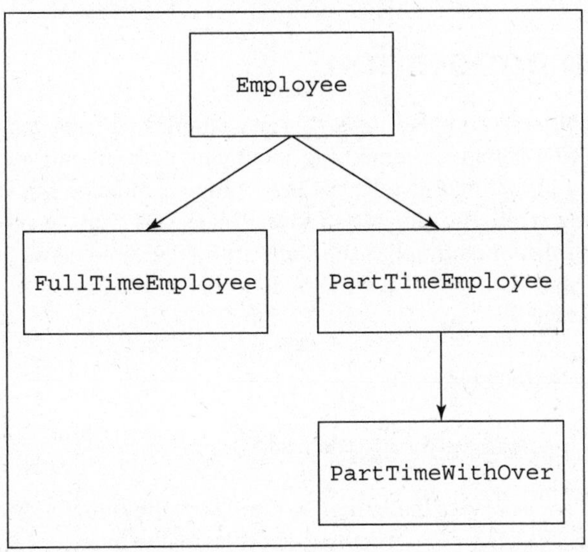

FIGURE 8-8: A tree of classes.

The PartTimeWithOver class extends the PartTimeEmployee class, but PartTimeWithOver picks and chooses what it wants to inherit from the PartTimeEmployee class. Because PartTimeWithOver has its own declaration for the findPaymentAmount method, the PartTimeWithOver class doesn't inherit a findPaymentAmount method from its parent. (See Figure 8-9.)

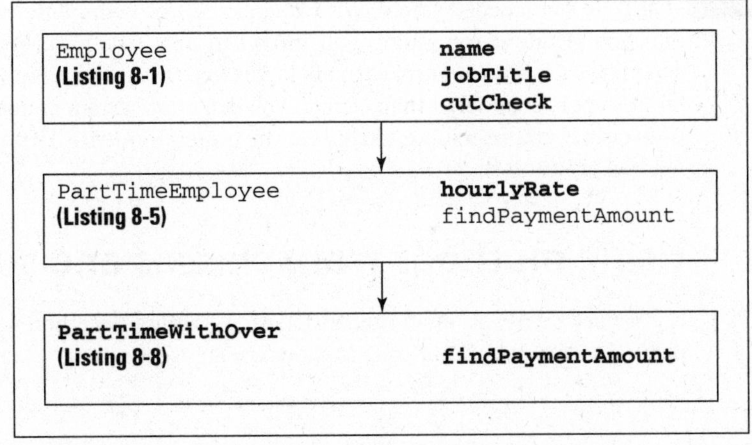

FIGURE 8-9: Method findPaymentAmount isn't inherited.

According to the official terminology, the `PartTimeWithOver` class *overrides* its parent class's `findPaymentAmount` method. If you create an object from the `PartTimeWithOver` class, that object has the `name`, `jobTitle`, `hourlyRate`, and `cutCheck` of the `PartTimeEmployee` class, but the object has the `findPaymentAmount` method that's defined in Listing 8-7.

A Java annotation

The word `@Override` in Listing 8-7 is an example of an *annotation*. A Java annotation tells your computer something about your code. In particular, the `@Override` annotation in Listing 8-7 tells the Java compiler to be on the lookout for a common coding error. The annotation says, "Make sure that the method immediately following this annotation has the same stuff (the same name, the same parameters, and so on) as one of the methods in the superclass. If not, then display an error message."

So if I accidentally type

```
public double findPaymentAmount(double hours) {
```

instead of `int hours` as in Listings 8-5 and 8-7, the compiler reminds me that my new `findPaymentAmount` method doesn't really override anything that's in Listing 8-5.

Java has other kinds of annotations (such as `@Deprecated` and `@SuppressWarnings`). You can read a bit about the `@SuppressWarnings` annotation in Chapter 9.

TECHNICAL STUFF

Java's annotations are optional. If you remove the word `@Override` from Listing 8-7, your code still runs correctly. But the `@Override` annotation gives your code some added safety. With `@Override`, the compiler checks to make sure that you're doing something you intend to do (namely, overriding one of the superclass's methods). And with apologies to George Orwell, some types of annotations are less optional than others. You can omit certain annotations from your code only if you're willing to replace the annotation with lots and lots of unannotated Java code.

Using methods from classes and subclasses

If you need clarification on this notion of overriding a method, look at the code in Listing 8-8. A run of that code is shown in Figure 8-10.

LISTING 8-8: Testing the Code from Listing 8-7

```
public class DoPayrollTypeF {

  public static void main(String args[]) {

    FullTimeEmployee ftEmployee = new FullTimeEmployee();

    ftEmployee.setName("Barry Burd");
    ftEmployee.setJobTitle("CEO");
    ftEmployee.setWeeklySalary(5000.00);
    ftEmployee.setBenefitDeduction(500.00);
    ftEmployee.cutCheck(ftEmployee.findPaymentAmount());

    PartTimeEmployee ptEmployee = new PartTimeEmployee();

    ptEmployee.setName("Chris Apelian");
    ptEmployee.setJobTitle("Computer Book Author");
    ptEmployee.setHourlyRate(7.53);
    ptEmployee.cutCheck(ptEmployee.findPaymentAmount(50));

    PartTimeWithOver ptoEmployee = new PartTimeWithOver();

    ptoEmployee.setName("Steve Surace");
    ptoEmployee.setJobTitle("Driver");
    ptoEmployee.setHourlyRate(7.53);
    ptoEmployee.cutCheck(ptoEmployee.findPaymentAmount(50));
  }
}
```

```
Pay to the order of Barry Burd (CEO) ***$4,500.00
Pay to the order of Chris Apelian (Computer Book Author) ***$376.50
Pay to the order of Steve Surace (Driver) ***$451.80
```

FIGURE 8-10: Running the code of Listing 8-8.

The code in Listing 8-8 writes checks to three employees. The first employee is a full-timer. The second is a part-time employee who hasn't yet gotten wind of the overtime payment scheme. The third employee knows about the overtime payment scheme and demands a fair wage.

With the subclasses, all three of these employees coexist in Listing 8-8. Sure, one subclass comes from the old `PartTimeEmployee` class, but that doesn't mean you can't create an object from the `PartTimeEmployee` class. In fact, Java is smart about this. Listing 8-8 has three calls to the `findPaymentAmount` method, and each call reaches out to a different version of the method:

- In the first call, `ftEmployee.findPaymentAmount`, the `ftEmployee` variable is an instance of the `FullTimeEmployee` class. So the method that's called is the one in Listing 8-3.
- In the second call, `ptEmployee.findPaymentAmount`, the `ptEmployee` variable is an instance of the `PartTimeEmployee` class. So the method that's called is the one in Listing 8-5.
- In the third call, `ptoEmployee.findPaymentAmount`, the `ptoEmployee` variable is an instance of the `PartTimeWithOver` class. So the method that's called is the one in Listing 8-7.

This code is fantastic. It's clean, elegant, and efficient. With all the money that you save on software, you can afford to pay everyone double for overtime hours. (Whether you do that or keep the money for yourself is another story.)

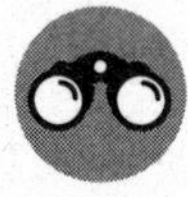

TRY IT OUT

Here are some things for you to try.

- In previous sections, you create House and `Apartment` subclasses of your `PlaceToLive` class. Create an `ApartmentWithFees` subclass of your `Apartment` class. In addition to the monthly rental price, someone living in an `ApartmentWithFees` pays a fixed amount every quarter (every three months). Create a separate class that displays the monthly cost of living in a House instance, an `Apartment` instance, and an `ApartmentWithFees` instance.
- What output do you see when you run the following code? What does this output tell you about variable declarations and method calling in Java?

```
public class Main {

    public static void main(String[] args) {
        MyThing myThing, myThing2;

        myThing = new MySubThing();
        myThing2 = new MyOtherThing();

        myThing.value = 7;
        myThing2.value = 44;
```

```
        myThing.display();
        myThing2.display();
    }
}

class MyThing {
    int value;

    public void display() {
        System.out.println("In MyThing, value is " + value);
    }
}

class MySubThing extends MyThing {

    @Override
    public void display() {
        System.out.println("in MySUBThing, value is " + value);
    }
}

class MyOtherThing extends MyThing {

    @Override
    public void display() {
        System.out.println("In MyOTHERThing, value is " + value);
    }
}
```

» Using constructors in subclasses

» Using Java's default constructor features

» Constructing a simple GUI from scratch

Chapter 9
Constructing New Objects

Ms. Jennie Burd

121 Schoolhouse Lane

Anywhere, Kansas

Dear Ms. Burd,

In response to your letter of June 21, I believe I can say with complete assurance that objects are not created spontaneously from nothing. Although I've never actually seen an object being created (and no one else in this office can claim to have seen an object in its moment of creation), I have every confidence that some process or another is responsible for the building of these interesting and useful thingamajigs. We here at ObjectsAndClasses.com support the unanimous opinions of both the scientific community and the private sector in matters of this nature. Furthermore, we agree with the recent finding of a Blue Ribbon Presidential Panel, which concludes beyond any doubt that spontaneous object creation would impede the present economic outlook.

Please be assured that I have taken all steps necessary to ensure the safety and well-being of you, our loyal customer. If you have any further questions, please do not hesitate to contact our complaint department. The department's manager is Mr. Blake Wholl. You can contact him by visiting our company's website.

Once again, let me thank you for your concern, and I hope you continue to patronize ObjectsAndClasses.com.

Yours truly,

Mr. Scott Brickenchicker

The one who couldn't get on the elevator in Chapter 4

Defining Constructors (What It Means to Be a Temperature)

Here's a statement that creates an object:

```
Account myAccount = new Account();
```

I know this works — I got it from one of my own examples in Chapter 7. Anyway, in Chapter 7 I say, "when Java executes `new Account()`, you're creating an object by calling the `Account` class's constructor." What does this mean?

Well, when you ask the computer to create a new object, the computer responds by performing certain actions. For starters, the computer finds a place in its memory to store information about the new object. If the object has fields, the fields should eventually have meaningful values.

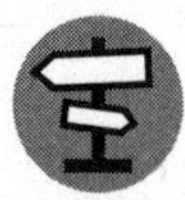
CROSS REFERENCE

To find out about fields, see Chapter 7.

One question is, when you ask the computer to create a new object, can you control what's placed in the object's fields? And what if you're interested in doing more than filling fields? Perhaps, when the computer creates a new object, you have a whole list of jobs for the computer to carry out. For instance, when the computer creates a new window object, you want the computer to realign the sizes of all buttons in that window.

Creating a new object can involve all kinds of tasks, so in this chapter you create constructors. A constructor tells the computer to perform a new object's start-up tasks.

What is a temperature?

"Good morning, and welcome to Object News. The local temperature in your area is a pleasant 73 degrees Fahrenheit."

Each temperature consists of two things: a number and a temperature scale. A number is just a `double` value, such as 32.0 or 70.52. But what's a temperature scale? Is it a string of characters, like `"Fahrenheit"` or `"Celsius"`? Not really, because some strings aren't temperature scales. There's no `"Quelploof"` temperature scale, and a program that can display the temperature `"73 degrees Quelploof`" is a bad program. So how can you limit the temperature scales to the small number of scales that people use? One way to do it is with Java's `enum` type.

What is a temperature scale? (Java's enum type)

Java provides lots of ways for you to group things together. In Chapter 11, you group things to form an array. And in Chapter 12, you group things together to form a collection. In this chapter, you group things into an `enum` type. (Of course, you can't group anything unless you can pronounce `enum`. The word *enum* is pronounced "ee-noom," like the first two syllables of the word *enumeration*.)

Creating a complicated `enum` type isn't easy, but to create a simple `enum` type, just write a bunch of words inside a pair of curly braces. Listing 9-1 defines an `enum` type. The name of the `enum` type is `TempScale`.

LISTING 9-1: The TempScale Type (an enum Type)

```
public enum TempScale {
    CELSIUS, FAHRENHEIT, KELVIN, RANKINE,
    NEWTON, DELISLE, RÉAUMUR, RØMER, LEIDEN
}
```

WARNING

In Listing 9-1, I'm showing off my physics prowess by naming not two, not four, but *nine* different temperature scales. Some readers' computers have trouble with the special characters in the words `RÉAUMUR` and `RØMER`. If you're one of those readers, simply delete the words `RÉAUMUR` and `RØMER` from the code. I promise: It won't mess up the example.

When you define an enum type, two important things happen:

- **You create values.**

  Just as 13 and 151 are int values, CELSIUS and FAHRENHEIT are TempScale values.

- **You can create variables to refer to those values.**

  In Listing 9-2, I declare the fields number and scale. Just as

  ```
  double number;
  ```

  declares that a number variable is of type double,

  ```
  TempScale scale;
  ```

  declares variable scale to be of type TempScale.

  "To be of type TempScale" means that you can have values CELSIUS, FAHRENHEIT, KELVIN, and so on. So, in Listing 9-2, I can give the scale variable the value FAHRENHEIT (or TempScale.FAHRENHEIT, to be more precise).

TECHNICAL STUFF

An enum type is a Java class in disguise. That's why Listing 9-1 contains an entire file devoted to one thing; namely, the declaration of an enum type (the TempScale type). Like the declaration of a class, an enum type declaration belongs in a file all its own. The code in Listing 9-1 belongs in a file named TempScale.java.

Okay, so then what is a temperature?

Each temperature consists of two things: a number and a temperature scale. The code in Listing 9-2 makes this fact abundantly clear.

LISTING 9-2: The Temperature Class

```
public class Temperature {
    private double number;

    private TempScale scale;

    public Temperature() {
        number = 0.0;
        scale = TempScale.FAHRENHEIT;
    }
```

```
    public Temperature(double number) {
        this.number = number;
        scale = TempScale.FAHRENHEIT;
    }

    public Temperature(TempScale scale) {
        number = 0.0;
        this.scale = scale;
    }

    public Temperature(double number, TempScale scale) {
        this.number = number;
        this.scale = scale;
    }

    public void setNumber(double number) {
        this.number = number;
    }

    public double getNumber() {
        return number;
    }

    public void setScale(TempScale scale) {
        this.scale = scale;
    }

    public TempScale getScale() {
        return scale;
    }
}
```

The code in Listing 9-2 has the usual setter and getter methods (accessor methods for the `number` and `scale` fields).

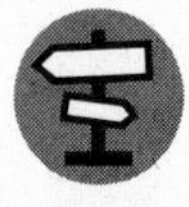

CROSS REFERENCE

For some good reading on setter and getter methods (also known as accessor methods), see Chapter 7.

On top of all of that, Listing 9-2 has four other method-like-looking things. Each of these method-like things has the name `Temperature`, which happens to be the same as the name of the class. None of these `Temperature` method-like things has a `return` type of any kind — not even `void`, which is the cop-out `return` type.

Each of these method-like things is called a *constructor*. A constructor is like a method, except that a constructor has a special purpose: to create new objects.

REMEMBER

Whenever the computer creates a new object, the computer executes the statements inside a constructor.

You can omit the word `public` in the first lines of Listings 9-1 and 9-2. If you omit `public`, other Java programs might not be able to use the features defined in the `TempScale` type and in the `Temperature` class. (Don't worry about the programs in this chapter: With or without the word `public`, all programs in this chapter can use the code in Listings 9-1 and 9-2. To find out which Java programs can use classes that aren't public, see Chapter 14.) If you *do* use the word `public` in the first line of Listing 9-1, Listing 9-1 *must* be in a file named `TempScale.java`, starting with a capital letter `T`. And if you *do* use the word `public` in the first line of Listing 9-2, Listing 9-2 *must* be in a file named `Temperature.java`, starting with a capital letter `T`. (For an introduction to public classes, see Chapter 7.)

What you can do with a temperature

Listing 9-3 gives form to some of the ideas that I describe in the preceding section. In Listing 9-3, you call the constructors that are declared back in Listing 9-2. Figure 9-1 shows what happens when you run all this code.

```
70.00 degrees FAHRENHEIT
32.00 degrees FAHRENHEIT
 0.00 degrees CELSIUS
 2.73 degrees KELVIN
```

FIGURE 9-1: Running the code from Listing 9-3.

LISTING 9-3: Using the Temperature Class

```
import static java.lang.System.out;

public class UseTemperature {

   public static void main(String args[]) {
      final String format = "%5.2f degrees %s\n";

      Temperature temp = new Temperature();
      temp.setNumber(70.0);
      temp.setScale(TempScale.FAHRENHEIT);
      out.printf(format, temp.getNumber(), temp.getScale());

      temp = new Temperature(32.0);
      out.printf(format, temp.getNumber(), temp.getScale());
```

```
        temp = new Temperature(TempScale.CELSIUS);
        out.printf(format, temp.getNumber(), temp.getScale());

        temp = new Temperature(2.73, TempScale.KELVIN);
        out.printf(format, temp.getNumber(), temp.getScale());
    }
}
```

In Listing 9-3, each statement of the kind

```
temp = new Temperature(blah,blah,blah);
```

calls one of the constructors from Listing 9-2. So, by the time the code in Listing 9-3 is done running, it creates four instances of the `Temperature` class. Each instance is created by calling a different constructor from Listing 9-2.

In Listing 9-3, the last of the four constructor calls has two parameters: `2.73` and `TempScale.KELVIN`. This isn't particular to constructor calls. A method call or a constructor call can have a bunch of parameters. You separate one parameter from another with a comma. Another name for "a bunch of parameters" is a *parameter list*.

The only rule you must follow is to match the parameters in the call with the parameters in the declaration. For example, in Listing 9-3, the fourth and last constructor call

```
new Temperature(2.73, TempScale.KELVIN)
```

has two parameters: the first of type `double` and the second of type `TempScale`. Java approves of this constructor call because Listing 9-2 contains a matching declaration. That is, the header

```
public Temperature(double number, TempScale scale)
```

has two parameters: the first of type `double` and the second of type `TempScale`. If a `Temperature` constructor call in Listing 9-3 had no matching declaration in Listing 9-2, Listing 9-3 would crash and burn. (To state things more politely, Java would display errors when you tried to compile the code in Listing 9-3.)

By the way, this business about multiple parameters isn't new. Over in Chapter 6, I write `keyboard.findWithinHorizon(".",0).charAt(0)`. In that line, the method call `findWithinHorizon(".",0)` has two parameters: a string and an `int` value. Luckily for me, the Java API has a method declaration for `findWithinHorizon` — a declaration whose first parameter is a string and whose second parameter is an `int` value.

HOW TO CHEAT: ENUM TYPES AND SWITCH STATEMENTS

Listings 9-2 and 9-3 contain long-winded names such as `TempScale.FAHRENHEIT` and `TempScale.CELSIUS`. Names such as `FAHRENHEIT` and `CELSIUS` belong to my `TempScale` type (the type defined in Listing 9-1). These names have no meaning outside of my `TempScale` context. (If you think I'm being egotistical with this "no meaning outside of my context" remark, try deleting the `TempScale.` part of `TempScale.FAHRENHEIT` in Listing 9-2. Suddenly, Java tells you that your code contains an error.)

Java is normally fussy about type names and dots. But when they created enum types, the makers of Java decided that enum types and `switch` statements deserved special treatment. You can use an enum value to decide which case to execute in a `switch` statement. When you do this, you don't use the enum type name in the case expressions. For example, the following Java code is correct:

```
TempScale scale = TempScale.RANKINE;
char letter;
switch (scale) {
case CELSIUS:
    letter = 'C';
    break;
case KELVIN:
    letter = 'K';
    break;
case RANKINE:
case RÉAUMUR:
case RØMER:
    letter = 'R';
    break;
default:
    letter = 'X';
    break;
}
```

In the first line of code, I write `TempScale.RANKINE` because this first line isn't inside a `switch` statement. But in the next several lines of code, I write `case CELSIUS`, `case KELVIN`, and `case RANKINE` without the word `TempScale`. In fact, if I create a case clause by writing `case TempScale.RANKINE`, Java complains with a loud, obnoxious error message.

Calling new Temperature(32.0): A case study

When the computer executes one of the `new Temperature` statements in Listing 9-3, the computer has to decide which of the constructors in Listing 9-2 to use. The computer decides by looking at the parameter list — the stuff in parentheses after the words `new Temperature`. For instance, when the computer executes

```
temp = new Temperature(32.0);
```

from Listing 9-3, the computer says to itself, "The number 32.0 in parentheses is a `double` value. One of the `Temperature` constructors in Listing 9-2 has just one parameter with type `double`. The constructor's header looks like this:

```
public Temperature(double number)
```

"So, I guess I'll execute the statements inside that particular constructor." The computer goes on to execute the following statements:

```
this.number = number;
scale = TempScale.FAHRENHEIT;
```

As a result, you get a brand-new object whose `number` field has the value `32.0` and whose `scale` field has the value `TempScale.FAHRENHEIT`.

In the two lines of code, you have two statements that set values for the fields `number` and `scale`. Take a look at the second of these statements, which is a bit easier to understand. The second statement sets the new object's `scale` field to `TempScale.FAHRENHEIT`. You see, the constructor's parameter list is `(double number)`, and that list doesn't include a `scale` value. So whoever programmed this code had to make a decision about what value to use for the `scale` field. The programmer could have chosen `FAHRENHEIT` or `CELSIUS`, but she could also have chosen `KELVIN`, `RANKINE`, or any of the other obscure scales named in Listing 9-1. (This programmer happens to live in New Jersey, in the United States, where people commonly use the old Fahrenheit temperature scale.)

Marching back to the first of the two statements, this first statement assigns a value to the new object's `number` field. The statement uses a cute trick that you can see in many constructors (and in other methods that assign values to objects' fields). To understand the trick, take a look at Listing 9-4. The listing shows you two ways that I could have written the same constructor code.

LISTING 9-4: Two Ways to Accomplish the Same Thing

```
//Use this constructor ...

    public Temperature(double whatever) {
        number = whatever;
        scale = TempScale.FAHRENHEIT;
    }

//... or use this constructor ...

    public Temperature(double number) {
        this.number = number;
        scale = TempScale.FAHRENHEIT;
    }

//... but don't put both constructors in your code.
```

Listing 9-4 has two constructors in it. In the first constructor, I use two different names: `number` and `whatever`. In the second constructor, I don't need two names. Rather than make up a new name for the constructor's parameter, I reuse an existing name by writing `this.number`.

Here's what's going on in Listing 9-2:

- In the statement `this.number = number`, the name *this.number* refers to the new object's `number` field — the field that's declared near the top of Listing 9-2. (See Figure 9-2.)

  In the statement `this.number = number`, *number* (on its own, without `this`) refers to the constructor's parameter. (Again, see Figure 9-2.)

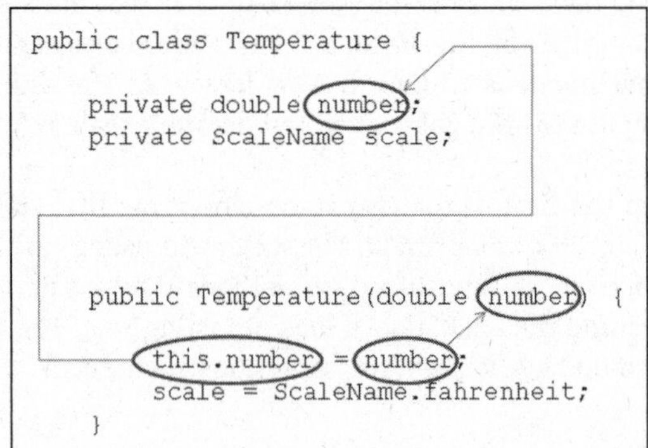

FIGURE 9-2: What `this.number` and `number` mean.

WHAT'S THIS ALL ABOUT?

Suppose your code contains a constructor — the first of the two constructors in Listing 9-4. The `whatever` parameter is passed a number like 32.0, for instance. Then the first statement in the constructor's body assigns that value, `32.0`, to the new object's `number` field. The code works. But in writing this code, you had to make up a new name for a parameter — the name *whatever*. And the only purpose for this new name is to hand a value to the object's `number` field. What a waste! To distinguish between the parameter and the `number` field, you gave a name to something that was just momentary storage for the `number` value.

Making up names is an art, not a science. I've gone through plenty of naming phases. Years ago, whenever I needed a new name for a parameter, I picked a confusing misspelling of the original variable name. (I'd name the parameter something like `numbr` or `nuhmber`.) I've also tried changing a variable name's capitalization to come up with a parameter name. (I'd use parameter names like `Number` or `nUMBER`.) In Chapter 8, I name all my parameters by adding the suffix *In* to their corresponding variable names. (The `jobTitle` variable matched up with the `jobTitleIn` parameter.) None of these naming schemes works well — I can never remember the quirky new names that I've created. The good news is that this parameter-naming effort isn't necessary. You can give the parameter the same name as the variable. To distinguish between the two, you use the Java keyword `this`.

In general, `this.`*`someName`* refers to a field belonging to the object that contains the code. In contrast, plain old *`someName`* refers to the closest place where *`someName`* happens to be declared. In the statement `this.number = number` (refer to Listing 9-2), that closest place happens to be the `Temperature` constructor's parameter list.

Some things never change

Chapter 7 introduces the `printf` method and explains that each `printf` call starts with a format string. The format string describes the way the other parameters are to be displayed.

In previous examples, this format string is always a quoted literal. For instance, the first `printf` call in Listing 7-7 (see Chapter 7) is

```
out.printf("$%4.2f\n", myInterest);
```

In Listing 9-3, I break with tradition and begin the `printf` call with a variable that I name *format.*

```
out.printf(format, temp.getNumber(), temp.getScale());
```

That's okay as long as my `format` variable is of type `String`. And indeed, in Listing 9-3, the first variable declaration is

```
final String format = "%5.2f degrees %s\n";
```

In this declaration of the `format` variable, take special note of the word `final`. This Java keyword indicates that the value of `format` can't be changed. If I add another assignment statement to Listing 9-3

```
format = "%6.2f (%s)\n";
```

the compiler barks back at me with the message `cannot assign a value to final variable`.

When I write the code in Listing 9-3, the use of the `final` keyword isn't absolutely necessary. But the `final` keyword provides some extra protection. When I initialize `format` to `"%5.2f degrees %s\n"`, I intend to use this same format just as it is, over and over again. I know darn well that I don't intend to change the `format` variable's value. Of course, in a 10,000-line program, I can become confused and try to assign a new value to `format` somewhere deep down in the code. To prevent me from accidentally changing the `format` string, I declare the `format` variable to be final. It's just good, safe programming practice.

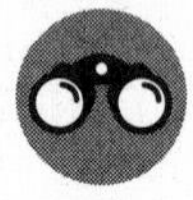

TRY IT OUT

There's always more stuff for you to try.

- Create a `Student` class with a name, an ID number, a grade point average (GPA), and a major area of study. The student's name is a `String`. The student's ID number is an `int` value. The GPA is a `double` value between 0.0 and 4.0. The `Major` is an enum type, with values such as `COMPUTER_SCIENCE`, `MATHEMATICS`, `LITERATURE`, `PHYSICS`, and `HISTORY`.

  Every student has a name and an ID number, but a brand-new student might not have a GPA or a major. Create constructors with and without GPA and `Major` parameters.

  As usual, create a separate class that makes use of your new `Student` class.

- Create an `AirplaneFlight` class with a flight number, a departure airport, the time of departure, an arrival airport, and a time of arrival. The flight number is an `int` value. The departure and arrival airport fields belong to an `Airport` enum type, with values corresponding to some of the official IATA airport codes. (For example, London Heathrow Airport's code is LHR; Los Angeles International Airport's code is LAX; check out `http://www.iata.org/publications/Pages/code-search.aspx` for a searchable database of airline codes.)

For the times of arrival and departure, use Java's `LocalTime` class. (For more on `LocalTime`, check out the `LocalTime` documents page at `https://docs.oracle.com/javase/8/docs/api/java/time/LocalTime.html`.) To create a `LocalTime` object that's set to 2:15 PM (also known as 14:15), execute

```
LocalTime twoFifteen = LocalTime.of(14, 15);
```

To create a `LocalTime` object that's set to the current time (according to the computer's system clock), execute

```
LocalTime currentTime = LocalTime.now();
```

Every flight has a number, a departure airport, and an arrival airport. But some flights might not have departure and arrival times. Create constructors with and without departure and arrival time parameters.

Create a separate class that makes use of your new `AirplaneFlight` class.

More Subclasses (Doing Something about the Weather)

In Chapter 8, I make a big fuss over the notion of subclasses. That's the right thing to do. Subclasses make code reusable, and reusable code is good code. With that in mind, it's time to create a subclass of the `Temperature` class (which I develop in this chapter's first section).

Building better temperatures

After perusing the code in Listing 9-3, you decide that the responsibility for displaying temperatures has been seriously misplaced. Listing 9-3 has several tedious repetitions of the lines to print temperature values. A 1970s programmer would tell you to collect those lines into one place and turn them into a method. (The 1970s programmer wouldn't have used the word *method*, but that's not important right now.) Collecting lines into methods is fine, but with today's object-oriented programming methodology, you think in broader terms. Why not get each `temperature` object to take responsibility for displaying itself? After all, if you develop a display method, you probably want to share the method with other people who use temperatures. So put the method right inside the declaration of a temperature object. That way, anyone who uses the code for temperatures has easy access to your display method.

Now replay the tape from Chapter 8. "Blah, blah, blah . . . don't want to modify existing code . . . blah, blah, blah . . . too costly to start again from scratch . . . blah, blah, blah . . . extend existing functionality." It all adds up to one thing:

> Don't abuse it. Instead, reuse it.

So you decide to create a subclass of the Temperature class — the class defined in Listing 9-2. Your new subclass complements the Temperature class's functionality by having methods to display values in a nice, uniform fashion. The new class, TemperatureNice, is shown in Listing 9-5.

LISTING 9-5: The TemperatureNice Class

```
import static java.lang.System.out;

public class TemperatureNice extends Temperature {

    public TemperatureNice() {
        super();
    }

    public TemperatureNice(double number) {
        super(number);
    }

    public TemperatureNice(TempScale scale) {
        super(scale);
    }

    public TemperatureNice(double number, TempScale scale) {
        super(number, scale);
    }

    public void display() {
        out.printf("%5.2f degrees %s\n", getNumber(), getScale());
    }
}
```

In the display method of Listing 9-5, notice the calls to the Temperature class's getNumber and getScale methods. Why do I do this? Well, inside the

TemperatureNice class's code, any direct references to the number and scale fields would generate error messages. It's true that every TemperatureNice object has its own number and scale fields. (After all, TemperatureNice is a subclass of the Temperature class, and the code for the Temperature class defines the number and scale fields.) But because number and scale are declared to be private inside the Temperature class, only code that's right inside the Temperature class can directly use these fields.

Don't put additional declarations of the number and scale fields inside the TemperatureNice class's code. If you do, you inadvertently create four different variables (two called number and another two called scale). You'll assign values to one pair of variables. Then you'll be shocked that when you display the other pair of variables, those values seem to have disappeared.

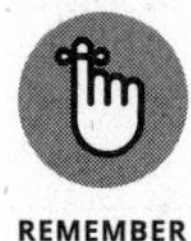

When an object's code contains a call to one of the object's own methods, you don't need to preface the call with a dot. For instance, in the last statement of Listing 9-5, the object calls its own methods with getNumber() and getScale(), not with *someObject*.getNumber() and somethingOrOther.getScale(). If going dotless makes you queasy, you can compensate by taking advantage of yet another use for the this keyword: Just write this.getNumber() and this.getScale() in the last line of Listing 9-5.

Constructors for subclasses

By far, the biggest news in Listing 9-5 is the way the code declares constructors. The TemperatureNice class has four of its own constructors. If you've gotten in gear thinking about subclass inheritance, you may wonder why these constructor declarations are necessary. Doesn't TemperatureNice inherit the parent Temperature class's constructors? No, subclasses don't inherit constructors.

Subclasses don't inherit constructors.

That's right. Subclasses don't inherit constructors. In one oddball case, a constructor may look like it's being inherited, but that oddball situation is a fluke, not the norm. In general, when you define a subclass, you declare new constructors to go with the subclass.

I describe the oddball case (in which a constructor looks like it's being inherited) later in this chapter, in the section "The default constructor."

So the code in Listing 9-5 has four constructors. Each constructor has the name TemperatureNice, and each constructor has its own uniquely identifiable parameter list. That's the boring part. The interesting part is that each constructor makes a call to something named super, which is a Java keyword.

In Listing 9-5, `super` stands for a constructor in the parent class:

- The statement `super()` in Listing 9-5 calls the parameterless `Temperature()` constructor that's in Listing 9-2. That parameterless constructor assigns `0.0` to the `number` field and `TempScale.FAHRENHEIT` to the `scale` field.
- The statement `super(number, scale)` in Listing 9-5 calls the constructor `Temperature(double number, TempScale scale)` that's in Listing 9-2. In turn, the constructor assigns values to the `number` and `scale` fields.
- In a similar way, the statements `super(number)` and `super(scale)` in Listing 9-5 call constructors from Listing 9-2.

The computer decides which of the `Temperature` class's constructors is being called by looking at the parameter list after the word `super`. For instance, when the computer executes

```
super(number, scale);
```

from Listing 9-5, the computer says to itself, "The `number` and `scale` fields in parentheses have types `double` and `TempScale`. But only one of the `Temperature` constructors in Listing 9-2 has two parameters with types `double` and `TempScale`. The constructor's header looks like this:

```
public Temperature(double number, TempScale scale)
```

"So, I guess I'll execute the statements inside that particular constructor."

Using all this stuff

In Listing 9-5, I define what it means to be in the `TemperatureNice` class. Now it's time to put this `TemperatureNice` class to good use. Listing 9-6 has code that uses `TemperatureNice`.

LISTING 9-6: Using the TemperatureNice Class

```
public class UseTemperatureNice {

    public static void main(String args[]) {

        TemperatureNice temp = new TemperatureNice();
        temp.setNumber(70.0);
        temp.setScale(TempScale.FAHRENHEIT);
        temp.display();
```

```
        temp = new TemperatureNice(32.0);
        temp.display();

        temp = new TemperatureNice(TempScale.CELSIUS);
        temp.display();

        temp = new TemperatureNice(2.73, TempScale.KELVIN);
        temp.display();
    }
}
```

The code in Listing 9-6 is much like its cousin code in Listing 9-3. The big differences are as follows:

- Listing 9-6 creates instances of the `TemperatureNice` class. That is, Listing 9-6 calls constructors from the `TemperatureNice` class, not the `Temperature` class.
- Listing 9-6 takes advantage of the `display` method in the `TemperatureNice` class. So the code in Listing 9-6 is much tidier than its counterpart in Listing 9-3.

A run of Listing 9-6 looks exactly like a run of the code in Listing 9-3 — it just gets to the finish line in a far more elegant fashion. (The run is shown previously in Figure 9-1.)

The default constructor

The main message in the previous section is that subclasses don't inherit constructors. So what gives with all the listings over in Chapter 8? In Listing 8-6, a statement says

```
FullTimeEmployee ftEmployee = new FullTimeEmployee();
```

But, here's the problem: The code defining `FullTimeEmployee` (refer to Listing 8-3) doesn't seem to have any constructors declared inside it. So, in Listing 8-6, how can you possibly call the `FullTimeEmployee` constructor?

Here's what's going on. When you create a subclass and don't put any explicit constructor declarations in your code, Java creates one constructor for you. It's called a *default constructor.* If you're creating the `public FullTimeEmployee` subclass, the default constructor looks like the one in Listing 9-7.

LISTING 9-7: A Default Constructor

```
public FullTimeEmployee() {
    super();
}
```

The constructor in Listing 9-7 takes no parameters, and its one statement calls the constructor of whatever class you're extending. (Woe be to you if the class that you're extending doesn't have a parameterless constructor.)

You've just read about default constructors, but watch out! Notice one thing that this talk about default constructors *doesn't* say: It doesn't say that you always get a default constructor. In particular, if you create a subclass and define any constructors yourself, Java doesn't add a default constructor for the subclass (and the subclass doesn't inherit any constructors, either).

So how can this trip you up? Listing 9-8 has a copy of the code from Listing 8-3, but with one constructor added to it. Take a look at this modified version of the `FullTimeEmployee` code.

LISTING 9-8: Look, I Have a Constructor!

```
public class FullTimeEmployee extends Employee {
    private double weeklySalary;
    private double benefitDeduction;

    public FullTimeEmployee(double weeklySalary) {
        this.weeklySalary = weeklySalary;
    }

    public void setWeeklySalary(double weeklySalaryIn) {
        weeklySalary = weeklySalaryIn;
    }

    public double getWeeklySalary() {
        return weeklySalary;
    }

    public void setBenefitDeduction(double benefitDedIn) {
        benefitDeduction = benefitDedIn;
    }

    public double getBenefitDeduction() {
        return benefitDeduction;
    }
```

```
    public double findPaymentAmount() {
        return weeklySalary - benefitDeduction;
    }
}
```

If you use the `FullTimeEmployee` code in Listing 9-8, a line like the following doesn't work:

```
FullTimeEmployee ftEmployee = new FullTimeEmployee();
```

It doesn't work because, having declared a `FullTimeEmployee` constructor that takes one `double` parameter, you no longer get a default parameterless constructor for free.

What do you do about this? If you declare any constructors, declare all constructors that you'll possibly need. Take the constructor in Listing 9-7 and add it to the code in Listing 9-8. Then the call `new FullTimeEmployee()` starts working again.

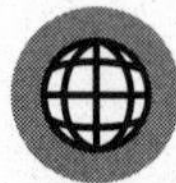

Under certain circumstances, Java automatically adds an invisible call to a parent class's constructor at the top of a constructor body. This automatic addition of a `super` call is a tricky bit of business that doesn't appear often, so when it does appear, it may seem quite mysterious. For more information, see this book's website (`www.allmycode.com/JavaForDummies`).

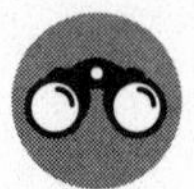

TRY IT OUT

In this section, I have three (count 'em — *three*) things for you to try:

- In a previous section, you create your own `Student` class. Create a subclass that has a method named `getString`.

  Like the `display` method in this chapter's `TemperatureNice` class, the `getString` method creates a nice-looking `String` representation of its object. But unlike the `TemperatureNice` class's `display` method, the `getString` method doesn't print that `String` representation on the screen. Instead, the `getString` method simply returns that `String` representation as its result.

  In a way, a `getString` method is much more versatile than a `display` method. With a `display` method, all you can do is show a `String` representation on the screen. But with a `getString` method, you can create a `String` representation and then do whatever you want with it.

  Create a separate class that creates some instances of your new subclass and puts their `getString` methods to good use.

- In a previous section, you create your own `AirplaneFlight` class. Create a subclass that has a method named `duration`. The `duration` method, which has no parameters, returns the amount of time between the flight's departure time and arrival time.

  To find the number of hours between two `LocalTime` objects (such as `twoFifteen` and `currentTime`), execute

  ```
  long hours = ChronoUnit.HOURS.between(twoFifteen, currentTime);
  ```

  To find the number of minutes between two `LocalTime` objects (such as `twoFifteen` and `currentTime`), execute

  ```
  long minutes = ChronoUnit.MINUTES.between(twoFifteen, currentTime);
  ```

- Create a new `TemperatureEvenNicer` class — a subclass of this section's `TemperatureNice` class. The `TemperatureEvenNicer` class has a `convertTo` method. If the variable `temp` refers to a Fahrenheit temperature and Java executes

  ```
  temp.convertTo(TempScale.CELSIUS);
  ```

  then the `temp` object changes to a Celsius temperature, with the number converted appropriately. The same kind of thing happens if Java executes

  ```
  temp.convertTo(TempScale.FAHRENHEIT);
  ```

  with `temp` already referring to a Celsius temperature.

A Constructor That Does More

Here's a quote from somewhere near the start of this chapter: "And what if you're interested in doing more than filling fields? Perhaps, when the computer creates a new object, you have a whole list of jobs for the computer to carry out." Okay, what if?

This section's example has a constructor that does more than just assign values to fields. The example is in Listings 9-9 and 9-10. The result of running the example's code is shown in Figure 9-3.

LISTING 9-9: Defining a Frame

```
import java.awt.FlowLayout;
import javax.swing.JFrame;
import javax.swing.JButton;

@SuppressWarnings("serial")
public class SimpleFrame extends JFrame {

    public SimpleFrame() {
        setTitle("Don't click the button!");
        setLayout(new FlowLayout());
        setDefaultCloseOperation(EXIT_ON_CLOSE);
        add(new JButton("Panic"));
        setSize(300, 100);
        setVisible(true);
    }
}
```

LISTING 9-10: Displaying a Frame

```
public class ShowAFrame {

    public static void main(String args[]) {
        new SimpleFrame();
    }
}
```

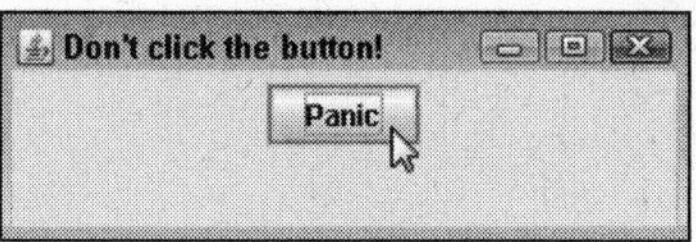

FIGURE 9-3: Don't panic.

Like my `DummiesFrame` examples, the code in Listings 9-9 and 9-10 displays a window on the computer screen. But unlike my `DummiesFrame` examples, all the method calls in Listings 9-9 and 9-10 refer to methods in Java's standard API (Application Programming Interface).

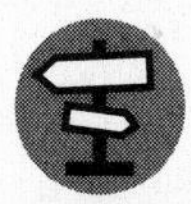

CROSS REFERENCE

To find my `DummiesFrame` examples, refer to Chapter 7.

The code in Listing 9-9 contains lots of names that are probably unfamiliar to you — names from Java's API. When I was first becoming acquainted with Java, I foolishly believed that knowing Java meant remembering all these names. Quite the contrary: These names are just carry-on baggage. The real Java is the way the language implements object-oriented concepts.

PACKAGES AND IMPORT DECLARATIONS

Java has a feature that lets you lump classes into groups of classes. Each lump of classes is called a *package*. In the Java world, programmers customarily give these packages long, dot-filled names. For instance, because I've registered the domain name *allmycode.com,* I may name a package `com.allmycode.utils.textUtils`. The Java API is actually a big collection of packages. The API has packages with names like `java.lang`, `java.util`, `java.awt`, and `javax.swing`.

With this information about packages, I can clear up some of the confusion about `import` declarations. Any `import` declaration that doesn't use the word `static` must start with the name of a package and must end with either of the following:

- The name of a class within that package
- An asterisk (indicating all classes within that package)

For example, the declaration

```
import java.util.Scanner;
```

is valid because `java.util` is the name of a package in the Java API, and `Scanner` is the name of a class in the `java.util` package. The dotted name `java.util.Scanner` is called the *fully qualified name* of the `Scanner` class. A class's fully qualified name includes the name of the package in which the class is defined. (You can find out all this stuff about `java.util` and `Scanner` by reading Java's API documentation. For tips on reading the documentation, see Chapter 3 and this book's website.)

Here's another example. The declaration

```
import javax.swing.*;
```

is valid because `javax.swing` is the name of a package in the Java API, and the asterisk refers to all classes in the `javax.swing` package. With this import declaration at the top of your Java code, you can use abbreviated names for classes in the `javax.swing` package — names like `JFrame`, `JButton`, `JMenuBar`, `JCheckBox`, and many others.

Here's one more example. A line like

```
import javax.*; //Bad!!
```

is *not* a valid `import` declaration. The Java API has no package with the one-word name `javax`. You may think that this line allows you to abbreviate all names beginning with `javax` (names like `javax.swing.JFrame`, and `javax.sound.midi`), but that's not the way the `import` declaration works. Because `javax` isn't the name of a package, the line `import javax.*` just angers the Java compiler.

Anyway, Listing 9-10's main method has only one statement: a call to the constructor in the `SimpleFrame` class. Notice how the object that this call creates isn't even assigned to a variable. That's okay because the code doesn't need to refer to the object anywhere else.

Up in the `SimpleFrame` class, there's only one constructor declaration. Far from just setting variables' values, this constructor calls method after method from the Java API.

All the methods called in the `SimpleFrame` class's constructor come from the parent class, `JFrame`. The `JFrame` class lives in the `javax.swing` package. This package and another package, `java.awt`, have classes that help you put windows, images, drawings, and other gizmos on a computer screen. (In the `java.awt` package, the letters *awt* stand for *a*bstract *w*indowing *t*oolkit.)

For a little gossip about the notion of a Java package, see the nearby sidebar, "Packages and import declarations." For lots of gossip about the notion of a Java package, see Chapter 14.

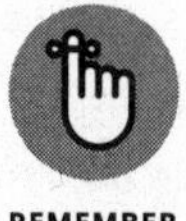
REMEMBER

In the Java API, what people normally call a *window* is an instance of the `javax.swing.JFrame` class.

Classes and methods from the Java API

Looking at Figure 9-3, you can probably tell that an instance of the `SimpleFrame` class doesn't do much. The frame has only one button, and when you click the button, nothing happens. I made the frame this way to keep the example from becoming too complicated. Even so, the code in Listing 9-9 uses several API classes and methods. The `setTitle`, `setLayout`, `setDefaultCloseOperation`, `add`, `setSize`, and `setVisible` methods all belong to the `javax.swing.JFrame` class. Here's a list of names used in the code:

- `setTitle`: Calling `setTitle` puts words in the frame's title bar. (The new `SimpleFrame` object is calling its own `setTitle` method.)
- `FlowLayout`: An instance of the `FlowLayout` class positions objects on the frame in a centered, typewriter fashion. Because the frame in Figure 9-3 has only one button on it, that button is centered near the top of the frame. If the frame had eight buttons, five of them may be lined up in a row across the top of the frame and the remaining three would be centered along a second row.
- `setLayout`: Calling `setLayout` puts the new `FlowLayout` object in charge of arranging components, such as buttons, on the frame. (The new `SimpleFrame` object is calling its own `setLayout` method.)

- setDefaultCloseOperation: Calling setDefaultCloseOperation tells Java what to do when you click the little × in the frame's upper-right corner. (On a Mac, you click the little red circle in the frame's upper-left corner.) Without this method call, the frame itself disappears, but the Java Virtual Machine (JVM) keeps running. To stop your program's run, you have to perform one more step. (You may have to look for a Terminate option in Eclipse, IntelliJ IDEA, or NetBeans.)

  Calling setDefaultCloseOperation(EXIT_ON_CLOSE) tells Java to shut itself down when you click the × in the frame's upper-right corner. The alternatives to EXIT_ON_CLOSE are HIDE_ON_CLOSE, DISPOSE_ON_CLOSE, and, my personal favorite, DO_NOTHING_ON_CLOSE. Use one of these alternatives when your program has more work to do after the user closes your frame.

- JButton: The JButton class lives in the javax.swing package. One of the class's constructors takes a String instance (such as "Panic") for its parameter. Calling this constructor makes that String instance into the label on the face of the new button.

- add: The new SimpleFrame object calls its add method. Calling the add method places the button on the object's surface (in this case, the surface of the frame).

- setSize: The frame becomes 300 pixels wide and 100 pixels tall. (In the javax.swing package, whenever you specify two dimension numbers, the width number always comes before the height number.)

- setVisible: When it's first created, a new frame is invisible. But when the new frame calls setVisible(true), the frame appears on your computer screen.

The SuppressWarnings annotation

Chapter 8 introduces the annotation — extra code that provides useful information about the nature of your program. In particular, Chapter 8 describes the Override annotation.

In this chapter, Listing 9-9 introduces another type of annotation: the SuppressWarnings annotation. When you use a SuppressWarnings annotation, you tell Java not to remind you that your program contains certain questionable code. In Listing 9-9, the line @SuppressWarnings("serial") tells Java not to remind you that you've omitted something called a serialVersionUID field. In other words, the SuppressWarnings annotation tells Java not to display a warning like the one in Figure 9-4.

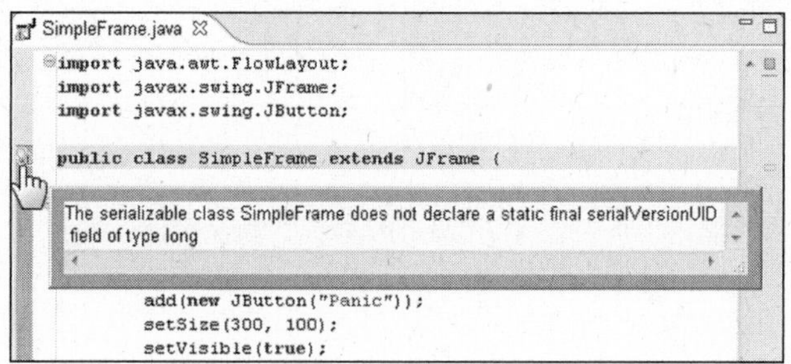

SimpleFrame.java
import java.awt.FlowLayout;
import javax.swing.JFrame;
import javax.swing.JButton;
public class SimpleFrame extends JFrame {
The serializable class SimpleFrame does not declare a static final serialVersionUID field of type long
add(new JButton("Panic"));
setSize(300, 100);
setVisible(true);

FIGURE 9-4: Without a Suppress Warnings annotation, Java warns you about a missing serialVersion UID field.

"And what," you ask, "is a `serialVersionUID` field?" It's something having to do with extending the `JFrame` class — something that you don't care about. Not having a `serialVersionUID` field generates a warning, not an error. So live dangerously! Just suppress the warning (with the annotation in Listing 9-9) and don't worry about `serialVersionUID` fields.

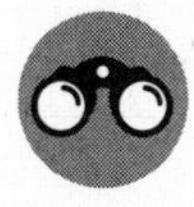

TRY IT OUT

- In JShell, type the following sequence of declarations and statements. What happens? Why?

```
jshell> import javax.swing.JFrame

jshell> JFrame frame

jshell> frame.setSize(100, 100)

jshell> frame = new JFrame()

jshell> frame.setSize(100, 100)

jshell> frame.setVisible(true)
```

- In Listing 9-9, change the statement

```
setLayout(new FlowLayout());
```

to

```
setLayout(new BorderLayout());
```

What difference does this change make when you run the program?

4 Smart Java Techniques

IN THIS PART . . .

Decide where declarations belong in your Java program.

Deal with bunches of things (bunches of rooms, bunches of sales, and even bunches of bunches).

Fully embrace Java's object-oriented features.

Create a windowed app and respond to mouse clicks.

Talk to your favorite database.

» Putting variables inside and outside methods

» Improving your batting average

Chapter 10
Putting Variables and Methods Where They Belong

Hello, again. You're listening to radio station WWW, and I'm your host, Sam Burd. It's the start again of the big baseball season, and today station WWW brought you live coverage of the Hankees-versus-Socks game. At this moment, I'm awaiting news of the game's final score.

If you remember from earlier this afternoon, the Socks looked like they were going to take those Hankees to the cleaners. Then, the Hankees were belting ball after ball, giving the Socks a run for their money. Those Socks! I'm glad I wasn't in their shoes.

Anyway, as the game went on, the Socks pulled themselves up. Now the Socks are nose-to-nose with the Hankees. We'll get the final score in a minute, but first, a few reminders. Stay tuned after this broadcast for the big Jersey's game. And don't forget to tune in next week when the Cleveland Gowns play the Bermuda Shorts.

Okay, here's the final score. Which team has the upper hand? Which team will come out a head? And the winner is . . . oh, no — it's a tie!

Defining a Class (What It Means to Be a Baseball Player)

As far as I'm concerned, a baseball player has a name and a batting average. Listing 10-1 puts my feeling about this into Java program form.

LISTING 10-1: The Player Class

```
import java.text.DecimalFormat;

public class Player {
  private String name;
  private double average;

  public Player(String name, double average) {
    this.name = name;
    this.average = average;
  }

  public String getName() {
    return name;
  }

  public double getAverage() {
    return average;
  }

  public String getAverageString() {
    DecimalFormat decFormat = new DecimalFormat();
    decFormat.setMaximumIntegerDigits(0);
    decFormat.setMaximumFractionDigits(3);
    decFormat.setMinimumFractionDigits(3);
    return decFormat.format(average);
  }
}
```

Here I go, picking apart the code in Listing 10-1. Luckily, earlier chapters cover lots of stuff in this code. The code defines what it means to be an instance of the `Player` class. Here's what's in the code:

- **Declarations of the fields `name` and `average`:** For bedtime reading about field declarations, see Chapter 7.
- **A constructor to make new instances of the `Player` class:** For the lowdown on constructors, see Chapter 9.

- **Getter methods for the fields `name` and `average`:** For chitchat about accessor methods (that is, setter and getter methods), see Chapter 7.
- **A method that returns the player's batting average in `String` form:** For the good word about methods, see Chapter 7. (I put a lot of good stuff in Chapter 7, didn't I?)

Another way to beautify your numbers

The `getAverageString` method in Listing 10-1 takes the value from the `average` field (a player's batting average), converts that value (normally of type `double`) into a `String`, and then sends that `String` value right back to the method caller. The use of `DecimalFormat`, which comes right from the Java API (Application Programming Interface), ensures that the `String` value looks like a baseball player's batting average. According to the `decFormat.setMaximum ...` and `decFormat.setMinimum ...` method calls, the `String` value has no digits to the left of the decimal point and has exactly three digits to the right of the decimal point.

Java's `DecimalFormat` class can be quite handy. For example, to display the values `345` and `-345` in an accounting-friendly format, you can use the following code:

```
DecimalFormat decFormat = new DecimalFormat();
decFormat.setMinimumFractionDigits(2);
decFormat.setNegativePrefix("(");
decFormat.setNegativeSuffix(")");
System.out.println(decFormat.format(345));
System.out.println(decFormat.format(-345));
```

In this little example's format string, everything before the semicolon dictates the way positive numbers are displayed, and everything after the semicolon determines the way negative numbers are displayed. So, with this format, the numbers 345 and −345 appear as follows:

```
345.00
(345.00)
```

To discover some other tricks with numbers, visit the `DecimalFormat` page of Java's API documentation (`https://docs.oracle.com/javase/8/docs/api/java/text/DecimalFormat.html`).

Using the Player class

Listings 10-2 and 10-3 have code that uses the `Player` class — the class that's defined back in Listing 10-1.

LISTING 10-2: Using the Player Class

```
import java.util.Scanner;
import java.io.File;
import java.io.IOException;
import javax.swing.JFrame;
import javax.swing.JLabel;
import java.awt.GridLayout;

@SuppressWarnings("serial")
public class TeamFrame extends JFrame {

  public TeamFrame() throws IOException {
    Player player;
    Scanner hankeesData = new Scanner(new File("Hankees.txt"));

    for (int num = 1; num <= 9; num++) {
      player = new Player(hankeesData.nextLine(), hankeesData.nextDouble());
      hankeesData.nextLine();
      addPlayerInfo(player);
    }

    setTitle("The Hankees");
    setLayout(new GridLayout(9, 2, 20, 3));
    setDefaultCloseOperation(EXIT_ON_CLOSE);
    pack();
    setVisible(true);

    hankeesData.close();
  }

  void addPlayerInfo(Player player) {
    add(new JLabel("   " + player.getName()));
    add(new JLabel(player.getAverageString()));
  }
}
```

LISTING 10-3: Displaying a Frame

```
import java.io.IOException;

public class ShowTeamFrame {

  public static void main(String args[]) throws IOException {
    new TeamFrame();
  }
}
```

For a run of the code in Listings 10-1, 10-2, and 10-3, see Figure 10-1.

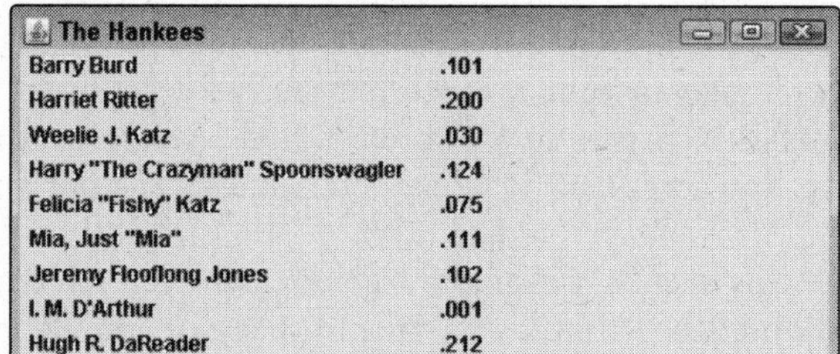

FIGURE 10-1: Would you bet money on these people?

To run this program yourself, you need the `Hankees.txt` file. This file contains data on your favorite baseball players. (See Figure 10-2.)

```
Barry Burd
.101
Harriet Ritter
.200
Weelie J. Katz
.030
Harry "The Crazyman" Spoonswagler
.124
Felicia "Fishy" Katz
.075
Mia, Just "Mia"
.111
Jeremy Flooflong Jones
.102
I. M. D'Arthur
.001
Hugh R. DaReader
.212
```

FIGURE 10-2: What a team!

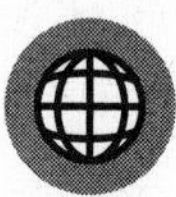

You don't have to create your own `Hankees.txt` file. The stuff that you download from this book's website comes with a `Hankees.txt` file, as shown in Figure 10-2. (Visit `www.allmycode.com/JavaForDummies`.)

WARNING

You may live in a country where the value of π is approximately 3,14159 (with a comma) instead of 3.14159 (with a period). If you do, the file shown in Figure 10-2 won't work for you. The program will crash with an `InputMismatchException`. To run this section's example, you have to change the periods in the `Hankees.txt` file into commas. Alternatively, you can add a statement such as `Locale.setDefault(Locale.US)` to your code. For details, see Chapter 8.

You must have the `Hankees.txt` file in a certain place on your hard drive. If you're using Eclipse, that "certain place" is a project directory within your Eclipse workspace. On the other hand, if you're running Java from the command line, that "place" may be the directory that contains the Listing 10-3 code. One way or another, you can't get away with not having the `Hankees.txt` file in the right place on your hard drive. If you don't have `Hankees.txt` in the right place, then when you try to run this section's example, you get an unpleasant `FileNotFound Exception` message.

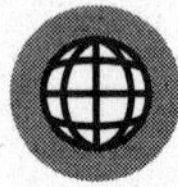

You can download stuff from this book's website, and get instructions for opening the book's examples in your favorite IDE (Eclipse, NetBeans, or IntelliJ IDEA). When you open this chapter's `10-01` project, the `Hankees.txt` file is exactly where it needs to be. You don't have to worry about putting the file where it belongs.

If you create this section's example from scratch, you have to think about the correct location of the `Hankees.txt` file. In that case, deciding where to put the `Hankees.txt` file depends on your computer. To read about all these topics, visit this book's website (`www.allmycode.com/JavaForDummies`).

REMEMBER

For this section's code to work correctly, you must have a line break after the last `.212` in Figure 10-2. For details about line breaks, see Chapter 8.

One class; nine objects

The code in Listing 10-2 calls the `Player` constructor nine times. This means that the code creates nine instances of the `Player` class. The first time through the loop, the code creates an instance with the name `Barry Burd`. The second time through the loop, the code abandons the `Barry Burd` instance and creates another instance with name `Harriet Ritter`. The third time through, the code abandons poor `Harriet Ritter` and creates an instance for `Weelie J. Katz`. The code has only one instance at a time but, all in all, the code creates nine instances.

Each `Player` instance has its own `name` and `average` fields. Each instance also has its own `Player` constructor and its own `getName`, `getAverage`, and `getAverageString` methods. Look at Figure 10-3 and think of the `Player` class with its nine incarnations.

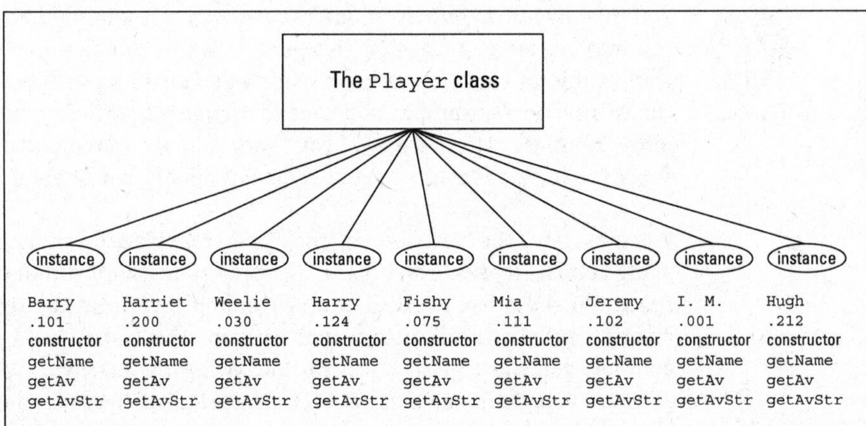

FIGURE 10-3: A class and its objects.

Don't get all GUI on me

The code in Listing 10-2 uses several names from the Java API. Some of these names are explained in Chapter 9. Others are explained right here:

- `JLabel`: A `JLabel` is an object with some text in it. One way to display text inside the frame is to add an instance of the `JLabel` class to the frame.

  In Listing 10-2, the `addPlayerInfo` method is called nine times, once for each player on the team. Each time `addPlayerInfo` is called, the method adds two new `JLabel` objects to the frame. The text for each `JLabel` object comes from a player object's getter method.

- `GridLayout`: A `GridLayout` arranges things in evenly spaced rows and columns. This constructor for the `GridLayout` class takes two parameters: the number of rows and the number of columns.

  In Listing 10-2, the call to the `GridLayout` constructor takes parameters `(9, 2, 20, 3)`. So in Figure 10-1, the display has nine rows (one for each player) and two columns (one for a name and another for an average). The horizontal gap between the two columns is 20 pixels wide, and the vertical gap between any two rows is 3 pixels tall.

- `pack`: When you pack a frame, you set the frame's size. That's the size the frame has when it appears on your computer screen. Packing a frame shrink-wraps the frame around whatever objects you've added inside the frame.

  In Listing 10-2, by the time you've reached the call to `pack`, you've already called `addPlayerInfo` nine times and added 18 labels to the frame. In executing the `pack` method, the computer picks a nice size for each label, given whatever text you've put inside the label. Then the computer picks a nice size for the whole frame, given that the frame has these 18 labels inside it.

When you plop stuff onto frames, you have quite a bit of leeway with the order in which you do things. For instance, you can set the layout before or after you've added labels and other stuff to the frame. If you call `setLayout` and then add labels, the labels appear in nice, orderly positions on the frame. If you reverse this order (add labels and then call `setLayout`), the calling of `setLayout` rearranges the labels in a nice, orderly fashion. It works fine either way.

In setting up a frame, the one thing that you shouldn't do is violate the following sequence:

```
Add things to the frame, then
pack();
setVisible(true);
```

If you call pack and then add more things to the frame, the pack method doesn't take into consideration the more recent things that you've added. If you call setVisible before you add things or call pack, the user sees the frame as it's being constructed. Finally, if you forget to set the frame's size (by calling pack or another sizing method), the frame that you see looks like the one in Figure 10-4. (Normally, I wouldn't show you an anomalous run like the one in Figure 10-4, but I've made the mistake so many times that I feel as if this puny frame is an old friend of mine.)

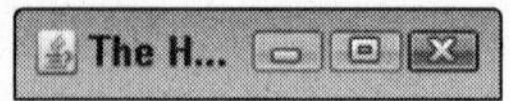

FIGURE 10-4: A shrunken frame.

Tossing an exception from method to method

Chapter 8 introduces input from a disk file, and along with that topic comes the notion of an exception. When you tinker with a disk file, you need to acknowledge the possibility of raising an IOException. That's the lesson from Chapter 8, and that's why the constructor in Listing 10-2 has a throws IOException clause.

But what about the main method in Listing 10-3? With no apparent reference to disk files in this main method, why does the method need its own throws IOException clause? Well, an exception is a hot potato. If you have one, you either have to eat it (as you can see in Chapter 13) or use a throws clause to toss it to someone else. If you toss an exception with a throws clause, someone else is stuck with the exception just the way you were.

The constructor in Listing 10-2 throws an IOException, but to whom is this exception thrown? Who in this chain of code becomes the bearer of responsibility for the problematic IOException? Well, who called the constructor in Listing 10-2? It was the main method in Listing 10-3 — that's who called the TeamFrame constructor. Because the TeamFrame constructor throws its hot potato to the main method in Listing 10-3, the main method has to deal with it. As shown in Listing 10-3, the main method deals with it by tossing the IOException again (by having a throws IOException clause of its own). That's how the throws clause works in Java programs.

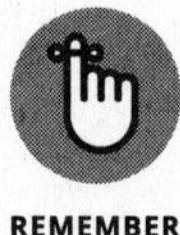

REMEMBER

If a method calls another method and the called method has a throws clause, the calling method must contain code that deals with the exception. To find out more about dealing with exceptions, read Chapter 13.

TECHNICAL STUFF

At this point in the book, the astute *For Dummies* reader may pose a follow-up question or two. "When a `main` method has a `throws` clause, someone else has to deal with the exception in that `throws` clause. But who called the `main` method? Who deals with the `IOException` in the `throws` clause of Listing 10-3?" The answer is that the Java Virtual Machine (or JVM, the thing that runs all your Java code) called the `main` method. So the JVM takes care of the `IOException` in Listing 10-3. If the program has any trouble reading the `Hankees.txt` file, the responsibility ultimately falls on the JVM. The JVM takes care of the situation by displaying an error message and then ending the run of your program. How convenient!

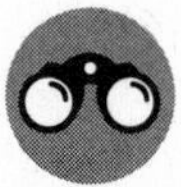
TRY IT OUT

Would you like some practice with the material in this section? If so, try this:

- The code in Listing 10-2 reads from a file named `Hankees.txt`. Delete that `Hankees.txt` file from your computer's hard drive, or temporarily move the file to a different directory. Then try to run the program in Listings 10-1 to 10-3. What horrible things happen when you do this?
- A line of men's clothing features shirts, pants, jackets, overcoats, neckties, and shoes. Create an `enum` to represent the six kinds of items. Then create a `MensClothingItem` class. Each instance of the class has a kind (one of the six `enum` values), and a name (such as *Casual Summer Design #7*).

  Write code to display a frame (like the frame in Figure 10-1). The frame has six rows to describe one complete men's wardrobe.
- Create an `enum` to represent the suits in a deck of playing cards (`CLUBS`, `DIAMONDS`, `HEARTS`, and `SPADES`). Create a `PlayingCard` class. Each playing card has a number (from 1 to 13) and a suit. In the numbering scheme, 11 stands for a Jack, 12 stands for a Queen, and 13 stands for a King. Write code that creates several cards and displays them on the screen (in either text-only format or as a frame like the one in Figure 10-1).

Making Static (Finding the Team Average)

Thinking about the code in Listings 10-1 through 10-3, you decide that you want to find the team's overall batting average. Not a bad idea! The Hankees in Figure 10-1 have an average of about .106, so the team needs some intensive training. While the players are out practicing on the ball field, you have a philosophical hurdle to overcome.

In Listings 10-1 through 10-3, you have three classes: a `Player` class and two other classes that help display data from the `Player` class. So in this class morass, where do the variables storing your overall, team-average tally go?

- It makes no sense to put tally variables in either of the displaying classes (`TeamFrame` and `ShowTeamFrame`). After all, the tally has something-or-other to do with players, teams, and baseball. The displaying classes are about creating windows, not about playing baseball.
- You're uncomfortable putting an overall team average in an instance of the `Player` class because an instance of the `Player` class represents just one player on the team. What business does a single player have storing overall team data? Sure, you could make the code work, but it wouldn't be an elegant solution to the problem.

Finally, you discover the keyword `static`. Anything that's declared to be `static` belongs to the whole class, not to any particular instance of the class. When you create the `static` field, `totalOfAverages`, you create just one copy of the field. This copy stays with the entire `Player` class. No matter how many instances of the `Player` class you create — one, nine, or none — you have just one `totalOfAverages` field. And, while you're at it, you create other `static` fields (`playerCount` and `decFormat`) and `static` methods (`findTeamAverage` and `findTeamAverageString`). To see what I mean, look at Figure 10-5.

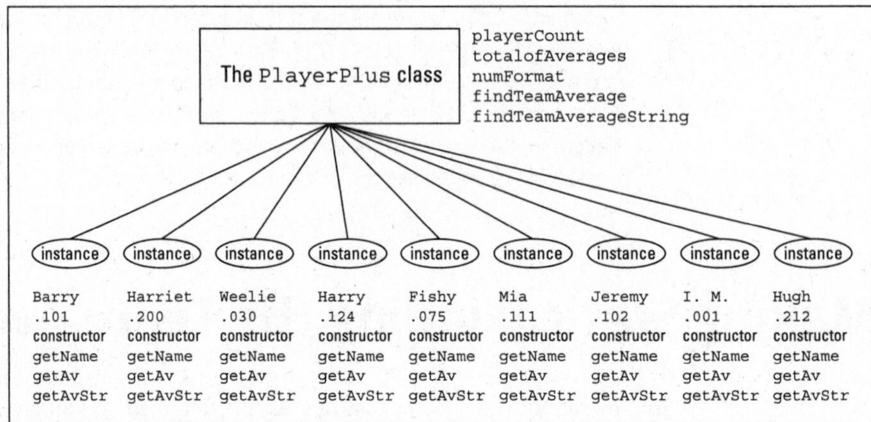

FIGURE 10-5: Some static and non-static fields and methods.

Going along with your passion for subclasses, you put code for team-wide tallies in a subclass of the `Player` class. The `PlayerPlus` subsclass code is shown in Listing 10-4.

LISTING 10-4: Creating a Team Batting Average

```
import java.text.DecimalFormat;

public class PlayerPlus extends Player {
  private static int playerCount = 0;
  private static double totalOfAverages = .000;
  private static DecimalFormat decFormat = new DecimalFormat();

  static {
    decFormat.setMaximumIntegerDigits(0);
    decFormat.setMaximumFractionDigits(3);
    decFormat.setMinimumFractionDigits(3);
  }

  public PlayerPlus(String name, double average) {
    super(name, average);
    playerCount++;
    totalOfAverages += average;
  }

  public static double findTeamAverage() {
    return totalOfAverages / playerCount;
  }

  public static String findTeamAverageString() {
    return decFormat.format(totalOfAverages / playerCount);
  }
}
```

Why is there so much static?

Maybe you've noticed — the code in Listing 10-4 is overflowing with the word `static`. That's because nearly everything in this code belongs to the entire `PlayerPlus` class and not to individual instances of the class. That's good because something like `playerCount` (the number of players on the team) shouldn't belong to individual players, and having each `PlayerPlus` object keep track of its own count would be silly. ("I know how many players I am. I'm just one player!") If you had nine individual `playerCount` fields, either each field would store the number 1 (which is useless) or you would have nine different copies of the count, which is wasteful and prone to error. By making `playerCount` static, you're keeping the `playerCount` in just one place, where it belongs.

The same kind of reasoning holds for the `totalOfAverages`. Eventually, the `totalOfAverages` field will store the sum of the players' batting averages. For all nine members of the Hankees, this adds up to .956. It's not until someone calls the findTeamAverage or findTeamAverageString method that the computer actually finds the overall Hankee team batting average.

You also want the methods findTeamAverage and findTeamAverageString to be static. Without the word *static*, there would be nine findTeamAverage methods — one for each instance of the PlayerPlus class. This wouldn't make much sense. Each instance would have the code to calculate totalOfAverages / playerCount on its own, and each of the nine calculations would yield the same answer.

In general, any task that all the instances have in common (and that yields the same result for each instance) should be coded as a static method.

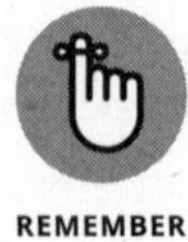

REMEMBER

Constructors are never static.

Meet the static initializer

In Listing 10-4, the decFormat field is static. This makes sense because decFormat makes totalOfAverages / playerCount look nice, and both fields in the expression totalOfAverages / playerCount are static. Thinking more directly, the code needs only one thing for formatting numbers. If you have several numbers to format, the same decFormat thing that belongs to the entire class can format each number. Creating a decFormat for each player is not only inelegant, but also wasteful.

But declaring decFormat to be static presents a little problem. To set up the formatting, you have to call methods like decFormat.setMaximumIntegerDigits(0). You can't just plop these method calls anywhere in the PlayerPlus class. For example, the following code is bad, invalid, illegal, and otherwise un-Java-like:

```
// THIS IS BAD CODE:
public class PlayerPlus extends Player {
  private static DecimalFormat decFormat = new DecimalFormat();

  decFormat.setMaximumIntegerDigits(0);       // Bad!
  decFormat.setMaximumFractionDigits(3);      // Bad!
  decFormat.setfsMinimumFractionDigits(3);    // Bad!
```

Look at the examples from previous chapters. In those examples, I never let a method call just dangle on its own, the way I do in the bad, bad code. In this chapter, in Listing 10-1, I don't call setMaximumIntegerDigits without putting the method call inside the getAverageString method's body. This no-dangling-method-calls business isn't an accident. Java's rules restrict the places in the code where you can issue calls to methods, and putting a lonely method call on its own immediately inside a class definition is a big no-no.

In Listing 10-4, where can you put the necessary setMax and setMin calls? You can put them inside the body of the findTeamAverageString method, much the way I put them inside the getAverageString method in Listing 10-1. But putting those method calls inside the findTeamAverageString method's body might defeat the purpose of having decFormat be static. After all, a programmer might call findTeamAverageString several times, calling decFormat.setMaximumIntegerDigits(0) each time. But that would be quite wasteful. The entire PlayerPlus class has only one decFormat field, and that decFormat field's MaximumIntegerDigits value is always 0. Don't keep setting MaximumIntegerDigits(0) over and over again.

The best alternative is to take the bad lines in this section's bad code and put them inside a *static initializer.* Then they become good lines inside good code. (See Listing 10-4.) A static initializer is a block that's preceded by the word static. Java executes the static initializer's statements once for the entire class. That's exactly what you want for something called "static."

Displaying the overall team average

You may be noticing a pattern. When you create code for a class, you generally write two pieces of code. One piece of code defines the class, and the other piece of code uses the class. (The ways to use a class include calling the class's constructor, referencing the class's non-private fields, calling the class's methods, and so on.) Listing 10-4, shown previously, contains code that defines the PlayerPlus class, and Listing 10-5 contains code that uses this PlayerPlus class.

LISTING 10-5: Using the Code from Listing 10-4

```
import java.util.Scanner;
import java.io.File;
import java.io.IOException;
import javax.swing.JFrame;
import javax.swing.JLabel;
import java.awt.GridLayout;


@SuppressWarnings("serial")
public class TeamFrame extends JFrame {

  public TeamFrame() throws IOException {
    PlayerPlus player;
    Scanner hankeesData = new Scanner(new File("Hankees.txt"));

    for (int num = 1; num <= 9; num++) {
      player =
```

(continued)

LISTING 10-5: (continued)

```
            new PlayerPlus(hankeesData.nextLine(), hankeesData.nextDouble());
        hankeesData.nextLine();

        addPlayerInfo(player);
      }

      add(new JLabel());
      add(new JLabel("  ------"));
      add(new JLabel("Team Batting Average:"));
      add(new JLabel(PlayerPlus.findTeamAverageString()));

      setTitle("The Hankees");
      setLayout(new GridLayout(11, 2, 20, 3));
      setDefaultCloseOperation(EXIT_ON_CLOSE);
      pack();
      setVisible(true);

      hankeesData.close();
    }

    void addPlayerInfo(PlayerPlus player) {
      add(new JLabel("  " + player.getName()));
      add(new JLabel(player.getAverageString()));
    }
}
```

To run the code in Listing 10-5, you need a class with a `main` method. The `ShowTeamFrame` class in Listing 10-3 works just fine.

Figure 10-6 shows a run of the code from Listing 10-5. This run depends on the availability of the `Hankees.txt` file from Figure 10-2. The code in Listing 10-5 is almost an exact copy of the code from Listing 10-2. (So close is the copy that if I could afford it, I'd sue myself for theft of intellectual property.) The only thing new in Listing 10-5 is the stuff shown in bold.

The Hankees	
Barry Burd	.101
Harriet Ritter	.200
Weelie J. Katz	.030
Harry "The Crazyman" Spoonswagler	.124
Felicia "Fishy" Katz	.075
Mia, Just "Mia"	.111
Jeremy Flooflong Jones	.102
I. M. D'Arthur	.001
Hugh R. DaReader	.212

Team Batting Average:	.106

FIGURE 10-6: A run of the code in Listing 10-5.

In Listing 10-5, the GridLayout has two extra rows: one row for spacing and another row for the Hankee team's average. Each of these rows has two Label objects in it.

- **The spacing row has a blank label and a label with a dashed line.** The blank label is a placeholder. When you add components to a GridLayout, the components are added row by row, starting at the left end of a row and working toward the right end. Without this blank label, the dashed-line label would appear at the left end of the row, under Hugh R. DaReader's name.
- **The other row has a label displaying the words *Team Batting Average,* and another label displaying the number *.106.*** The method call that gets the number .106 is interesting. The call looks like this:

  ```
  PlayerPlus.findTeamAverageString()
  ```

  Take a look at that method call. That call has the following form:

  ```
  ClassName.methodName()
  ```

  That's new and different. In earlier chapters, I say that you normally preface a method call with an object's name, not a class's name. So why do I use a class name here? The answer: When you call a static method, you preface the method's name with the name of the class that contains the method. The same holds true whenever you reference another class's static field. This makes sense. ***Remember:*** The whole class that defines a static field or method owns that field or method. So, to refer to a static field or method, you preface the field or method's name with the class's name.

TIP

When you're referring to a static field or method, you can cheat and use an object's name in place of the class name. For instance, in Listing 10-5, with judicious rearranging of some other statements, you can use the expression player.findTeamAverageString().

The static keyword is yesterday's news

This section makes a big noise about static fields and methods, but static things have been part of the picture since early in this book. For example, Chapter 3 introduces System.out.println. The name System refers to a class, and out is a static field in that class. That's why, in Chapter 4 and beyond, I use the static keyword to import the out field:

```
import static java.lang.System.out;
```

In Java, `static` fields and methods show up all over the place. When they're declared in someone else's code and you're making use of them in your code, you hardly ever have to worry about them. But when you're declaring your own fields and methods and must decide whether to make them `static`, you have to think a little harder.

TECHNICAL STUFF

In this book, my first serious use of the word *static* is way back in Listing 3-1. I use the `static` keyword as part of every main method (and lots of `main` methods are in this book's listings). So why does `main` have to be static? Well, remember that non-static things belong to objects, not classes. If the `main` method isn't static, you can't have a `main` method until you create an object. But, when you start up a Java program, no objects have been created yet. The statements that are executed in the `main` method start creating objects. So, if the `main` method isn't static, you have a big chicken-and-egg problem.

Could cause static; handle with care

When I first started writing Java programs, I had recurring dreams about getting a certain error message. The message was `non-static variable or method cannot be referenced from a static context`. So often did I see this message, so thoroughly was I perplexed, that the memory of this message became burned into my subconscious existence.

These days, I know why I got that error message so often. I can even make the message occur if I want. But I still feel a little shiver whenever I see this message on my screen.

Before you can understand why the message occurs and how to fix the problem, you need to get some terminology under your belt. If a field or method isn't static, it's called *non-static*. (Real surprising, hey?) Given that terminology, there are at least two ways to make the dreaded message appear:

- » Put *`Class.nonstaticThing`* somewhere in your program.
- » Put *`nonstaticThing`* somewhere inside a `static` method.

In either case, you're getting yourself into trouble. You're taking something that belongs to an object (the non-static thing) and putting it in a place where no objects are in sight.

Take, for instance, the first of the two situations I just described. To see this calamity in action, go back to Listing 10-5. Toward the end of the listing, change `player.getName()` to `Player.getName()`. That does the trick. What could `Player.getName` possibly mean? If anything, the expression `Player.getName` means "call the getName method that belongs to the entire Player class." But look back at Listing 10-1. The getName method isn't static. Each instance of the Player (or PlayerPlus) class has a getName method. None of the getName methods belongs to the entire class. So the call Player.getName doesn't make any sense. (Maybe the computer is pulling punches when it displays the inoffensive cannot be referenced ... message. Perhaps a harsh, nonsensical expression message would be more fitting.)

For a taste of the second situation (in the bullet list earlier in this section), go back to Listing 10-4. While no one's looking, quietly remove the word *static* from the declaration of the decFormat field (near the top of the listing). This removal turns decFormat into a non-static field. Suddenly, each player on the team has a separate decFormat field.

Well, things are just hunky-dory until the computer reaches the findTeamAverageString method. That static method has four decFormat.SuchAndSuch statements in it. Once again, you're forced to ask what a statement of this kind could possibly mean. Method findTeamAverageString belongs to no instance in particular. (The method is static, so the entire PlayerPlus class has one findTeamAverageString method.) But with the way you've just butchered the code, plain old decFormat without reference to a particular object has no meaning. So again, you're referencing the non-static field, decFormat, from inside a static method's context. For shame, for shame, for shame!

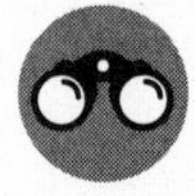

TRY IT OUT

I don't know about you, but I can always use some practice with static variables and methods:

- In a previous section, you create a class to represent items in a line of men's clothing. Create a subclass that includes the name of the designer *(Dummies House of Fashion),* the color of the item, and the cost of the item.

  The designer's name will be static because all items in the line have the same designer. The color can be a static field from Java's own Color class. (See https://docs.oracle.com/javase/8/docs/api/java/awt/Color.html.)

  Write code to display a frame (like the frame in Figure 10-1). The frame has eight rows. The first row displays the name of the designer. The next six rows describe one complete men's wardrobe. The last row shows the wardrobe's total cost.

- In a previous section, you create a class to represent a playing card. Add a static field to your PlayingCard class. The field keeps track of the number of times the class's constructor has been called, and thus has a count of the number of playing cards.

» What's the output of the following code? Make some predictions, and then run the code to see whether your predictions are correct:

```
import static java.lang.System.out;

public class Main {

  public static void main(String[] args) {

    out.println("bigValue: " + MutableInteger.bigValue);
    // out.println("bigValue: " + IntegerHolder.value); ILLEGAL

    MutableInteger holder1 = new MutableInteger(42);
    MutableInteger holder2 = new MutableInteger(7);

    out.println("holder1: " + holder1.value);
    out.println("holder2: " + holder2.value);

    out.println();
    holder1.value++;
    holder2.value++;
    MutableInteger.bigValue++;

    out.println("bigValue: " + MutableInteger.bigValue);
    out.println("holder1: " + holder1.value);
    out.println("holder2: " + holder2.value);

    out.println();
    holder1.bigValue++;
    out.println("bigValue according to holder1: " + holder1.bigValue);
    out.println("bigValue according to holder2: " + holder2.bigValue);
  }
}

class MutableInteger {
  int value;
  static int bigValue = 1_000_000;

  public MutableInteger(int value) {
    this.value = value;
  }
}
```

Experiments with Variables

One summer during my college days, I was sitting on the front porch, loafing around, talking with someone I'd just met. I think her name was Janine. "Where are you from?" I asked. "Mars," she answered. She paused to see whether I'd ask a follow-up question.

As it turned out, Janine was from Mars, Pennsylvania, a small town about 20 miles north of Pittsburgh. Okay, so what's my point? The point is that the meaning of a name depends on the context. If you're just north of Pittsburgh and ask, "How do I get to Mars from here?" you may get a sensible, nonchalant answer. But if you ask the same question standing on a street corner in Manhattan, you'll probably arouse some suspicion. (Okay, knowing Manhattan, people would probably just ignore you.)

Of course, the people who live in Mars, Pennsylvania, are very much aware that their town has an oddball name. Fond memories of teenage years at Mars High School don't prevent a person from knowing about the big red planet. On a clear evening in August, you can still have the following conversation with one of the local residents:

> *You:* How do I get to Mars?
>
> *Local resident:* You're in Mars, pal. What particular part of Mars are you looking for?
>
> *You:* No, I don't mean Mars, Pennsylvania. I mean the planet Mars.
>
> *Local resident:* Oh, the planet! Well, then, catch the 8:19 train leaving for Cape Canaveral . . . No, wait — that's the local train. That'd take you through West Virginia. . . .

So the meaning of a name depends on where you're using the name. Although most English-speaking people think of Mars as a place with a carbon dioxide atmosphere, some folks in Pennsylvania think about all the shopping they can do in Mars. And those folks in Pennsylvania really have two meanings for the name *Mars*. In Java, those names may look like this: `Mars` and `planets.Mars`.

Putting a variable in its place

Your first experiment is shown in Listings 10-6 and 10-7. The listings' code highlights the difference between variables that are declared inside and outside methods.

LISTING 10-6: Two Meanings for Mars

```
import static java.lang.System.out;

class EnglishSpeakingWorld {
    String mars = "   red planet";

    void visitPennsylvania() {
        out.println("visitPA is running:");

        String mars = "   Janine's home town";

        out.println(mars);
        out.println(this.mars);
    }
}
```

LISTING 10-7: Calling the Code of Listing 10-6

```
import static java.lang.System.out;

public class GetGoing {

    public static void main(String args[]) {
        out.println("main is running:");
        EnglishSpeakingWorld e = new EnglishSpeakingWorld();

        //out.println(mars);   cannot resolve symbol
        out.println(e.mars);
        e.visitPennsylvania();
    }
}
```

Figure 10-7 shows a run of the code in Listings 10-6 and 10-7. Figure 10-8 shows a diagram of the code's structure. In the `GetGoing` class, the `main` method creates an instance of the `EnglishSpeakingWorld` class. The variable `e` refers to the new instance. The new instance is an object with a variable named `mars` inside it. That `mars` variable has the value `"red planet"`. The `"red planet"` `mars` variable is a field.

```
main is running:
   red planet
visitPA is running:
   Janine's home town
   red planet
```

FIGURE 10-7: A run of the code in Listings 10-6 and 10-7.

Another way to describe that `mars` field is to call it an *instance variable* because that `mars` variable (the variable whose value is `"red planet"`) belongs to an *instance* of the `EnglishSpeakingWorld` class. In contrast, you can refer to `static` fields (like the `playerCount`, `totalOfAverages`, and `decFormat` fields in Listing 10-4) as *class variables*. For example, `playerCount` in Listing 10-4 is a class variable because one copy of `playerCount` belongs to the entire `PlayerPlus` class.

Now look at the `main` method in Listing 10-7. Inside the `GetGoing` class's `main` method, you aren't permitted to write `out.println(mars)`. In other words, a bare-faced reference to any `mars` variable is a definite no-no. The `mars` variable that I mention in the preceding paragraph belongs to the `EnglishSpeakingWorld` object, not the `GetGoing` class.

However, inside the `GetGoing` class's `main` method, you can certainly write `e.mars` because the `e` variable refers to your `EnglishSpeakingWorld` object. That's nice.

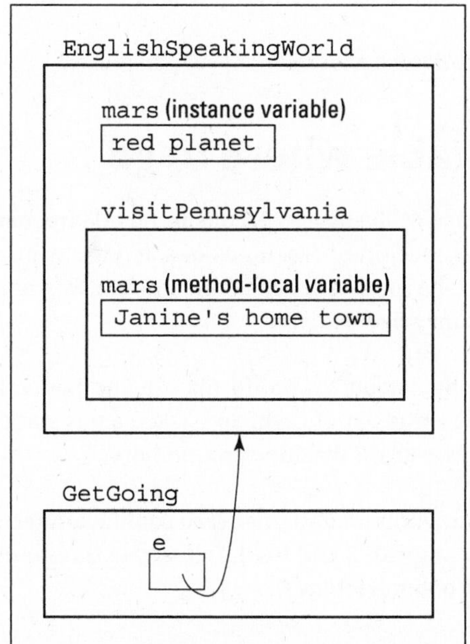

FIGURE 10-8: The structure of the code in Listings 10-6 and 10-7.

Near the bottom of the code, the `visitPennsylvania` method is called. When you're inside `visitPennsylvania`, you have another declaration of a `mars` variable, whose value is `"Janine's home town"`. This particular `mars` variable is called a *method-local variable* because it belongs to just one method: the `visitPennsylvania` method.

Now you have two variables, both with the name *mars*. One `mars` variable, a field, has the value `"red planet"`. The other `mars` variable, a method-local variable, has the value `"Janine's home town"`. In the code, when you use the word *mars*, to which of the two variables are you referring?

The answer is, when you're visiting Pennsylvania, the variable with value `"Janine's home town"` wins. When in Pennsylvania, think the way the Pennsylvanians think. When you're executing code inside the `visitPennsylvania` method, resolve any variable name conflicts by going with method-local variables — variables declared right inside the `visitPennsylvania` method.

What if you're in Pennsylvania and need to refer to that 2-mooned celestial object? More precisely, how does code inside the `visitPennsylvania` method refer to the field with value `"red planet"`? The answer is, use `this.mars`. The word *this* points to whatever object contains all this code (and not to any methods inside the code). That object, an instance of the `EnglishSpeakingWorld` class, has a big, fat `mars` field, and that field's value is `"red planet"`. So that's how you can force code to see outside the method it's in — you use the Java keyword `this`.

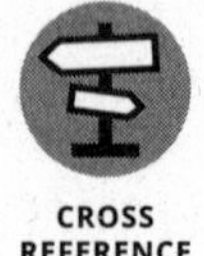

CROSS REFERENCE

For more information on the keyword `this`, see Chapter 9.

Telling a variable where to go

Years ago, when I lived in Milwaukee, Wisconsin, I made frequent use of the local bank's automatic teller machines. Machines of this kind were just beginning to become standardized. The local teller machine system was named *TYME*, which stood for Take Your Money Everywhere.

I remember traveling by car out to California. At one point, I got hungry and stopped for a meal, but I was out of cash. So I asked a gas station attendant, "Do you know where there's a TYME machine around here?"

So you see, a name that works well in one place could work terribly, or not at all, in another place. In Listings 10-8 and 10-9, I illustrate this point (with more than just an anecdote about teller machines).

LISTING 10-8: Tale of Atomic City

```
import static java.lang.System.out;

class EnglishSpeakingWorld2 {
    String mars;
```

```
    void visitIdaho() {
        out.println("visitID is running:");

        mars = "   red planet";
        String atomicCity = "   Population: 25";

        out.println(mars);
        out.println(atomicCity);
    }

    void visitNewJersey() {
        out.println("visitNJ is running:");

        out.println(mars);
        //out.println(atomicCity);   cannot resolve symbol
    }
}
```

LISTING 10-9: Calling the Code of Listing 10-8

```
public class GetGoing2 {

    public static void main(String args[]) {
        EnglishSpeakingWorld2 e = new EnglishSpeakingWorld2();

        e.visitIdaho();
        e.visitNewJersey();
    }
}
```

Figure 10-9 shows a run of the code in Listings 10-8 and 10-9. Figure 10-10 shows a diagram of the code's structure. The code for `EnglishSpeakingWorld2` has two variables. The `mars` variable, which isn't declared inside a method, is a field. The other variable, `atomicCity`, is a method-local variable and is declared inside the `visitIdaho` method.

```
visitID is running:
   red planet
   Population: 25
visitNJ is running:
   red planet
```

FIGURE 10-9: A run of the code in Listings 10-8 and 10-9.

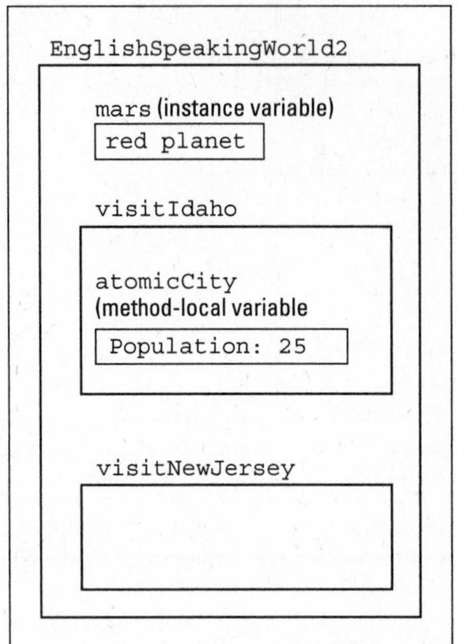

FIGURE 10-10: The structure of the code in Listings 10-8 and 10-9.

In Listing 10-8, notice where each variable can and can't be used. When you try to use the `atomicCity` variable inside the `visitNewJersey` method, you get an error message. Literally, the message says `cannot resolve symbol`. Figuratively, the message says, "Hey, buddy, Atomic City is in Idaho, not New Jersey." Technically, the message says that the method-local variable `atomicCity` is available only in the `visitIdaho` method because that's where the variable was declared.

Back inside the `visitIdaho` method, you're free to use the `atomicCity` variable as much as you want. After all, the `atomicCity` variable is declared inside the `visitIdaho` method.

And what about Mars? Have you forgotten about your old friend, that lovely 80-degrees-below-0 planet? Well, both the `visitIdaho` and `visitNewJersey` methods can access the `mars` variable. That's because the `mars` variable is a field. That is, the `mars` variable is declared in the code for the `EnglishSpeakingWorld2` class but not inside any particular method. (In my stories about the names for things, remember that people who live in both states, Idaho and New Jersey, have heard of the planet Mars.)

The life cycle of the `mars` field has three separate steps:

- When the `EnglishSpeakingWorld2` class first flashes into existence, the computer sees `String mars` and creates space for the `mars` field.

- When the `visitIdaho` method is executed, the method assigns the value `"red planet"` to the `mars` field. (The `visitIdaho` method also prints the value of the `mars` field.)
- When the `visitNewJersey` method is executed, the method prints the `mars` value once again.

In this way, the `mars` field's value is passed from one method to another.

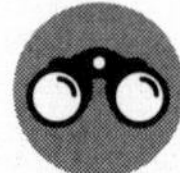
TRY IT OUT

Try out these programs. See what you think.

- What's the output of the following code? Why?

```
public class Main1 {
  static String name = "George";

  public static void main(String[] args) {

    System.out.println(name);

    String name = "Barry";
    System.out.println(name);
  }
}
```

- What's the output of the following code? Why?

```
public class Main2 {
  String name = "George";

  public static void main(String[] args) {
    new Main2();
  }

  Main2() {
    System.out.println(name);

    String name = "Barry";
    System.out.println(name);

    System.out.println(this.name);
  }
}
```

» What's the output of the following code? Why?

```
public class Main3 {
  static String name = "George";

  public static void main(String[] args) {
    String name = "Barry";
    new OtherClass();
  }
}

class OtherClass {

  OtherClass() {
    String name = "Leonard";
    System.out.println(name);
    System.out.println(Main3.name);
  }
}
```

» What's the output of the following code? Why?

```
public class Main4 {
  String name = "George";

  public static void main(String[] args) {
    new Main4();
  }

  Main4() {
    String name = "Barry";
    new YetAnotherClass(this);
  }
}

class YetAnotherClass {

  YetAnotherClass(Main4 whoCreatedMe) {
    String name = "Leonard";
    System.out.println(name);
    // System.out.println(Main4.name); ILLEGAL
    System.out.println(whoCreatedMe.name);
  }
}
```

Passing Parameters

A method can communicate with another part of your Java program in several ways. One way is through the method's parameter list. Using a parameter list, you pass on-the-fly information to a method as the method is being called.

Imagine that the information you pass to the method is stored in one of your program's variables. What, if anything, does the method actually do with that variable? The following sections present a few interesting case studies.

Pass by value

According to my web research, the town of Smackover, Arkansas, has 2,232 people in it. But my research isn't current. Just yesterday, Dora Kermongoos celebrated a joyous occasion over at Smackover General Hospital — the birth of her healthy, blue-eyed baby girl. (The girl weighs 7 pounds, 4 ounces, and is 21 inches tall.) Now the town's population has risen to 2,233.

Listing 10-10 has a very bad program in it. The program is supposed to add 1 to a variable that stores Smackover's population, but the program doesn't work. Take a look at Listing 10-10 and see why.

LISTING 10-10: This Program Doesn't Work

```
public class TrackPopulation {

    public static void main(String args[]) {
        int smackoverARpop = 2232;

        birth(smackoverARpop);
        System.out.println(smackoverARpop);
    }

    static void birth(int cityPop) {
        cityPop++;
    }
}
```

When you run the program in Listing 10-10, the program displays the number 2,232 onscreen. After nine months of planning and anticipation and Dora's whopping seven hours in labor, the Kermongoos family's baby girl wasn't registered in the system. What a shame!

The improper use of parameter passing caused the problem. In Java, when you pass a parameter that has one of the eight primitive types, that parameter is *passed by value.*

CROSS REFERENCE

For a review of Java's eight primitive types, see Chapter 4.

Here's what this means in plain English: Any changes that the method makes to the value of its parameter don't affect the values of variables back in the calling code. In Listing 10-10, the `birth` method can apply the ++ operator to `cityPop` all it wants — the application of ++ to the `cityPop` parameter has absolutely no effect on the value of the `smackoverARpop` variable back in the main method.

Technically, what's happening is the copying of a value. (See Figure 10-11.) When the `main` method calls the `birth` method, the value stored in `smackoverARpop` is copied to another memory location — a location reserved for the `cityPop` parameter's value. During the `birth` method's execution, 1 is added to the `cityPop` parameter. But the place where the original 2232 value was stored — the memory location for the `smackoverARpop` variable — remains unaffected.

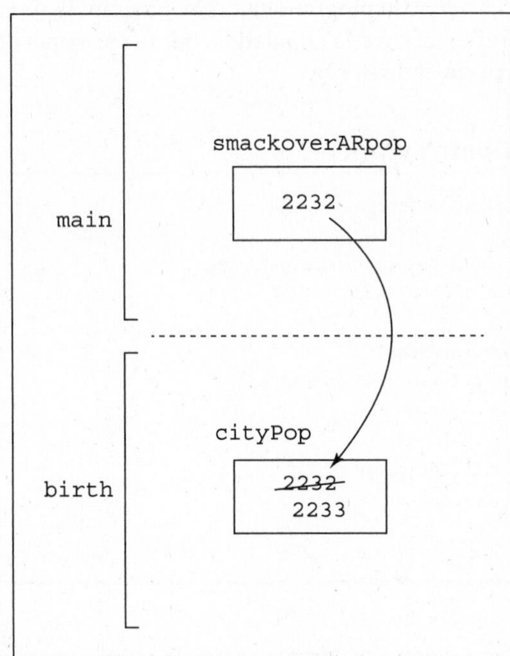

FIGURE 10-11: Pass by value, under the hood.

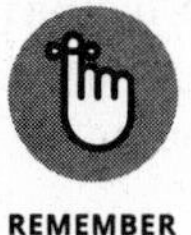

When you do parameter passing with any of the eight primitive types, the computer uses *pass by value*. The value stored in the calling code's variable remains unchanged. This happens even if the calling code's variable and the called method's parameter happen to have exactly the same name.

Returning a result

You must fix the problem that the code in Listing 10-10 poses. After all, a young baby Kermongoos can't go through life untracked. To record this baby's existence, you have to add 1 to the value of the `smackoverARpop` variable. You can do this in plenty of ways, and the way presented in Listing 10-11 isn't the simplest. Even so, the way shown in Listing 10-11 illustrates a point: Returning a value from a method call can be an acceptable alternative to parameter passing. Look at Listing 10-11 to see what I mean.

LISTING 10-11: This Program Works

```
public class TrackPopulation2 {

    public static void main(String args[]) {
        int smackoverARpop = 2232;

        smackoverARpop = birth(smackoverARpop);
        System.out.println(smackoverARpop);
    }

    static int birth(int cityPop) {
        return cityPop + 1;
    }
}
```

After running the code in Listing 10-11, the number you see on your computer screen is the correct number, 2,233.

The code in Listing 10-11 has no new features in it (unless you call *working correctly* a new feature). The most important idea in Listing 10-11 is the `return` statement, which also appears in Chapter 7. Even so, Listing 10-11 presents a nice contrast to the approach in Listing 10-10, which had to be discarded.

Pass by reference

In the previous section or two, I take great pains to emphasize a certain point — that when a parameter has one of the eight primitive types, the parameter is passed by value. If you read this, you probably missed the emphasis on the parameter's having one of the eight primitive types. The emphasis is needed because passing objects (reference types) doesn't quite work the same way.

When you pass an object to a method, the object is *passed by reference*. What this means to you is that statements in the called method *can* change any values that are stored in the object's variables. Those changes *do* affect the values that are seen by whatever code called the method. Listings 10-12 and 10-13 illustrate the point.

LISTING 10-12: What Is a City?

```
class City {
    int population;
}
```

LISTING 10-13: Passing an Object to a Method

```
public class TrackPopulation3 {

    public static void main(String args[]) {
        City smackoverAR = new City();
        smackoverAR.population = 2232;
        birth(smackoverAR);
        System.out.println(smackoverAR.population);
    }

    static void birth(City aCity) {
        aCity.population++;
    }
}
```

When you run the code in Listings 10-12 and 10-13, the output that you get is the number 2,233. That's good because the code has things like ++ and the word *birth* in it. The deal is, adding 1 to `aCity.population` inside the `birth` method actually changes the value of `smackoverAR.population`, as it's known in the `main` method.

To see how the `birth` method changes the value of `smackoverAR.population`, look at Figure 10-12. When you pass an object to a method, the computer doesn't make a copy of the entire object. Instead, the computer makes a copy of a reference to that object. (Think of it the way it's shown in Figure 10-12. The computer makes a copy of an arrow that points to the object.)

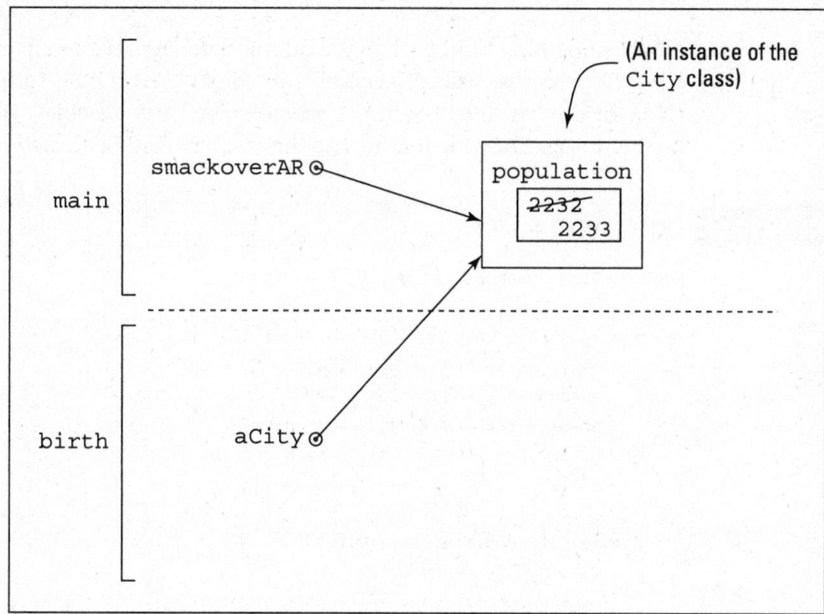

FIGURE 10-12: Pass by reference, under the hood.

In Figure 10-12, you see just one instance of the City class, with a population variable inside it. Now keep your eye on that object as you read the following steps:

1. Just before the birth method is called, the smackoverAR variable refers to that object — the instance of the City class.
2. When the birth method is called and smackoverAR is passed to the birth method's aCity parameter, the computer copies the reference from smackoverAR to aCity. Now aCity refers to that same object — the instance of the City class.
3. When the statement aCity.population++ is executed inside the birth method, the computer adds 1 to the object's population field. Now the program's one and only City instance has 2233 stored in its population field.
4. The flow of execution goes back to the main method. The value of smackoverAR.population is printed. But smackoverAR refers to that one instance of the City class. So smackoverAR.population has the value 2233. The Kermongoos family is so proud.

Returning an object from a method

Believe it or not, the previous sections on parameter passing left one nook and cranny of Java methods unexplored. When you call a method, the method can return something right back to the calling code. In previous chapters and sections, I return primitive values, such as `int` values, or nothing (otherwise known as *void*). In this section, I return a whole object. It's an object of type `City` from Listing 10-12. The code that makes this happen is in Listing 10-14.

LISTING 10-14: Here, Have a City

```
public class TrackPopulation4 {

    public static void main(String args[]) {
        City smackoverAR = new City();
        smackoverAR.population = 2232;
        smackoverAR = doBirth(smackoverAR);
        System.out.println(smackoverAR.population);
    }

    static City doBirth(City aCity) {
        City myCity = new City();
        myCity.population = aCity.population + 1;
        return myCity;
    }
}
```

If you run the code in Listing 10-14, you get the number 2,233. That's good. The code works by telling the `doBirth` method to create another `City` instance. In the new instance, the value of `population` is `2233`. (See Figure 10-13.)

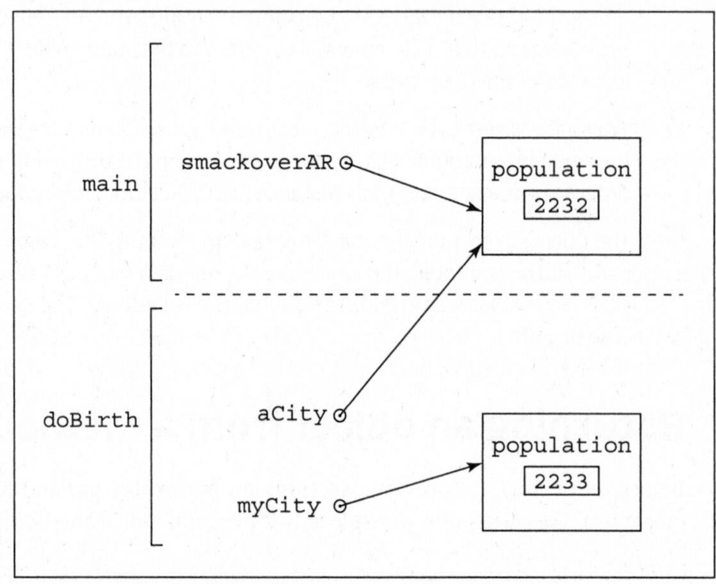

FIGURE 10-13: The `doBirth` method creates a City instance.

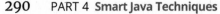

After the doBirth method is executed, that City instance is returned to the main method. Then, back in the main method, that instance (the one that doBirth returns) is assigned to the smackoverAR variable. (See Figure 10-14.) Now smackoverAR refers to a brand-new City instance — an instance whose population is 2,233.

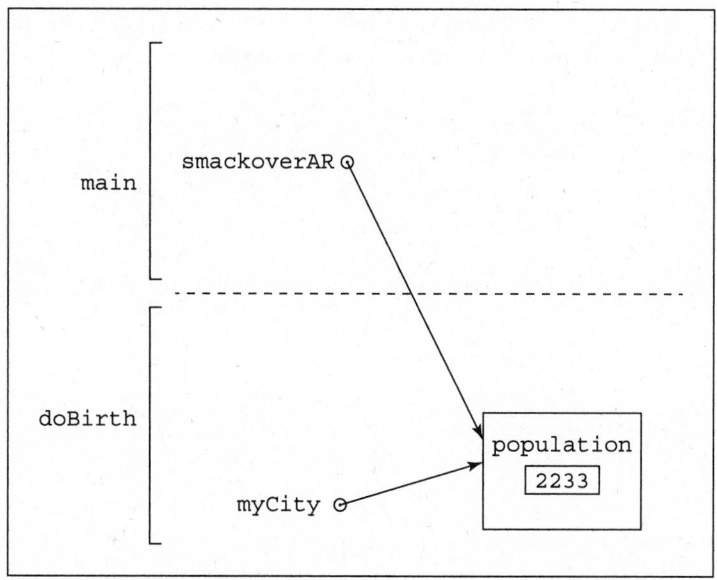

FIGURE 10-14: The new City instance is assigned to the smackoverAR variable.

In Listing 10-14, notice the type consistency in the calling and returning of the doBirth method:

- The smackoverAR variable has type City. The smackoverAR variable is passed to the aCity parameter, which is also of type City.
- The myCity variable is of type City. The myCity variable is sent back in the doBirth method's return statement. That's consistent, because the doBirth method's header begins with static City doBirth(*blah, blah, blah . . .* — a promise to return an object of type City.
- The doBirth method returns an object of type City. Back in the main method, the object that the call to doBirth returns is assigned to the smackoverAR variable, and (you guessed it) the smackoverAR variable is of type City.

Aside from being quite harmonious, all this type agreement is absolutely necessary. If you write a program in which your types don't agree with one another, the compiler spits out an unsympathetic `incompatible types` message.

Epilogue

Dora Kermongoos and her newborn baby daughter are safe, healthy, and resting happily in their Smackover, Arkansas, home.

IN THIS CHAPTER

- » Dealing with several values at once
- » Searching for things
- » Creating values as you get a program running

Chapter 11

Using Arrays to Juggle Values

Welcome to the Java Motel! No haughty bellhops, no overpriced room service, none of the usual silly puns. Just a clean double room that's a darn good value!

Getting Your Ducks All in a Row

The Java Motel, with its ten comfortable rooms, sits in a quiet place off the main highway. Aside from a small, separate office, the motel is just one long row of ground-floor rooms. Each room is easily accessible from the spacious front parking lot.

Oddly enough, the motel's rooms are numbered 0 through 9. I could say that the numbering is a fluke — something to do with the builder's original design plan. But the truth is that starting with 0 makes the examples in this chapter easier to write.

Anyway, you're trying to keep track of the number of guests in each room. Because you have ten rooms, you may think about declaring ten variables:

```
int guestsInRoomNum0, guestsInRoomNum1, guestsInRoomNum2,
    guestsInRoomNum3, guestsInRoomNum4, guestsInRoomNum5,
    guestsInRoomNum6, guestsInRoomNum7, guestsInRoomNum8,
    guestsInRoomNum9;
```

Doing it this way may seem a bit inefficient — but inefficiency isn't the only thing wrong with this code. Even more problematic is the fact that you can't loop through these variables. To read a value for each variable, you have to copy the `nextInt` method ten times.

```
guestsInRoomNum0 = diskScanner.nextInt();
guestsInRoomNum1 = diskScanner.nextInt();
guestsInRoomNum2 = diskScanner.nextInt();
// ... and so on.
```

Surely a better way exists.

That better way involves an array. An *array* is a row of values, like the row of rooms in a 1-floor motel. To picture the array, just picture the Java Motel:

- First, picture the rooms, lined up next to one another.
- Next, picture the same rooms with their front walls missing. Inside each room you can see a certain number of guests.
- If you can, forget that the two guests in Room 9 are putting piles of bills into a big briefcase. Ignore the fact that the guests in Room 6 haven't moved away from the TV set in a day-and-a-half. Instead of all these details, see only numbers. In each room, see a number representing the count of guests in that room. (If free-form visualization isn't your strong point, look at Figure 11-1.)

In the lingo of this chapter, the entire row of rooms is called an *array.* Each room in the array is called a *component* of the array (also known as an array *element*). Each component has two numbers associated with it:

- The room number (a number from 0 to 9), which is called an *index* of the array
- A number of guests, which is a *value* stored in a component of the array

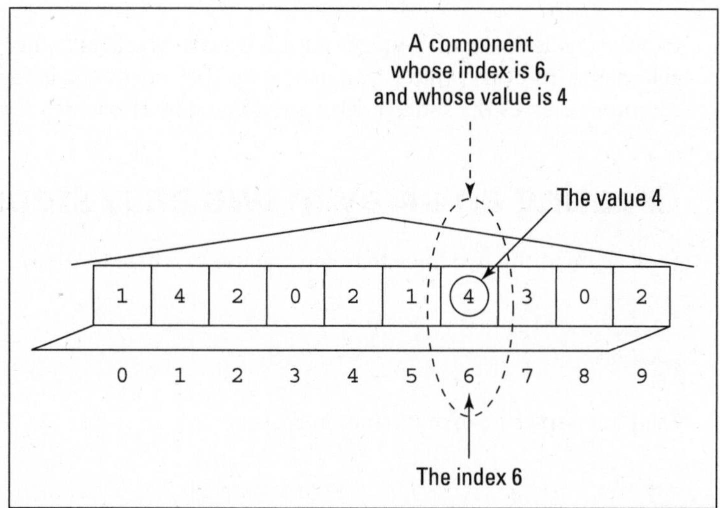

FIGURE 11-1: An abstract snapshot of rooms in the Java Motel.

Using an array saves you from all the repetitive nonsense in the sample code shown at the beginning of this section. For instance, to declare an array with ten values in it, you can write one fairly short statement:

```
int guests[] = new int[10];
```

If you're especially verbose, you can expand this statement so that it becomes two separate statements:

```
int guests[];
guests = new int[10];
```

In either of these code snippets, notice the use of the number 10. This number tells the computer to make the `guests` array have ten components. Each component of the array has a name of its own. The starting component is named *guests[0]*, the next is named *guests[1]*, and so on. The last of the ten components is named *guests[9]*.

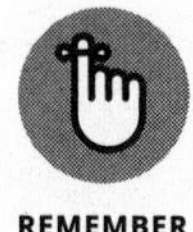

REMEMBER

In creating an array, you always specify the number of components. The array's indices start with 0 and end with the number that's one less than the total number of components.

The snippets that I show you give you two ways to create an array. The first way uses one line. The second way uses two lines. If you take the single-line route, you can put that line inside or outside a method. The choice is yours. On the other hand, if you use two separate lines, the second line, `guests = new int[10]`, should be inside a method.

TIP

In an array declaration, you can put the square brackets before or after the variable name. In other words, you can write `int guests[]` or `int[] guests`. The computer creates the same `guests` variable no matter which form you use.

Creating an array in two easy steps

Look again at the two lines that you can use to create an array:

```
int guests[];
guests = new int[10];
```

Each line serves its own distinct purpose:

- `int guests[]`: This first line is a declaration. The declaration reserves the array name (a name like *guests*) for use in the rest of the program. In the Java Motel metaphor, this line says, "I plan to build a motel here and put a certain number of guests in each room." (See Figure 11-2.)

  Never mind what the declaration `int guests[]` actually does. It's more important to notice what the declaration `int guests[]` *doesn't* do. The declaration doesn't reserve ten memory locations. Indeed, a declaration like `int guests[]` doesn't really create an array. All the declaration does is set up the `guests` variable. At that point in the code, the `guests` variable still doesn't refer to a real array. (In other words, the motel has a name, but the motel hasn't been built yet.)

- `guests = new int[10]`: This second line is an assignment statement. The assignment statement reserves space in the computer's memory for ten `int` values. In terms of real estate, this line says, "I've finally built the motel. Go ahead and put guests in each room." (Again, see Figure 11-2.)

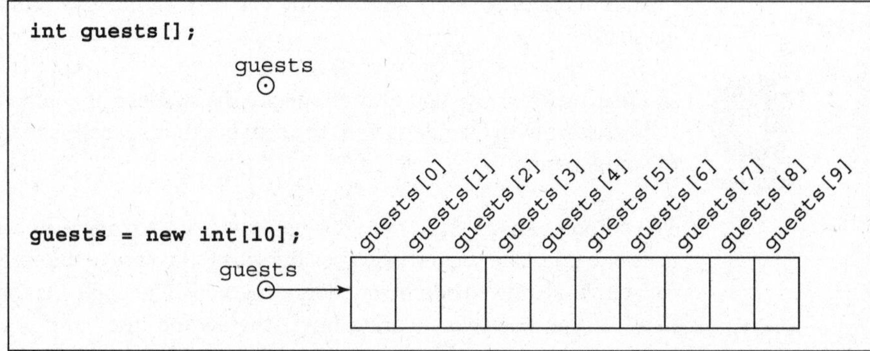

FIGURE 11-2: Two steps in creating an array.

Storing values

After you've created an array, you can put values into the array's components. For instance, you want to store the fact that Room 6 contains four guests. To put the value 4 in the component with index 6, you write `guests[6] = 4`.

Now business starts to pick up. A big bus pulls up to the motel. On the side of the bus is a sign that says *Noah's Ark*. Out of the bus come 25 couples, each walking, stomping, flying, hopping, or slithering to the motel's small office. Only 10 of the couples can stay at the Java Motel, but that's okay because you can send the other 15 couples down the road to the old C-Side Resort and Motor Lodge.

Anyway, to register ten couples into the Java Motel, you put a couple (two guests) in each of your ten rooms. Having created an array, you can take advantage of the array's indexing and write a `for` loop, like this:

```
for (int roomNum = 0; roomNum < 10; roomNum++) {
    guests[roomNum] = 2;
}
```

This loop takes the place of ten assignment statements. Notice how the loop's counter goes from 0 to 9. Compare this with Figure 11-2 and remember that the indices of an array go from zero to one less than the number of components in the array.

However, given the way the world works, your guests won't always arrive in neat pairs, and you'll have to fill each room with a different number of guests. You probably store information about rooms and guests in a database. If you do, you can still loop through an array, gathering numbers of guests as you go. The code to perform such a task may look like this:

```
resultset = statement.executeQuery("select GUESTS from RoomData");
for (int roomNum = 0; roomNum < 10; roomNum++) {
    resultset.next();
    guests[roomNum] = resultset.getInt("GUESTS");
}
```

But because this book doesn't cover databases until Chapter 17, you may be better off reading numbers of guests from a plain-text file. A sample file named `GuestList.txt` is shown in Figure 11-3.

```
1 4 2 0 2 1 4 3 0 2
```

FIGURE 11-3: The `GuestList.txt` file.

After you've made a file, you can call on the Scanner class to get values from the file. The code is shown in Listing 11-1, and the resulting output is in Figure 11-4.

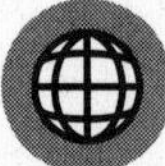

This book's website (www.allmycode.com/JavaForDummies) has tips for readers who need to create data files. This includes instructions for Windows, Linux, and Macintosh environments.

LISTING 11-1: Filling an Array with Values

```
import static java.lang.System.out;
import java.util.Scanner;
import java.io.File;
import java.io.IOException;

public class ShowGuests {

    public static void main(String args[]) throws IOException {
        int guests[] = new int[10];
        Scanner diskScanner = new Scanner(new File("GuestList.txt"));

        for(int roomNum = 0; roomNum < 10; roomNum++) {
            guests[roomNum] = diskScanner.nextInt();
        }

        out.println("Room\tGuests");

        for(int roomNum = 0; roomNum < 10; roomNum++) {
            out.print(roomNum);
            out.print("\t");
            out.println(guests[roomNum]);
        }
        diskScanner.close();
    }
}
```

```
Room    Guests
0       1
1       4
2       2
3       0
4       2
5       1
6       4
7       3
8       0
9       2
```

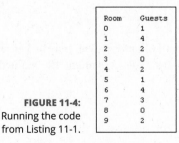

FIGURE 11-4: Running the code from Listing 11-1.

The code in Listing 11-1 has two `for` loops: The first loop reads numbers of guests, and the second loop writes numbers of guests.

TIP

Every array has a built-in length field. An array's *length* is the number of components in the array. So, in Listing 11-1, if you print the value of `guests.length`, you get 10.

Tab stops and other special things

In Listing 11-1, some calls to `print` and `println` use the `\t` escape sequence. It's called an *escape sequence* because you escape from displaying the letter `t` on the screen. Instead, the characters `\t` stand for a tab. The computer moves forward to the next tab stop before printing any more characters. Java has a few of these handy escape sequences. Some of them are shown in Table 11-1.

TABLE 11-1 Escape Sequences

Sequence	Meaning
`\b`	backspace
`\t`	horizontal tab
`\n`	line feed
`\f`	form feed
`\r`	carriage return
`\"`	double quote "
`\'`	single quote '
`\\`	backslash \

Using an array initializer

Besides what you see in Listing 11-1, you have another way to fill an array in Java: with an *array initializer*. When you use an array initializer, you don't even have to tell the computer how many components the array has. The computer figures this out for you.

Listing 11-2 shows a new version of the code to fill an array. The program's output is the same as the output of Listing 11-1. (It's the stuff shown in Figure 11-4.) The only difference between Listings 11-1 and 11-2 is the bold text in Listing 11-2. That bold doodad is an array initializer.

LISTING 11-2: Using an Array Initializer

```
import static java.lang.System.out;

public class ShowGuests {

    public static void main(String args[]) {
        int guests[] = {1, 4, 2, 0, 2, 1, 4, 3, 0, 2};

        out.println("Room\tGuests");

        for (int roomNum = 0; roomNum < 10; roomNum++) {
            out.print(roomNum);
            out.print("\t");
            out.println(guests[roomNum]);
        }
    }
}
```

TIP

An array initializer can contain expressions as well as literals. In plain English, this means that you can put all kinds of things between the commas in the initializer. For instance, an initializer like `{1 + 3, keyboard.nextInt(), 2, 0, 2, 1, 4, 3, 0, 2}` works just fine.

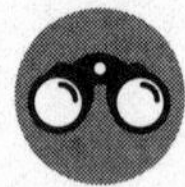

TRY IT OUT

Use my `DummiesFrame` (from Chapter 7) to create a GUI program based on the ideas in Listings 11-1 and 11-2. In your program, the frame has only one input row: a *Room number* row. If the user types **3** in the *Room number* row and then clicks the button, the program displays the number of guests in Room 3.

Stepping through an array with the enhanced for loop

Java has an enhanced `for` loop — a `for` loop that doesn't use counters or indices. Listing 11-3 shows you how to do it.

WARNING

The material in this section applies to Java 5.0 and later Java versions. But this section's material doesn't work with older versions of Java — versions such as 1.3, 1.4, and so on. For a bit more about Java's version numbers, see Chapter 2.

LISTING 11-3: Get a Load o' That for Loop!

```
import static java.lang.System.out;

public class ShowGuests {

    public static void main(String args[]) {
        int guests[] = {1, 4, 2, 0, 2, 1, 4, 3, 0, 2};
        int roomNum = 0;

        out.println("Room\tGuests");

        for (int numGuests : guests) {
            out.print(roomNum++);
            out.print("\t");
            out.println(numGuests);
        }
    }
}
```

Listings 11-1 and 11-3 have the same output. It's in Figure 11-4.

An *enhanced* `for` *statement* has three parts:

```
for (variable-type variable-name : range-of-values)
```

The first two parts are *variable-type* and *variable-name*. The loop in Listing 11-3 defines a variable named `numGuests`, and `numGuests` has type `int`. During each loop iteration, the variable `numGuests` takes on a new value. Look at Figure 11-4 to see these values. The initial value is `1`. The next value is `4`. After that comes `2`. And so on.

Where is the loop finding all these numbers? The answer lies in the loop's *range-of-values*. In Listing 11-3, the loop's *range-of-values* is `guests`. So, during the initial loop iteration, the value of `numGuests` is `guests[0]` (which is `1`). During the next iteration, the value of `numGuests` is `guests[1]` (which is `4`). After that comes `guests[2]` (which is `2`). And so on.

WARNING

Java's enhanced `for` loop requires a word of caution. Each time through the loop, the variable that steps through the range of values stores a *copy* of the value in the original range. The variable does *not* point to the range itself.

For example, if you add an assignment statement that changes the value of `numGuests` in Listing 11-3, this statement has no effect on any of the values stored in the guests array. To drive this point home, imagine that business is bad and I've filled my hotel's guests array with zeros. Then I execute the following code:

```
for (int numGuests : guests) {
    numGuests += 1;
    out.print(numGuests + " ");
}

out.println();

for (int numGuests : guests) {
    out.print(numGuests + " ");
}
```

The numGuests variable takes on values stored in the guests array. But the numGuests += 1 statement doesn't change the values stored in this guests array. The code's output looks like this:

```
1 1 1 1 1 1 1 1 1 1
0 0 0 0 0 0 0 0 0 0
```

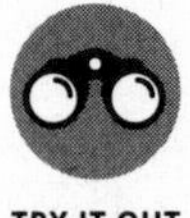

TRY IT OUT

Write a program that stores five double values in an array and then displays the average of the values in the array.

Searching

You're sitting behind the desk at the Java Motel. Look! Here comes a party of five. These people want a room, so you need software that checks whether a room is vacant. If one is, the software modifies the GuestList.txt file (refer to Figure 11-3) by replacing the number 0 with the number 5. As luck would have it, the software is on your hard drive. The software is shown in Listing 11-4.

LISTING 11-4: Do You Have a Room?

```
import static java.lang.System.out;
import java.util.Scanner;
import java.io.File;
import java.io.IOException;
import java.io.PrintStream;

public class FindVacancy {

    public static void main(String args[]) throws IOException {
```

```
        int guests[] = new int[10];
        int roomNum;

        Scanner diskScanner = new Scanner(new File("GuestList.txt"));
        for (roomNum = 0; roomNum < 10; roomNum++) {
            guests[roomNum] = diskScanner.nextInt();
        }
        diskScanner.close();

        roomNum = 0;
        while (roomNum < 10 && guests[roomNum] != 0) {
            roomNum++;
        }

        if (roomNum == 10) {
            out.println("Sorry, no v cancy");
        } else {
            out.print("How many people for room ");
            out.print(roomNum);
            out.print("? ");

            Scanner keyboard = new Scanner(System.in);
            guests[roomNum] = keyboard.nextInt();
            keyboard.close();

            PrintStream listOut = new PrintStream("GuestList.txt");
            for (roomNum = 0; roomNum < 10; roomNum++) {
                listOut.print(guests[roomNum]);
                listOut.print(" ");
            }
            listOut.close();
        }
    }
}
```

Figures 11-5 through 11-7 show the running of the code in Listing 11-4. Back in Figure 11-3, the motel starts with two vacant rooms — Rooms 3 and 8. (Remember, the rooms start with Room 0.) The first time that you run the code in Listing 11-4, the program tells you that Room 3 is vacant and puts five people into the room. The second time you run the code, the program finds the remaining vacant room (Room 8) and puts a party of ten in the room. (What a party!) The third time you run the code, you have no more vacant rooms. When the program discovers this, it displays the message `Sorry, no v cancy`, omitting at least one letter in the tradition of all motel neon signs.

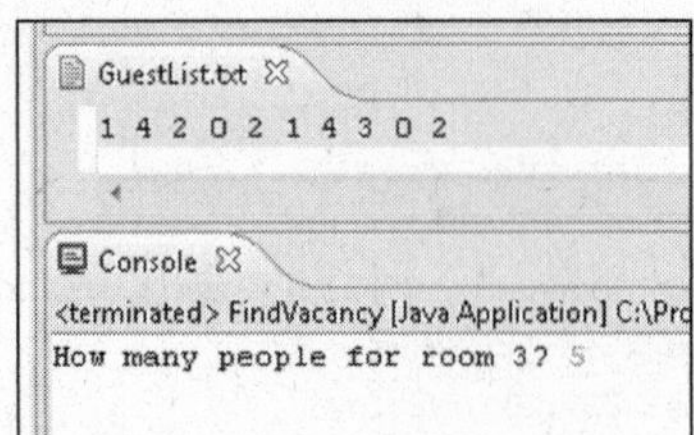

FIGURE 11-5: Filling a vacancy.

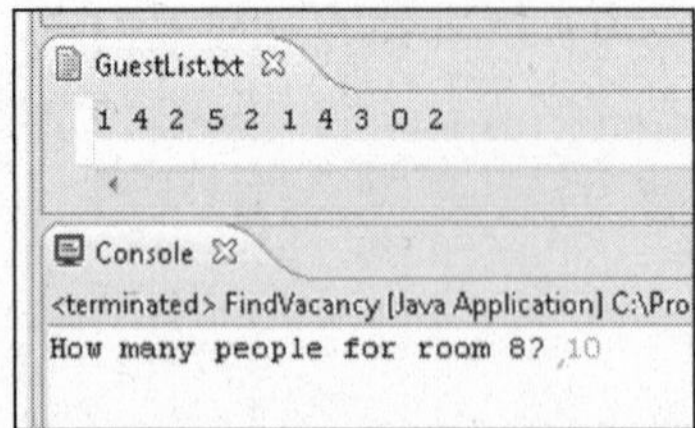

FIGURE 11-6: Filling the last vacant room.

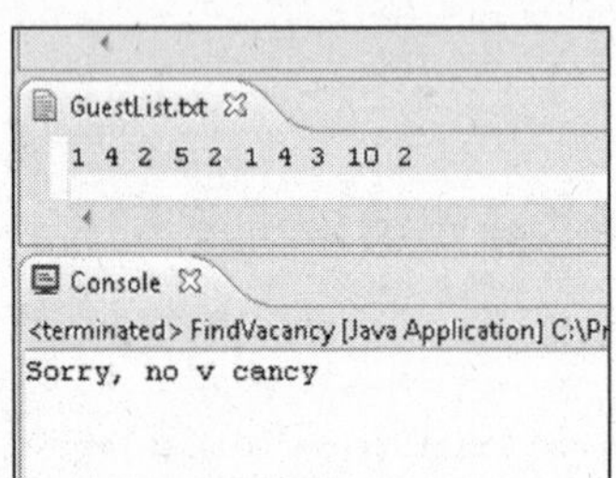

FIGURE 11-7: Sorry, Bud. No rooms.

WARNING

A run of the code in Listing 11-4 writes a brand-new `GuestList.txt` file. This can be confusing because each Java IDE has its own way of displaying the `GuestList.txt file`'s content. Some IDEs don't automatically display the newest `GuestList.txt` file, so after running the code from Listing 11-4, you may not immediately see a change. (For example, in Figure 11-5, Room 3 is empty. But after a run of the code, Figure 11-6 shows Room 3 having five guests.) Even if you don't see a change, consecutive runs of Listing 11-4 change the `GuestList.txt` file. Poke around within your favorite IDE to find out how to make the IDE refresh the `GuestList.txt` file's display.

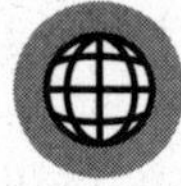

In Listing 11-4, the condition `roomNum < 10 && guests[roomNum] != 0` can be really tricky. If you move things around and write **guests[roomNum] != 0 && roomNum < 10**, you can get yourself into lots of trouble. For details, see this book's website (`www.allmycode.com/JavaForDummies`).

Writing to a file

The code in Listing 11-4 uses tricks from other chapters and sections of this book. The code's only brand-new feature is the use of `PrintStream` to write to a disk file. Think about any example in this book that calls `System.out.print`, `out.println`, or their variants. What's really going on when you call one of these methods?

The thing called `System.out` is an object. The object is defined in the Java API. In fact, `System.out` is an instance of a class named `java.io.PrintStream` (or just `PrintStream` to its close friends). Now each object created from the `PrintStream` class has methods named `print` and `println`. Just as each `Account` object in Listing 7-3 has a `display` method, and just as the `DecimalFormat` object in Listing 10-1 has a `format` method, so the `PrintStream` object named `out` has `print` and `println` methods. When you call `System.out.println`, you're calling a method that belongs to a `PrintStream` instance.

Okay, so what of it? Well, `System.out` always stands for some text area on your computer screen. If you create your own `PrintStream` object and you make that object refer to a disk file, that `PrintStream` object refers to the disk file. When you call that object's `print` method, you write text to a file on your hard drive.

In Listing 11-4, when you say

```
PrintStream listOut = new PrintStream("GuestList.txt");


listOut.print(guests[roomNum]);
listOut.print(" ");
```

you're telling Java to write text to a file on your hard drive — the `GuestList.txt` file.

That's how you update the count of guests staying in the hotel. When you call `listOut.print` for the number of guests in Room 3, you may print the number 5. So, between Figures 11-5 and 11-6, a number in the `GuestList.txt` file changes from 0 to 5. Then in Figure 11-6, you run the program a second time. When the program gets data from the newly written `GuestList.txt` file, Room 3 is no longer vacant. This time, the program suggests Room 8.

TIP

This is more of an observation than a tip. Say that you want to *read* data from a file named `Employees.txt`. To do this, you make a scanner. You call `new Scanner(new File("Employees.txt"))`. If you accidentally call `new Scanner("Employees.txt")` without the `new File` part, the call doesn't connect to your `Employees.txt` file. But notice how you prepare to *write* data to a file. You make a `PrintStream` instance by calling `new PrintStream("GuestList.txt")`. You don't use `new File` anywhere in the call. If you goof and accidentally include `new File`, the Java compiler becomes angry, jumps out, and bites you.

When to close a file

Notice the placement of new Scanner calls, new PrintStream calls, and close calls in Listing 11-4. As in all the examples, each new Scanner call has a corresponding close call. And in Listing 11-4, the new PrintStream call has its own close call (the listOut.close() call). But in Listing 11-4, I'm careful to place these calls tightly around their corresponding nextInt and print calls. For example, I don't set up diskScanner at the very start of the program, and I don't wait until the very end of the program to close diskScanner. Instead, I perform all my diskScanner tasks one after the other in quick succession:

```
Scanner diskScanner = new Scanner(new File("GuestList.txt"));   //construct
for (roomNum = 0; roomNum < 10; roomNum++) {
    guests[roomNum] = diskScanner.nextInt();                    //read
}
diskScanner.close();                                            //close
```

I do the same kind of thing with the keyboard and listOut objects.

I do this quick dance with input and output because my program uses GuestList.txt twice — once for reading numbers and a second time for writing numbers. If I'm not careful, the two uses of GuestList.txt might conflict with one another. Consider the following program:

```
// THIS IS BAD CODE
import java.io.File;
import java.io.IOException;
import java.io.PrintStream;
import java.util.Scanner;

public class BadCode {

    public static void main(String args[]) throws IOException {
        int guests[] = new int[10];

        Scanner diskScanner = new Scanner(new File("GuestList.txt"));
        PrintStream listOut = new PrintStream("GuestList.txt");

        guests[0] = diskScanner.nextInt();
        listOut.print(5);

        diskScanner.close();
        listOut.close();
    }
}
```

Like many methods and constructors of its kind, the `PrintStream` constructor doesn't pussyfoot around with files. If it can't find a `GuestList.txt` file, the constructor creates a `GuestList.txt` file and prepares to write values into it. But, if a `GuestList.txt file` already exists, the `PrintStream` constructor deletes the existing file and prepares to write to a new, empty `GuestList.txt` file. In the `BadCode` class, the new `PrintStream` constructor call deletes whatever `GuestList.txt` file already exists. This deletion comes before the call to `diskScanner.nextInt()`. So `diskScanner.nextInt()` can't read whatever was originally in the `GuestList.txt` file. That's bad!

To avoid this disaster, I carefully separate the two uses of the `GuestList.txt` file in Listing 11-4. Near the top of the listing, I construct `diskScanner`, and then read from the original `GuestList.txt` file, and then close `diskScanner`. Later, toward the end of the listing, I construct `listOut`, and then write to a new `GuestList.txt` file, and then close `listOut`. With writing separated completely from reading, everything works correctly.

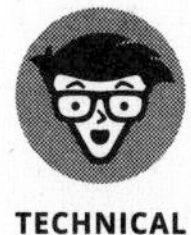
TECHNICAL STUFF

The `keyboard` variable in Listing 11-4 doesn't refer to `GuestList.txt`, so `keyboard` doesn't conflict with the other input or output variables. No harm would come from following my regular routine — putting `keyboard = new Scanner(System.in)` at the start of the program and putting `keyboard.close()` at the end of the program. But to make Listing 11-4 as readable and as uniform as possible, I place the `keyboard` constructor and the `close` call very tightly around the `keyboard.nextInt` call.

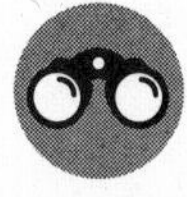
TRY IT OUT

Use my `DummiesFrame` (from Chapter 7) to create a GUI program based on the ideas in Listing 11-4. In your program, the frame has only one input row. If room 3 is vacant, the input row's label is *How many people for room 3?* If the user types 5 in the *How many people for room 3* row and then clicks the button, the program puts 5 people in room 3.

Arrays of Objects

The Java Motel is open for business, now with improved guest registration software! The people who brought you this chapter's first section are always scratching their heads, looking for the best ways to improve their services. Now, with some ideas from object-oriented programming, they've started thinking in terms of a `Room` class.

"And what," you ask, "would a `Room` instance look like?" That's easy. A `Room` instance has three properties: the number of guests in the room, the room rate, and a smoking/nonsmoking stamp. Figure 11-8 illustrates the situation.

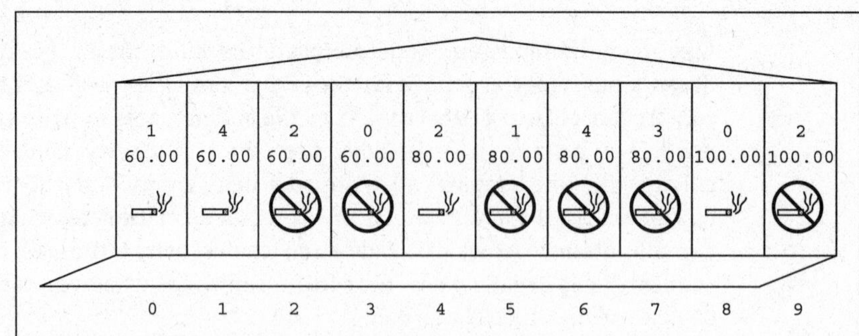

FIGURE 11-8: Another abstract snapshot of rooms in the Java Motel.

Listing 11-5 shows the code that describes the `Room` class. As promised, each instance of the `Room` class has three fields: the `guests`, `rate`, and `smoking` fields. (A `false` value for the boolean field, `smoking`, indicates a nonsmoking room.) In addition, the entire `Room` class has a `static` field named `currency`. On my computer in the United States, this `currency` object makes room rates look like dollar amounts.

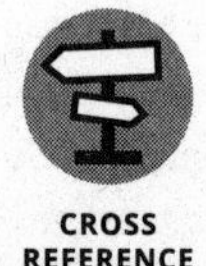

CROSS REFERENCE

To find out what *static* means, see Chapter 10.

LISTING 11-5: So This Is What a Room Looks Like!

```
import static java.lang.System.out;
import java.util.Scanner;
import java.text.NumberFormat;

public class Room {
    private int guests;
    private double rate;
    private boolean smoking;
    private static NumberFormat currency = NumberFormat.getCurrencyInstance();

    public void readRoom(Scanner diskScanner) {
        guests = diskScanner.nextInt();
        rate = diskScanner.nextDouble();
        smoking = diskScanner.nextBoolean();
    }

    public void writeRoom() {
        out.print(guests);
        out.print("\t");
        out.print(currency.format(rate));
        out.print("\t");
        out.println(smoking ? "yes" : "no");
    }
}
```

Listing 11-5 has a few interesting quirks, but I'd rather not describe them until after you see all the code in action. That's why, at this point, I move right on to the code that calls the Listing 11-5 code. After you read about arrays of rooms (shown in Listing 11-6), check out my description of the Listing 11-5 quirks.

WARNING

This warning is a deliberate repeat of an idea from Chapter 4, Chapter 7, and from who-knows-what-other chapter: *Be careful* when you use type `double` or type `float` to store money values. Calculations with `double` or `float` can be inaccurate. For more information (and more finger wagging), see Chapters 4 and 7.

TIP

This tip has absolutely nothing to do with Java. If you're the kind of person who prefers a smoking room (with boolean field `smoking = true` in Listing 11-5), find someone you like — someone who can take three consecutive days off work. Have that person sit with you and comfort you for 72 straight hours while you refrain from smoking. You might become temporarily insane while the nicotine leaves your body, but eventually you'll be okay. And your friend will feel like a real hero.

Using the Room class

Now you need an array of rooms. The code to create such a thing is in Listing 11-6. The code reads data from the `RoomList.txt` file. (Figure 11-9 shows the contents of the `RoomList.txt` file.)

Figure 11-10 shows a run of the code in Listing 11-6.

LISTING 11-6: Would You Like to See a Room?

```
import static java.lang.System.out;
import java.util.Scanner;
import java.io.File;
import java.io.IOException;

public class ShowRooms {
    public static void main(String args[]) throws IOException {

        Room rooms[];
        rooms = new Room[10];

        Scanner diskScanner = new Scanner(new File("RoomList.txt"));
        for (int roomNum = 0; roomNum < 10; roomNum++) {
            rooms[roomNum] = new Room();
            rooms[roomNum].readRoom(diskScanner);
        }
```

(continued)

LISTING 11-6: *(continued)*

```
        out.println("Room\tGuests\tRate\tSmoking?");
        for (int roomNum = 0; roomNum < 10; roomNum++) {
            out.print(roomNum);
            out.print("\t");
            rooms[roomNum].writeRoom();
        }
        diskScanner.close();
    }
}
```

```
1
60.00
true
4
60.00
true
2
60.00
false
0
60.00
false
2
80.00
true
1
80.00
false
4
80.00
false
3
80.00
false
0
100.00
true
2
100.00
false
```

FIGURE 11-9: A file of Room data.

```
Room    Guests  Rate    Smoking?
0       1       $60.00  yes
1       4       $60.00  yes
2       2       $60.00  no
3       0       $60.00  no
4       2       $80.00  yes
5       1       $80.00  no
6       4       $80.00  no
7       3       $80.00  no
8       0       $100.00 yes
9       2       $100.00 no
```

FIGURE 11-10: A run of the code in Listing 11-6.

Say what you want about the code in Listing 11-6. As far as I'm concerned, only one issue in the whole listing should concern you. And what, you ask, is that issue? Well, to create an array of *objects* — as opposed to an array made up of primitive values — you have to do three things: Make the array variable, make the array itself, and then construct each individual object in the array. This is different from creating an array of `int` values or an array containing any other primitive type values. When you create an array of primitive type values, you do only the first two of these three things.

To help make sense of all this, follow along in Listing 11-6 and Figure 11-11 as you read the following points:

- `Room rooms[];`: This declaration creates a `rooms` variable. This variable is destined to refer to an array (but doesn't yet refer to anything).
- `rooms = new Room[10];`: This statement reserves ten slots of storage in the computer's memory. The statement also makes the `rooms` variable refer to the group of storage slots. Each slot is destined to refer to an object (but doesn't yet refer to anything).
- `rooms[roomNum] = new Room();`: This statement is inside a `for` loop. The statement is executed once for each of the ten room numbers. For example, the first time through the loop, this statement says `rooms[0] = new Room()`. That first time around, the statement makes the slot `rooms[0]` refer to an actual object (an instance of the `Room` class).

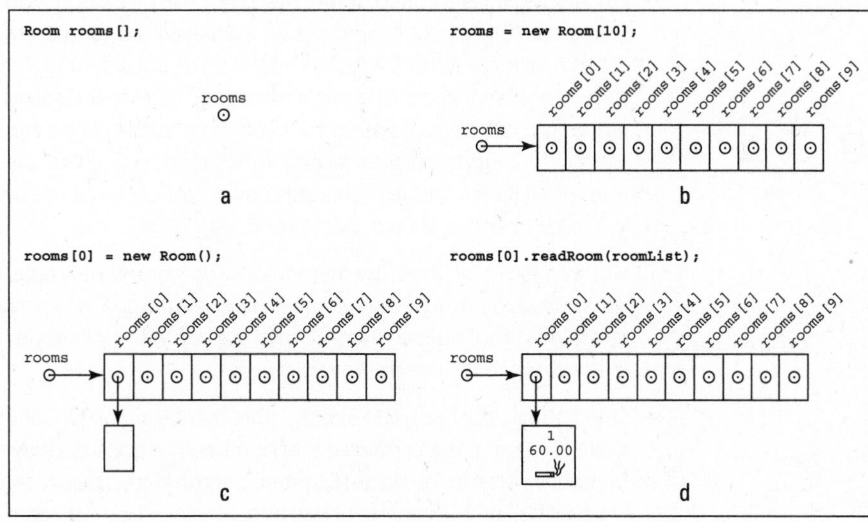

FIGURE 11-11: Steps in creating an array of objects.

Although it's technically not considered a step in array making, you still have to fill each object's fields with values. For instance, the first time through the loop, the readRoom call says rooms[1].readRoom(diskScanner), which means, "Read data from the RoomList.txt file into the rooms[1] object's fields (the guests, rate, and smoking fields)." Each time through the loop, the program creates a new object and reads data into that new object's fields.

You can squeeze the steps together just as you do when creating arrays of primitive values. For instance, you can do the first two steps in one fell swoop, like this:

```
Room rooms[] = new Room[10];
```

You can also use an array initializer. (For an introduction to array initializers, see the section "Using an array initializer," earlier in this chapter.)

Yet another way to beautify your numbers

You can make numbers look nice in plenty of ways. If you take a peek at some earlier chapters, for example, you can see that Listing 7-7 uses printf, and Listing 10-1 uses a DecimalFormat. But in Listing 11-5, I display a currency amount. I use the NumberFormat class with its getCurrencyInstance method.

If you compare the formatting statements in Listings 10-1 and 11-5, you don't see much difference.

- **One listing uses a constructor; the other listing calls getCurrency Instance.** The getCurrencyInstance method is a good example of what's called a factory method. A *factory method* is a convenient tool for creating commonly used objects. People always need code that displays currency amounts. So the getCurrencyInstance method creates a currency format without forcing you to write a complicated DecimalFormat constructor call. In the United States, this complicated constructor call would be new DecimalFormat ("$###0.00;($###0.00)").

  Like a constructor, a factory method returns a brand-new object. But unlike a constructor, a factory method has no special status. If you create your own factory method, you can name it anything you want. When you call a factory method, you don't use the keyword new.

- **One listing uses DecimalFormat;** the other listing uses NumberFormat. A decimal number is a certain kind of number. (In fact, a decimal number is a number written in the base-10 system.) Accordingly, the DecimalFormat class is a subclass of the NumberFormat class. The DecimalFormat methods are more specific, so for most purposes, I use DecimalFormat. But it's harder to use the DecimalFormat class's `getCurrencyInstance` method. For programs that involve money, I tend to use `NumberFormat`.

- **Both listings use `format` methods.** In the end, you just write something like `currency.format(rate)` or `decFormat.format(average)`. After that, Java does the work for you.

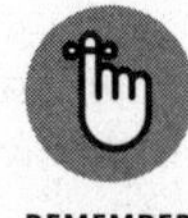

REMEMBER

From Chapter 4 onward, I issue gentle warnings against using types such as `double` and `float` for storing currency values. For the most accurate currency calculations, use `int`, `long`, or — best of all — `BigDecimal`.

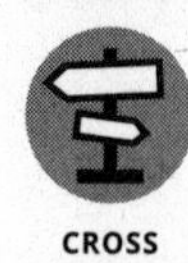

CROSS REFERENCE

You can read more about the dangers of `double` types and currency values in Chapter 7.

The conditional operator

Listing 11-5 uses an interesting doodad called the *conditional operator.* This conditional operator takes three expressions and returns the value of just one of them. It's like a mini `if` statement. When you use the conditional operator, it looks something like this:

```
conditionToBeTested ? expression1 : expression2
```

The computer evaluates the *conditionToBeTested* condition. If the condition is true, the computer returns the value of *expression1*. But, if the condition is false, the computer returns the value of *expression2*.

So, in the code

```
smoking ? "yes" : "no"
```

the computer checks whether `smoking` has the value `true`. If so, the whole 3-part expression stands for the first string, `"yes"`. If not, the whole expression stands for the second string, `"no"`.

In Listing 11-5, the call to `out.println` causes either `"yes"` or `"no"` to display. Which string gets displayed depends on whether `smoking` has the value `true` or `false`.

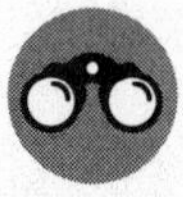

TRY IT OUT

How do you learn Java? You learn it the same way you get to Carnegie Hall — Practice! Practice! Practice!

- In Chapter 9, you create a `Student` class. Each student has a name and an ID number. For this programming challenge, imagine that each student has five grades — one for each of the five courses the student takes. Each grade is a `double` value from 0.0 to 4.0 (4.0 is the best). A student's grade point average (GPA) is the average of the student's five grade values.

In this chapter's `Student` class, one of the fields is an array of five `double` values. Your program finds the student's GPA and displays it (along with the student's name and ID number) on the screen.

- Here's a challenging exercise: Write a primitive word processor program. To show you what your program might do, I've created a sample run. In this run, I've set the user's input in boldface text.

```
>
>
>
>
>

Line to replace (or -1 to quit): 0
Type the new line: There once was an old man with glasses

> There once was an old man with glasses
>
>
>
>

Line to replace (or -1 to quit): 1
Type the new line: Who learned about objects and classes.

> There once was an old man with glasses
> Who learned about objects and classes.
>
>
>

Line to replace (or -1 to quit): 3
Type the new line: Go climb a tree.

> There once was an old man with glasses
> Who learned about objects and classes.
>
> Go climb a tree.
>
```

```
Line to replace (or -1 to quit): 2
Type the new line: "At last, I see!

> There once was an old man with glasses
> Who learned about objects and classes.
> "At last, I see!
> Go climb a tree.
>

Line to replace (or -1 to quit): 4
Type the new line: I'll teach these ideas to the masses!"

> There once was an old man with glasses
> Who learned about objects and classes.
> "At last, I see!
> Go climb a tree.
> I'll teach these ideas to the masses!"

Line to replace (or -1 to quit): 3
Type the new line: It's not only for me.

> There once was an old man with glasses
> Who learned about objects and classes.
> "At last, I see!
> It's not only for me.
> I'll teach these ideas to the masses!"

Line to replace (or -1 to quit): -1
```

Command Line Arguments

Once upon a time, most programmers used a text-based development interface. To run the `Displayer` example in Chapter 3, they didn't select Run from a menu in a fancy integrated development environment. Instead, they typed a command in a plain-looking window, usually with white text on a black background. Figure 11-12 illustrates the point. In Figure 11-12, I type the words **java Displayer** and the computer responds with my Java program's output (the words `You'll love Java!`).

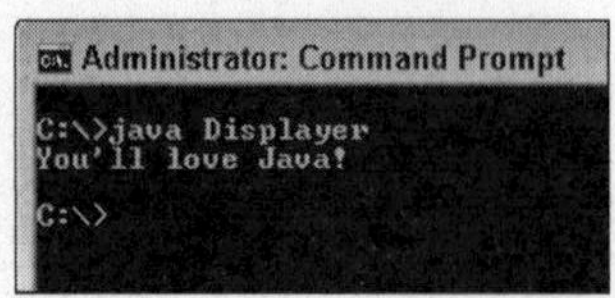

FIGURE 11-12: How dull!

The plain-looking window goes by the various names, depending on the kind of operating system that you use. In Windows, a text window of this kind is a *command prompt window.* On a Macintosh and in Linux, this window is the *terminal.* Some versions of Linux and UNIX call this window a *shell.*

Anyway, back in ancient times, you could write a program that sucked up extra information when you typed the command to launch the program. Figure 11-13 shows you how this worked.

```
Administrator: Command Prompt
C:\>java MakeRandomNumsFile MyNumberedFile.txt 5

C:\>type MyNumberedFile.txt
1
9
10
6
3

C:\>_
```

FIGURE 11-13: When you launch `MakeRandomNumsFile`, you type some extra information.

In Figure 11-13, the programmer types **java MakeRandomNumsFile** to run the `MakeRandomNumsFile` program. But the programmer follows **java MakeRandomNumsFile** with two extra pieces of information: **MyNumberedFile.txt** and **5**. When the `MakeRandomNumsFile` program runs, the program sucks up two extra pieces of information and uses them to do whatever the program has to do. In Figure 11-13, the program sucks up `MyNumberedFile.txt 5`, but on another occasion the programmer might type **SomeStuff 28** or **BunchONumbers 2000**. The extra information can be different each time you run the program.

The next question is, "How does a Java program know that it's supposed to snarf up extra information each time it runs?" Since you first started working with Java, you've been seeing this `String args[]` business in the header of every `main` method. Well, it's high time you found out what that's all about. The parameter `args[]` is an array of `String` values. These `String` values are called *command line arguments.*

REMEMBER

Some programmers write

```
public static void main(String args[])
```

and other programmers write

```
public static void main(String[] args)
```

Either way, `args` is an array of `String` values.

Using command line arguments in a Java program

Listing 11-7 shows you how to use command line arguments in your code.

LISTING 11-7: Generate a File of Numbers

```
import java.util.Random;
import java.io.PrintStream;
import java.io.IOException;

public class MakeRandomNumsFile {

   public static void main(String args[]) throws IOException {

      Random generator = new Random();

      if (args.length < 2) {
         System.out.println("Usage: MakeRandomNumsFile filename number");
         System.exit(1);
      }

      PrintStream printOut = new PrintStream(args[0]);
      int numLines = Integer.parseInt(args[1]);

      for (int count = 1; count <= numLines; count++) {
         printOut.println(generator.nextInt(10) + 1);
      }

      printOut.close();
   }
}
```

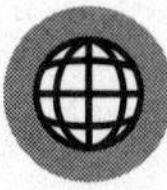

If a particular program expects some command line arguments, you can't start the program running the same way you'd start most of the other programs in this book. The way you feed command line arguments to a program depends on the IDE that you're using — Eclipse, NetBeans, or whatever. That's why this book's website (`www.allmycode.com/JavaForDummies`) has instructions for feeding arguments to programs using various IDEs.

When the code in Listing 11-7 begins running, the `args` array gets its values. With the run shown in Figure 11-13, the array component `args[0]` automatically takes on the value `"MyNumberedFile.txt"`, and `args[1]` automatically becomes `"5"`. So the program's assignment statements end up having the following meaning:

```
PrintStream printOut = new PrintStream("MyNumberedFile.txt");
int numLines = Integer.parseInt("5");
```

The program creates a file named `MyNumberedFile.txt` and sets `numLines` to `5`. So later in the code, the program randomly generates five values and puts those values into `MyNumberedFile.txt`. One run of the program gives me the file shown in Figure 11-14.

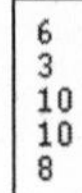

FIGURE 11-14: A file from a run of the code in Listing 11-7.

TIP

After running the code in Listing 11-7, where can you find the new file (`MyNumberedFile.txt`) on your hard drive? The answer depends on a lot of different things, so I don't want to commit to one particular answer. If you use an IDE with programs divided into projects, then the new file is somewhere in the project's folder. One way or another, you can change Listing 11-7 to specify a full path name — a name like `"c:\\Users\\`*`MyName`*`\\Documents\\MyNumberedFile.txt"` or `"/Users/`*`MyName`*`/Documents/MyNumberedFile.txt"`.

REMEMBER

In Windows, file path names contain backslash characters. And in Java, when you want to indicate a backslash inside a double-quoted `String` literal, you use a double backslash instead. That's why `"c:\\Users\\MyName\\Documents\\MyNumberedFile.txt"` contains pairs of backslashes. In contrast, file paths in the Linux and Macintosh operating systems contain forward slashes. To indicate a forward slash in a Java String, use only one forward slash.

Notice how each command line argument in Listing 11-7 is a `String` value. When you look at `args[1]`, you don't see the number 5 — you see the string `"5"` with a digit character in it. Unfortunately, you can't use that `"5"` to do any counting. To get an `int` value from `"5"`, you have to apply the `parseInt` method. (Again, see Listing 11-7.)

The `parseInt` method lives inside a class named *Integer*. So, to call `parseInt`, you preface the name *parseInt* with the word *Integer*. The `Integer` class has all kinds of handy methods for doing things with `int` values.

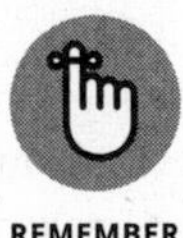

REMEMBER

In Java, *Integer* is the name of a class, and *int* is the name of a primitive (simple) type. The two things are related, but they're not the same. The `Integer` class has methods and other tools for dealing with `int` values.

Checking for the right number of command line arguments

What happens if the user makes a mistake? What if the user forgets to type the number **5** on the first line in Figure 11-13?

Then the computer assigns `"MyNumberedFile.txt"` to `args[0]`, but it doesn't assign anything to `args[1]`. This is bad. If the computer ever reaches the statement

```
int numLines = Integer.parseInt(args[1]);
```

the program crashes with an unfriendly `ArrayIndexOutOfBoundsException`.

What do you do about this? In Listing 11-7, you check the length of the `args` array. You compare `args.length` with `2`. If the `args` array has fewer than two components, you display a message on the screen and exit from the program. Figure 11-15 shows the resulting output.

FIGURE 11-15: The code in Listing 11-7 tells you how to run it.

```
Usage: MakeRandomNumsFile filename number
```

WARNING

Despite the checking of `args.length` in Listing 11-7, the code still isn't crash-proof. If the user types **five** instead of **5**, the program takes a nosedive with a `NumberFormatException`. The second command line argument can't be a word. The argument has to be a number (and a whole number, at that). I can add statements to Listing 11-7 to make the code more bulletproof, but checking for the `NumberFormatException` is better done in Chapter 13.

When you're working with command line arguments, you can enter a `String` value with a blank space in it. Just enclose the value in double quote marks. For instance, you can run the code of Listing 11-7 with arguments `"My Big Fat File.txt" 7`.

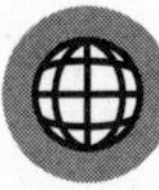

The sun is about to set on this book's discussion of arrays. But before you leave the subject of arrays, think about this: An array is a row of things, and not every kind of thing fits into just one row. Take the first few examples in this chapter involving the motel. The motel rooms, numbered 0 through 9, are in one long line.

But what if you move up in the world? You buy a big hotel with 50 floors and with 100 rooms on each floor. Then the data is square shaped. You have 50 rows, and each row contains 100 items. Sure, you can think of the rooms as if they're all in one long row, but why should you have to do that? How about having a 2-dimensional array? It's a square-shaped array in which each component has two indices: a row number and a column number. Alas, I have no space in this book to show you a 2-dimensional array (and I can't afford a big hotel's prices, anyway). But if you visit this book's website (`www.allmycode.com/JavaForDummies`), you can read all about it.

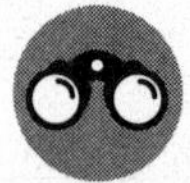
TRY IT OUT

You can never get too much practice:

- Write a program whose command line arguments include three `int` values. As its output, the program displays the largest of the three `int` values.
- In a previous section, you create a simple word processing program. Improve the program by adding two command line arguments:
  - **The first argument is the name of an input file.** The input file contains five lines of text, some or all of which may be blank. At the start of its run, the program reads lines from the input file and displays them on the screen.
  - **The second argument is the name of another file — an output file.** At the end of its run, the program writes the edited text to the output file.

» Dealing with a bunch of objects at once

» Using Java's cool functional programming features

» Developing code for multicore processors

Chapter 12
Using Collections and Streams (When Arrays Aren't Good Enough)

Chapter 11 is about arrays. With an array, you can manage a bunch of things all at once. In a hotel-management program, you can keep track of all the rooms. You can quickly find the number of people in a room or find one of the vacant rooms.

However, arrays don't always fit the bill. In this chapter, you find out where arrays fall short and how collections can save the day.

Understanding the Limitations of Arrays

Arrays are nice, but they have some serious limitations. Imagine that you store customer names in some predetermined order. Your code contains an array, and the array has space for 100 names:

```
String name[] = new String[100];
for (int i = 0; i < 100; i++) {
```

```
    name[i] = new String();
}
```

All is well until, one day, customer number 101 shows up. As your program runs, you enter data for customer 101, hoping desperately that the array with 100 components can expand to fit your growing needs.

No such luck. Arrays don't expand. Your program crashes with an ArrayIndexOutOfBoundsException.

"In my next life, I'll create arrays of length 1,000," you say to yourself. And when your next life rolls around, you do just that:

```
String name[] = new String[1000];
for (int i = 0; i < 1000; i++) {
    name[i] = new String();
}
```

But during your next life, an economic recession occurs. Instead of having 101 customers, you have only 3 customers. Now you're wasting space for 1,000 names when space for 3 names would do.

And what if no economic recession occurs? You're sailing along with your array of size 1,000, using a tidy 825 spaces in the array. The components with indices 0 through 824 are being used, and the components with indices 825 through 999 are waiting quietly to be filled.

One day, a brand-new customer shows up. Because your customers are stored in order (alphabetically by last name, numerically by Social Security number, whatever), you want to squeeze this customer into the correct component of your array. The trouble is that this customer belongs very early on in the array, at the component with index 7. What happens then?

You take the name in component number 824 and move it to component 825. Then you take the name in component 823 and move it to component 824. Take the name in component 822 and move it to component 823. You keep doing this until you've moved the name in component 7. Then you put the new customer's name into component 7. What a pain! Sure, the computer doesn't complain. (If the computer has feelings, it probably likes this kind of busywork.) But as you move around all these names, you waste processing time, you waste power, and you waste all kinds of resources.

"In my next life, I'll leave three empty components between every two names." And of course, your business expands. Eventually you find that three aren't enough.

Collection Classes to the Rescue

The issues in the preceding section aren't new. Computer scientists have been working on these issues for a long time. They haven't discovered any magic one-size-fits-all solution, but they've discovered some clever tricks.

The Java API has a bunch of classes known as *collection* classes. Each collection class has methods for storing bunches of values, and each collection class's methods use some clever tricks. For you, the bottom line is as follows: Certain collection classes deal as efficiently as possible with the issues raised in the preceding section. If you have to deal with such issues when writing code, you can use these collection classes and call the classes' methods. Rather than fret about a customer whose name belongs in position 7, you can just call a class's `add` method. The method inserts the name at a position of your choice and deals reasonably with whatever ripple effects have to take place. In the best circumstances, the insertion is very efficient. In the worst circumstances, you can rest assured that the code does everything the best way it can.

Using an ArrayList

One of the most versatile of Java's collection classes is the `ArrayList`. Listing 12-1 shows you how it works.

LISTING 12-1: Working with a Java Collection

```
import static java.lang.System.out;
import java.util.Scanner;
import java.io.File;
import java.io.IOException;
import java.util.ArrayList;

public class ShowNames {

    public static void main(String args[]) throws IOException {

        ArrayList<String> people = new ArrayList<>();
        Scanner diskScanner = new Scanner(new File("names.txt"));

        while (diskScanner.hasNext()) {
            people.add(diskScanner.nextLine());
        }

        people.remove(0);
        people.add(2, "Jim Newton");
```

(continued)

LISTING 12-1: *(continued)*

```
        for (String name : people) {
            out.println(name);
        }

        diskScanner.close();
    }
}
```

Figure 12-1 shows you a sample names.txt file. The code in Listing 12-1 reads that names.txt file and prints the stuff in Figure 12-2.

```
Barry Burd
Harriet Ritter
Weelie J. Katz
Harry "The Crazyman" Spoonswagler
Felicia "Fishy" Katz
Mia, Just "Mia"
Jeremy Flooflong Jones
I. M. D'Arthur
Hugh R. DaReader
```

FIGURE 12-1: Several names in a file.

```
Harriet Ritter
Weelie J. Katz
Jim Newton
Harry "The Crazyman" Spoonswagler
Felicia "Fishy" Katz
Mia, Just "Mia"
Jeremy Flooflong Jones
I. M. D'Arthur
Hugh R. DaReader
```

FIGURE 12-2: The code in Listing 12-1 changes some of the names.

All the interesting things happen when you execute the remove and add methods. The variable named people refers to an ArrayList object. When you call that object's remove method,

```
people.remove(0);
```

you eliminate a value from the list. In this case, you eliminate whatever value is in the list's initial position (the position numbered 0). So in Listing 12-1, the call to remove takes the name Barry Burd out of the list.

That leaves only eight names in the list, but then the next statement,

```
people.add(2, "Jim Newton");
```

inserts a name into position number 2. (After Barry is removed, position number 2 is the position occupied by Harry Spoonswagler, so Harry moves to position 3, and Jim Newton becomes the number 2 man.)

Notice that an ArrayList object has two different add methods. The method that adds Jim Newton has two parameters: a position number and a value to be added. Another add method

```
people.add(diskScanner.nextLine());
```

takes only one parameter. This statement takes whatever name it finds on a line of the input file and appends that name to the end of the list. (The add method with only one parameter always appends its value to what's currently the end of the ArrayList object.)

The last few lines of Listing 12-1 contain an enhanced for loop. Like the loop in Listing 11-3, the enhanced loop in Listing 12-1 has the following form:

```
for (variable-type variable-name : range-of-values)
```

In Listing 12-1, the *variable-type* is String, the *variable-name* is name, and the *range-of-values* includes the things stored in the people collection. During an iteration of the loop, name refers to one of the String values stored in people. (So if the people collection contains nine values, the for loop goes through nine iterations.) During each iteration, the statement inside the loop displays a name on the screen.

Using generics

Look again at Listing 12-1, shown earlier, and notice the funky ArrayList declaration:

```
ArrayList<String> people = new ArrayList<>();
```

Starting with Java 5.0, each collection class is *generified.* That ugly-sounding word means that every collection declaration should contain some angle-bracketed stuff, such as <String>. The thing that's sandwiched between < and > tells Java what kinds of values the new collection may contain. For example, in Listing 12-1, the words ArrayList<String> people tell Java that people is a bunch of strings. That is, the people list contains String objects (not Room objects, not Account objects, not Employee objects, nothing other than String objects).

REMEMBER

You can't use generics in any version of Java before Java 5.0, and the code in Listing 12-1 goes kablooey in any version before Java 7. For more about generics, see the nearby sidebar, "All about generics." And for more about Java's version numbers, see Chapter 2.

In Listing 12-1, the words `ArrayList<String> people` say that the `people` variable can refer only to a collection of `String` values. So, from that point on, any reference to an item from the `people` collection is treated exclusively as a `String`. If you write

```
people.add(new Room());
```

the compiler coughs up your code and spits it out because a `Room` (created in Chapter 11) isn't the same as a `String`. (This coughing and spitting happens even if the compiler has access to the `Room` class's code — the code in Chapter 11.) But the statement

```
people.add("George Gow");
```

is just fine. Because `"George Gow"` has type `String`, the compiler smiles happily.

ALL ABOUT GENERICS

One of the original design goals for Java was to keep the language as simple as possible. James Gosling, the language's creator, took some unnecessarily complicated features of C++ and tossed them out the window. The result was a language that was elegant and sleek. Some people said the language was *too* sleek. So, after several years of discussion and squabbling, Java became a bit more complicated. By the year 2004, Java had `enum` types, enhanced `for` loops, static import, and some other interesting new features. But the most talked-about new feature was the introduction of generics:

```
ArrayList<String> people = new ArrayList<String>();
```

The use of anything like `<String>` was new in Java 5.0. In old-style Java, you'd write

```
ArrayList people = new ArrayList();
```

In those days, an `ArrayList` could store almost anything you wanted to put in it: a number, an `Account`, a `Room`, a `String` — anything. The `ArrayList` class was versatile, but with this versatility came some headaches. If you could put anything into an `ArrayList`, you couldn't easily predict what you would get out of an `ArrayList`. In particular, you couldn't easily write code that assumed you had stored certain types of values in the `ArrayList`. Here's an example:

```
ArrayList things = new ArrayList();
things.add(new Account());
Account myAccount = things.get(0);
//DON'T USE THIS. IT'S BAD CODE.
```

In the third line, the call to get(0) grabs the earliest value in the things collection. The call to get(0) is okay, but then the compiler chokes on the attempted assignment to myAccount. You get a message on the third line saying that whatever you get from the things list can't be stuffed into the myAccount variable. You get this message because by the time the compiler reaches the third line, it has forgotten that the item added on the second line was of type Account!

The introduction of generics fixes this problem:

```
ArrayList<Account> things = new ArrayList<Account>();
things.add(new Account());
Account myAccount = things.get(0);
//USE THIS CODE INSTEAD. IT'S GOOD CODE.
```

Adding <Account> in two places tells the compiler that things stores Account instances — nothing else. So, in the third line in the preceding code, you get a value from the things collection. Then, because things stores only Account objects, you can make myAccount refer to that new value.

Java 5.0 added generics to Java. But soon after the birth of Java 5.0, programmers noticed how clumsy the code for generics can be. After all, you can create generics within generics. An ArrayList can contain a bunch of arrays, each of which can be an ArrayList. So you can write

```
ArrayList<ArrayList<String>[]> mess = new ArrayList<ArrayList
    <String>[]>();
```

All the repetition in that mess declaration gives me a headache! To avoid this ugliness, Java 7 and later versions have a diamond operator: <>. The diamond operator tells Java to reuse whatever insanely complicated stuff you put in the previous part of the generic declaration. In this example, the <> tells Java to reuse <ArrayList<String> []>, even though you write <ArrayList<String> []> only once. Here's how the streamlined Java 7 code looks:

```
ArrayList<ArrayList<String>[]> mess = new ArrayList<>();
```

In Java 7 and later, you can write either of these mess declarations: the original, nasty declaration with two occurrences of ArrayList<String> [] or the streamlined (only mildly nasty) declaration with the diamond operator and only one ArrayList<String> [] occurrence.

Yes, the streamlined code is still complicated. But without all the ArrayList<String> [] repetition, the streamlined code is less cumbersome. The Java 7 diamond operator takes away one chance for you to copy something incorrectly and have a big error in your code.

Wrapper classes

In Chapter 4, I point out that Java has two kinds of types: primitive types and reference types. (If you didn't read those sections, or you don't remember them, don't feel guilty. You'll be okay.) Things like `int`, `double`, `char`, and `boolean` are primitive types, and things like `String`, `JFrame`, `ArrayList`, and `Account` are reference types.

The distinction between primitive types and reference types has been a source of contention since Java's birth in 1995. Even now, Oracle's wizards are hatching plans to get around the stickier consequences of having two kinds of types. One of those consequences is the fact that collections, such as the `ArrayList`, can't contain values of a primitive type. For example, it's okay to write

```
ArrayList<String> people = new ArrayList<>();
```

but it's not okay to write

```
ArrayList<int> numbers = new ArrayList<>(); // BAD! BAD!
```

because `int` is a primitive type. So, if you want to store values like `3`, `55`, and `21` in an `ArrayList`, what do you do? Rather than store `int` values in the `ArrayList`, you store Java's `Integer` values:

```
ArrayList<Integer> list = new ArrayList<>();
```

In previous chapters, you see the `Integer` class in connection with the `parseInt` method:

```
int numberOfCows = Integer.parseInt("536");
```

The `Integer` class has many methods, such as `parseInt`, for dealing with `int` values. The class also has fields such as `MAX_VALUE` and `MIN_VALUE`, which stand for the largest and smallest values that `int` variables may have.

The `Integer` class is an example of a *wrapper class*. Each of Java's eight primitive types has a corresponding wrapper class. You can use methods and fields in Java's `Double`, `Character`, `Boolean`, `Long`, `Float`, `Short`, and `Byte` wrapper classes. For example, the `Double` class has methods named `parseDouble`, `compareTo`, `toHexString`, and fields named `MAX_VALUE` and `MAX_EXPONENT`.

The `Integer` class wraps the primitive `int` type with useful methods and values. In addition, you can create an `Integer` instance that wraps a single `int` value:

```
Integer myInteger = new Integer(42);
```

In this line of code, the `myInteger` variable has one `int` value inside it: the `int` value `42`. In Paul's words, wrapping the `int` value `42` into an `Integer` object `myInteger` is "something like putting lots of extra breading on okra. It makes `42` more digestible for finicky eaters like collections."

Instances of the other wrapper classes work the same way. For example, an instance of the `Double` class wraps up a single primitive `double` value.

```
Double averageNumberOfTomatoes = new Double(1.41421356237);
```

Here's a program that stores five `Integer` values in an `ArrayList`:

```
import java.util.ArrayList;

public class Main {

    public static void main(String[] args) {
        ArrayList<Integer> list = new ArrayList<>();
        fillTheList(list);
        for (Integer n : list) {
            System.out.println(n);
        }
    }

    public static void fillTheList(ArrayList<Integer> list) {
        list.add(85);
        list.add(19);
        list.add(0);
        list.add(103);
        list.add(13);
    }
}
```

In the code, notice calls like `list.add(85)` that have `int` value parameters. At this point, little Billy gets excited and says, "Look, Mom! I added the primitive `int` value `85` to my `ArrayList`!" No, Billy. That's not what's really going on.

In this code, the `list` collection contains `Integer` values, not `int` values. A primitive `int` value is a lot like an instance of the `Integer` class. But a primitive `int` value isn't exactly the same as an `Integer` instance.

What's going on is called *autoboxing*. Before Java 5.0, you had to write

```
list.add(new Integer(85));
```

if you wanted to add an Integer to an ArrayList. But Java 5.0 and later Java versions can automatically wrap an int value inside a box. An int value in a parameter list becomes an Integer in ArrayList. Java's autoboxing feature makes programs easier to read and write.

Testing for the presence of more data

Here's a pleasant surprise. When you write a program like the one shown previously in Listing 12-1, you don't have to know how many names are in the input file. Having to know the number of names may defeat the purpose of using the easily expandable ArrayList class. Rather than loop until you read exactly nine names, you can loop until you run out of data.

The Scanner class has several nice methods, such as hasNextInt, hasNextDouble, and plain old hasNext. Each of these methods checks for more input data. If there's more data, the method returns true. Otherwise, the method returns false.

Listing 12-1 uses the general-purpose hasNext method. This hasNext method returns true as long as there's anything more to read from the program's input. After the program scoops up that last Hugh R. DaReader line in Figure 12-1, the subsequent hasNext call returns false. This false condition ends execution of the while loop and plummets the computer toward the remainder of the Listing 12-1 code.

The hasNext method is quite handy. In fact, hasNext is so handy that it's part of a bigger concept known as an *iterator*, and iterators are baked into all of Java's collection classes.

Using an iterator

An iterator spits out a collection's values, one after another. To obtain a value from the collection, you call the iterator's next method. To find out whether the collection has any more values in it, you call the iterator's hasNext method. Listing 12-2 uses an iterator to display people's names.

LISTING 12-2: Iterating through a Collection

```
import static java.lang.System.out;
import java.util.Iterator;
import java.util.Scanner;
import java.io.File;
import java.io.IOException;
import java.util.ArrayList;
```

```
public class ShowNames {

    public static void main(String args[]) throws IOException {

        ArrayList<String> people = new ArrayList<>();
        Scanner diskScanner = new Scanner(new File("names.txt"));

        while (diskScanner.hasNext()) {
            people.add(diskScanner.nextLine());
        }

        people.remove(0);
        people.add(2, "Jim Newton");

        Iterator<String> iterator = people.iterator();
        while (iterator.hasNext()) {
            out.println(iterator.next());
        }

        diskScanner.close();
    }
}
```

You can replace the enhanced `for` loop at the end of Listing 12-1 with the boldface code in Listing 12-2. When you do, you get the same output as before. (You get the output in Figure 12-2.) In Listing 12-2, the first boldface line of code creates an iterator from the `people` collection. The second and third lines call the iterator's `hasNext` and `next` methods to grab all objects stored in the `people` collection — one for each iteration of the loop. These lines display each of the `people` collection's values.

Which is better? An enhanced `for` loop or an iterator? Java programmers prefer the enhanced `for` loop because the `for` loop involves less baggage — no `iterator` object to carry from one line of code to the next. But as you see later in this chapter, the most programming-enhanced feature can be upgraded, streamlined, tweaked, and otherwise reconstituted. There's no end to the way you can improve upon your code.

Java's many collection classes

The `ArrayList` class that I use in many of this chapter's examples is only the tip of the Java collections iceberg. The Java library contains many collections classes, each with its own advantages. Table 12-1 contains an abbreviated list.

TABLE 12-1 **Some Collection Classes**

Class Name	Characteristic
`ArrayList`	A resizable array.
`LinkedList`	A list of values, each having a field that points to the next one in the list.
`Stack`	A structure that grows from bottom to top. The structure is optimized for access to the topmost value. You can easily add a value to the top or remove the value from the top.
`Queue`	A structure that grows at one end. The structure is optimized for adding values to one end (the rear) and removing values from the other end (the front).
`PriorityQueue`	A structure, like a queue, that lets certain (higher-priority) values move toward the front.
`HashSet`	A collection containing no duplicate values.
`HashMap`	A collection of key/value pairs.

Each collection class has its own set of methods (in addition to the methods that it inherits from `AbstractCollection`, the ancestor of all collection classes).

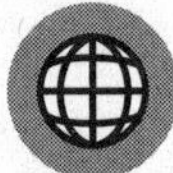

To find out which collection classes best meet your needs, visit the Java API documentation pages at `http://docs.oracle.com/javase/8/docs/api`.

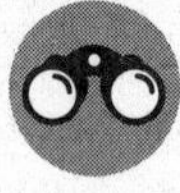

TRY IT OUT

Once again, I'd like to put you to work:

- Create an `ArrayList` containing `Integer` values. Then step through the values in the list to find the largest value among all values in the list. For example, if the list contains the numbers 85, 19, 0, 103, and 13, display the number 103.
- Create an `ArrayList` containing `String` values in alphabetical order. When the user types an additional word on the keyboard, the program inserts the new word into the `ArrayList` in the proper (alphabetically ordered) place.

  For example, imagine that the list starts off containing the words `"cat"`, `"dog"`, `"horse"`, and `"zebra"` (in that order). After the user types the word `fish` on the keyboard (and presses Enter), the list contains the words `"cat"`, `"dog"`, `"fish"`, `"horse"`, and `"zebra"` (in that order).

  To write this program, you may find the `String` class's `compareToIgnoreCase` method and the `ArrayList` class's `size` method useful. You can find out about these methods by visiting `https://docs.oracle.com/javase/8/docs/api/java/lang/String.html#compareToIgnoreCase-java.lang.String-` and `http://docs.oracle.com/javase/8/docs/api/java/util/ArrayList.html#size--`.

» In Chapter 11, you create a simple word processor. Your program stores lines of text in an array, so the number of lines is limited by the size of the array.

In this chapter, you can improve on your work from Chapter 11 by storing lines of text in an `ArrayList`. An `ArrayList` has no fixed size, so the number of lines can grow to meet the user's needs.

Your improved word processor supports three kinds of commands:

- The command `i 21` tells your program to insert the 21st line of text into the document. (If there's already a 21st line of text, the new line goes between the existing 20th and 21st lines.)
- The command `r 13` tells your program to replace the 13th line of text in the document. (If there's already a 13th line of text, that old line of text goes away.)
- The command `d 7` tells your program to delete the seventh line of text. (If there's already an eighth line of text, that existing line becomes the seventh line of text.)

This word processor program may be quite challenging. Work slowly and carefully and don't be discouraged. If you don't get it at first, put the project aside and come back to it later.

Functional Programming

From 1953 to 1957, John Backus and others developed the FORTRAN programming language, which contained the basic framework for thousands of 20th century programming languages. The framework has come to be known as *imperative programming* because of its do-this-then-do-that nature.

A few years after the rise of FORTRAN, John McCarthy created another language, named *Lisp*. Unlike FORTRAN, the underlying framework for Lisp is *functional programming*. In a purely functional program, you avoid writing "do this, then do that." Instead, you write things like "Here's how you'll be transforming this into that when you get around to doing the transformation."

For one reason or another, imperative programming became the dominant mode. As a result, Java is fundamentally an imperative programming language. But recently, functional programming has emerged as a powerful and useful way of thinking about code.

To help you understand functional programming, I start this section with an analogy. Then, in the rest of this chapter, I present some Java examples.

The analogy that I use to describe functional programming is very rough. A friend of mine called this analogy a stretch because it applies to many different programming frameworks, not only to functional programming. One way or another, I think the analogy is helpful.

Here's the analogy: Imagine a programming problem as a cube, and imagine an imperative programming solution as a way of slicing up the cube into manageable pieces. (See Figure 12-3.)

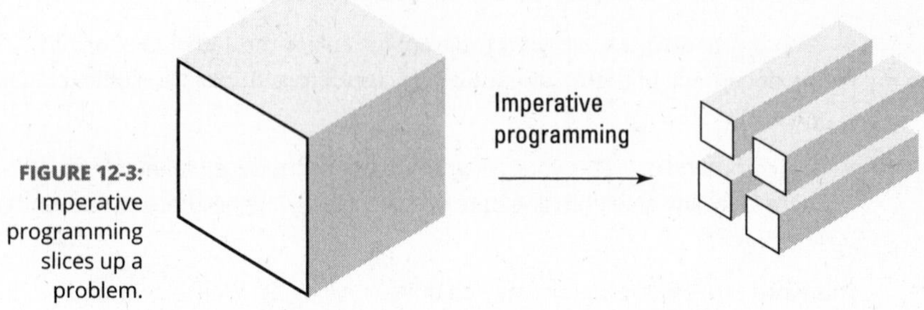

Imperative
programming

FIGURE 12-3: Imperative programming slices up a problem.

All was well until 2007, when, for the first time, computers sold to consumers had multicore processors. A *multicore* processor can perform more than one instruction at a time. Figure 12-4 shows what happens when you try to squeeze an imperative program into a multicore processor.

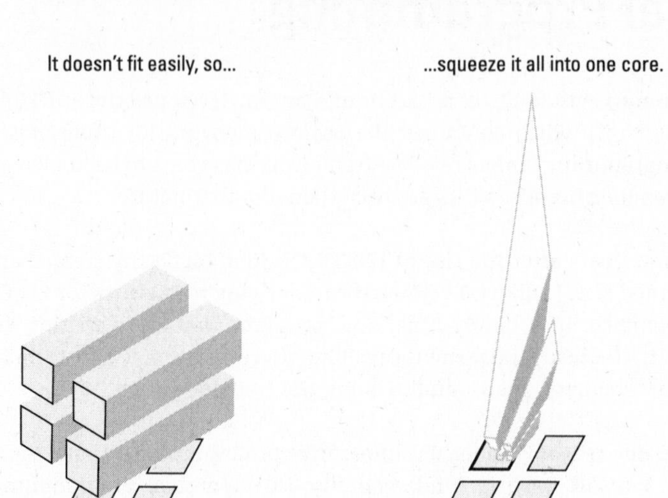

It doesn't fit easily, so...
...squeeze it all into one core.

FIGURE 12-4: An imperative program's pieces don't fit neatly into a multicore chip.

To get the most out of a four-core processor, you divide your code into four pieces — one piece for each core. But with imperative programming, your program's pieces don't fit neatly into your processor's cores.

TECHNICAL STUFF

In imperative programming, your code's pieces interact with one another. All the pieces might be updating the current price of Oracle stock shares (ticker symbol: ORCL). The simultaneous updates become tangled. It's like several high school boys asking the same girl to the senior prom — nothing good ever comes of it. You've experienced the same phenomenon if you've ever clicked a website's Purchase button, only to learn that the item you're trying to purchase is out of stock. Someone else completed a purchase while you were filling in your credit card information. Too many customers were grabbing for the same goods at the same time.

Figure 12-3 suggests that, with imperative programming, you divide your code into several pieces. Functional programming also divides code into pieces, but it does so along different lines. (See Figure 12-5.) And here's the good news: With functional programming, the pieces of the code fit neatly into the processor's cores. (See Figure 12-6.)

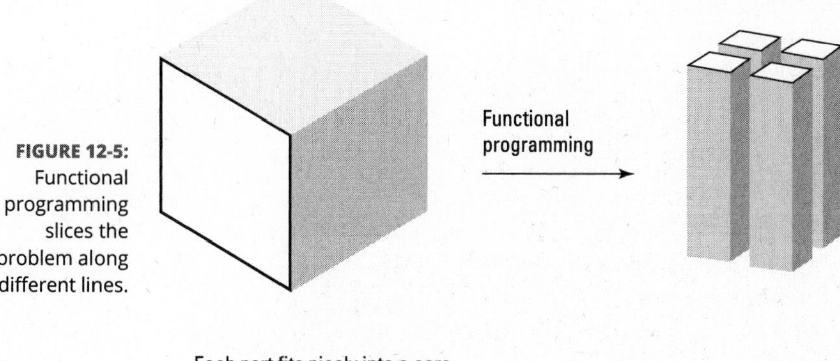
Functional
programming

FIGURE 12-5: Functional programming slices the problem along different lines.

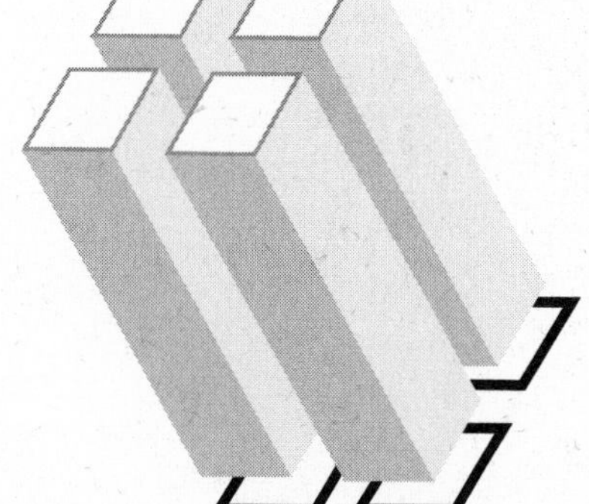
Each part fits nicely into a core.

FIGURE 12-6: A functional program's pieces fit neatly into a multicore chip.

Solving a problem the old-fashioned way

In Chapter 11, you use arrays to manage the Java Motel. But that venture is behind you now. You've given up the hotel business. (You tell people that you decided to move on. But in all honesty, the hotel was losing a lot of money. According to the United States bankruptcy court, the old Java Motel is currently in Chapter 11.)

Since leaving the hotel business, you've transitioned into online sales. Nowadays, you run a website that sells books, DVDs, and other content-related items. (Barry Burd's *Java For Dummies*, 7th Edition, is currently your best seller, but that's beside the point.)

In your world, the sale of a single item looks something like the stuff in Listing 12-3. Each sale has an item and a price.

LISTING 12-3: The Sale Class

```
public class Sale {
    private String item;
    private double price;

    public String getItem() {
      return item;
    }

    public void setItem(String item) {
      this.item = item;
    }

    public double getPrice() {
      return price;
    }

    public void setPrice(double price) {
      this.price = price;
    }

    public Sale(String item, double price) {
        this.item = item;
        this.price = price;
    }
}
```

To make use of the Sale class, you create a small program. The program totals up the sales on DVDs. The program is shown in Listing 12-4.

LISTING 12-4: Using the Sale Class

```
import java.text.NumberFormat;
import java.util.ArrayList;

public class TallySales {

    public static void main(String[] args) {
        ArrayList<Sale> sales = new ArrayList<Sale>();
        NumberFormat currency = NumberFormat.getCurrencyInstance();

        fillTheList(sales);

        double total = 0;
        for (Sale sale : sales) {
            if (sale.getItem().equals("DVD")) {
                total += sale.getPrice();
            }
        }

        System.out.println(currency.format(total));
    }

    static void fillTheList(ArrayList<Sale> sales) {
        sales.add(new Sale("DVD", 15.00));
        sales.add(new Sale("Book", 12.00));
        sales.add(new Sale("DVD", 21.00));
        sales.add(new Sale("CD", 5.25));
    }
}
```

In Chapter 11, you step through an array by using an enhanced for statement. Listing 12-4 has its own enhanced for statement. But in Listing 12-4, the enhanced for statement steps through the values in a collection. Each such value is a sale. The loop repeatedly checks a sale to find out whether the item sold is a DVD. If so, the code adds the sale's price to the running total. The program's output is $36.00 — the running total displayed as a currency amount.

The scenario in Listing 12-4 isn't unusual. You have a collection of items (a collection of sales, perhaps). You step through the items in the collection, finding the items that meet certain criteria (the sale of a DVD, for example). You grab a certain value (such as the sale price) of each item that meets your criteria. Then you do something useful with the values that you've grabbed (for example, adding the values together).

Here are some other examples:

- Step through your list of employees. Find each employee whose performance evaluation scored 3 or higher. Give each such employee a $100 bonus and then determine the total amount of money you'll pay in bonuses.
- Step through your list of customers. For each customer who has shown interest in buying a smartphone, send the customer an email about this month's discount plans.
- Step through the list of planets that have been discovered. For each M-class planet, find the probability of finding intelligent life on that planet. Then find the average of all such probabilities.

This scenario is so common that it's worth finding better and better ways to deal with the scenario. One way to deal with it is to use some of the functional programming features in Java.

Streams

The earlier section "Using an iterator" introduces iterators. You use an iterator's `next` method to spit out a collection's values. Java takes this concept one step further with the notion of a stream. A *stream* is like an iterator except that, with a stream, you don't have to call a `next` method. After being created, a stream spits out a collection's values automatically. To get values from a stream, you don't call a stream's `next` method. In fact, a typical stream has no `next` method.

How does this work as part of a Java program? How do you create a stream that spits out values? How does the stream know when to start spitting, and where does the stream aim when it spits? For answers to these and other questions, read the next several sections.

Lambda expressions

In the 1930s, mathematician Alonzo Church used the Greek letter *lambda* (λ) to represent a certain mathematical construct that's created on the fly.* Over the next several decades, the idea survived quietly in mathematics and computer science journals. These days, in Java, the term *lambda expression* represents a short piece of code that serves as both a method declaration and a method call, all created on the fly.

Your first lambda expression

Here's an example of a lambda expression:

```
(sale) -> sale.getItem().equals("DVD")
```

Figure 12-7 describes the lambda expression's meaning.

A lambda expression is a concise way of defining a method and calling the method without even giving the method a name. The lambda expression in Figure 12-7 does (roughly) what the following code does:

```
boolean itemIsDVD(Sale sale) {
    if sale.getItem().equals("DVD") {
        return true;
    } else {
        return false;
    }
}

itemIsDVD(sale);
```

The lambda expression in Figure 12-7 takes objects from a stream and calls a method resembling `itemIsDVD` on each object. The result is a bunch of `boolean` values — `true` for each sale of a DVD and `false` for a sale of something other than a DVD.

---

*I attended a lecture given by Alonzo Church many years ago at the University of Illinois. He was the world's most meticulous presenter. Every detail of his lecture was carefully planned and scrupulously executed. He handed out paper copies of his notes, and I spent half the lecture staring at the notes, trying to decide whether the notes were hand-written or typed.

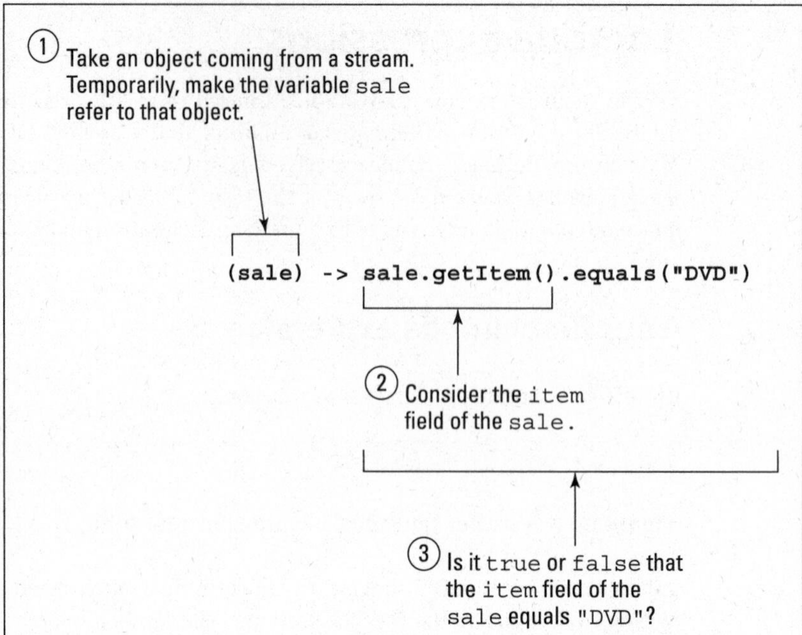

1 Take an object coming from a stream. Temporarily, make the variable sale refer to that object.
(sale) -> sale.getItem().equals("DVD")
2 Consider the item field of the sale.
3 Is it true or false that the item field of the sale equals "DVD"?

FIGURE 12-7: Does the item that's being sold happen to be a DVD?

TIP

With or without lambda expressions, you can rewrite the `itemIsDVD` method with a 1-line body:

```
boolean itemIsDVD(Sale sale) {
    return sale.getItem().equals("DVD");
}
```

A lambda expression with two parameters

Consider the following lambda expression:

```
(price1, price2) -> price1 + price2
```

Figure 12-8 describes the new lambda expression's meaning.

The lambda expression in Figure 12-8 does (roughly) what the following code does:

```
double sum(double price1, double price2) {
    return price1 + price2;
}

sum(price1, price2);
```

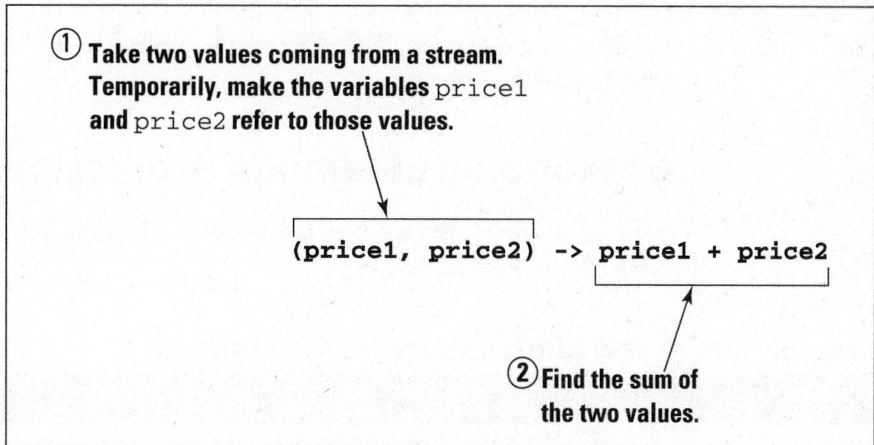

① Take two values coming from a stream.
Temporarily, make the variables price1
and price2 refer to those values.
(price1, price2) -> price1 + price2
② Find the sum of
the two values.

FIGURE 12-8: Add two prices.

The lambda expression in Figure 12-8 takes values from a stream and calls a method resembling `sum` to combine the values. The result is the total of all prices.

The black sheep of lambda expressions

Here's an interesting lambda expression:

```
(sale) -> System.out.println(sale.getPrice())
```

This lambda expression does (roughly) what the following code does:

```
void display(Sale sale) {
    System.out.println(sale.getPrice());
}

display(sale);
```

The lambda expression takes objects from a stream and calls a method resembling `display` on each object. In the `display` method's header, the word `void` indicates that the method doesn't return a value. When you call the `display` method (or you use the equivalent lambda expression), you don't expect to get back a value. Instead, you expect the code to do something in response to the call (something like displaying text on the computer's screen).

To draw a sharp distinction between returning a value and "doing something," functional programmers have a name for "doing something without returning a value" — they call that something a *side effect*. In functional programming, a side effect is considered a second-class citizen, a last resort, a tactic that you use when you can't simply return a result. Unfortunately, displaying information on a screen (something that so many computer programs do) is a side effect. Any program that displays output (on a screen, on paper, or as tea leaves in a cup) isn't a purely functional program.

A taxonomy of lambda expressions

Java divides lambda expressions into about 45 different categories. Table 12-2 lists a few of the categories.

TABLE 12-2 A Few Kinds of Lambda Expressions

Name	Description	Example
`Function`	Accepts one parameter; produces a result of any type	`(sale) -> sale. price`
`Predicate`	Accepts one parameter; produces a `boolean` valued result	`(sale) -> sale.item. equals("DVD")`
`BinaryOperator`	Accepts two parameters of the same type; produces a result of the same type	`(price1, price2) -> price1 + price2`
`Consumer`	Accepts one parameter; produces no result	`(sale) -> System.out. println (sale. price)`

REMEMBER

The categories in Table 12-2 aren't mutually exclusive. For example, every `Predicate` is a `Function`. (Every `Predicate` accepts one parameter and returns a result. The result happens to be `boolean`.)

Using streams and lambda expressions

Java has fancy methods that make optimal use of streams and lambda expressions. With streams and lambda expressions, you can create an assembly line that elegantly solves this chapter's sales problem. Unlike the code in Listing 12-4, the new assembly-line solution uses concepts from functional programming.

The assembly line consists of several methods. Each method takes the data, transforms the data in some way or other, and hands its results to the next method in line. Figure 12-9 illustrates the assembly line for this chapter's sales problem.

In Figure 12-9, each box represents a bunch of raw materials as they're transformed along an assembly line. Each arrow represents a method (or, metaphorically, a worker on the assembly line).

For example, in the transition from the second box to the third box, a worker method (the `filter` method) sifts out sales of items that aren't DVDs. Imagine Lucy Ricardo standing between the second and third boxes, removing each book or CD from the assembly line and tossing it carelessly onto the floor.

The parameter to Java's `filter` method is a `Predicate` — a lambda expression whose result is `boolean`. (See Tables 12-2 and 12-3.) The `filter` method in Figure 12-9 sifts out items that don't pass the lambda expression's `true / false` test.

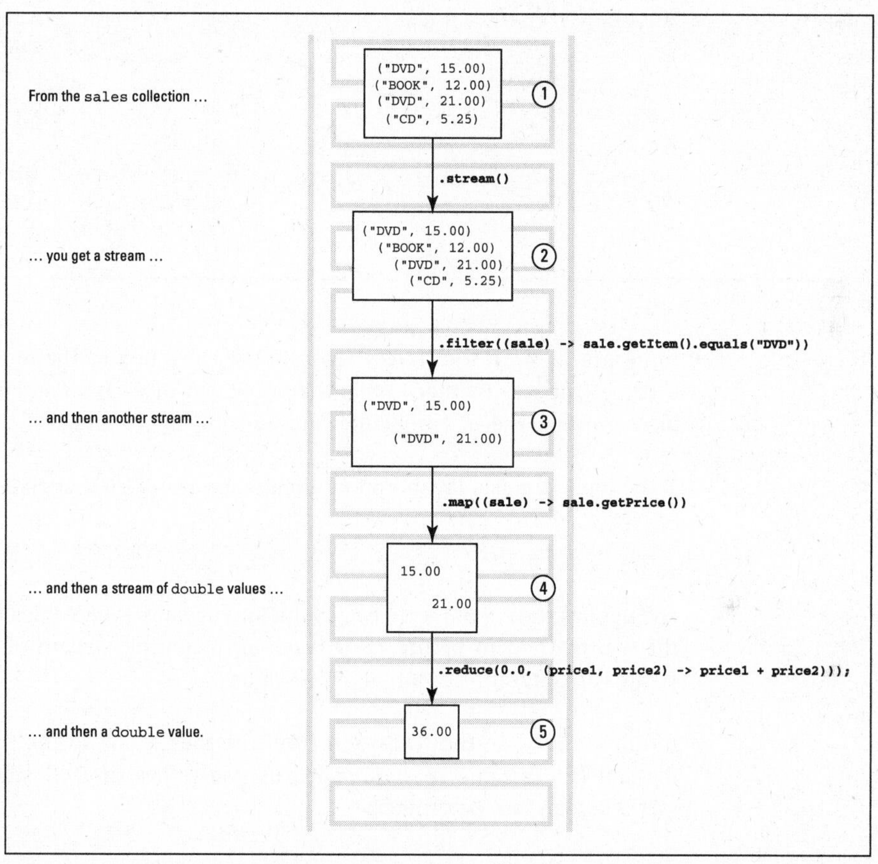

FIGURE 12-9: A functional programming assembly line.

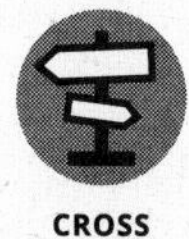

For some help understanding the words in the third column of Table 12-3 (`Predicate`, `Function` and `BinaryOperator`), see the earlier section "A taxonomy of lambda expressions."

TABLE 12-3 **Some Functional Programming Methods**

Method Name	Member Of	Parameter(s)	Result Type	Result Value
`stream`	`Collection` (for example, an `ArrayList` object)	(none)	`Stream`	A stream that spits out elements of the collection
`filter`	`Stream`	`Predicate`	`Stream`	A new stream containing values for which the lambda expression returns `true`
`map`	`Stream`	`Function`	`Stream`	A new stream containing the results of applying the lambda expression to the incoming stream
`reduce`	`Stream`	`BinaryOperator`	The type used by the `BinaryOperator`	The result of combining all the values in the incoming stream

In Figure 12-9, in the transition from the third box to the fourth box, a worker method (the `map` method) pulls the `price` out of each `sale`. From that worker's place onward, the assembly line contains only `price` values.

To be more precise, Java's `map` method takes a `Function` such as

```
(sale) -> sale.getPrice()
```

and applies the `Function` to each value in a stream. (See Tables 12-2 and 12-3.) So the `map` method in Figure 12-9 takes an incoming stream of `sale` objects and creates an outgoing stream of `price` values.

In Figure 12-9, in the transition from the fourth box to the fifth box, a worker method (the `reduce` method) adds up the prices of DVD sales. Java's `reduce` method takes two parameters:

- The first parameter is an initial value.

  In Figure 12-9, the initial value is `0.0`.

- The second parameter is a `BinaryOperator`. (See Tables 12-2 and 12-3.)

  In Figure 12-9, the `reduce` method's `BinaryOperator` is

  ```
  (price1, price2) -> price1 + price2
  ```

The reduce method uses its BinaryOperator to combine the values from the incoming stream. The initial value serves as the starting point for all the combining. So, in Figure 12-9, the reduce method does two additions. (See Figure 12-10.)

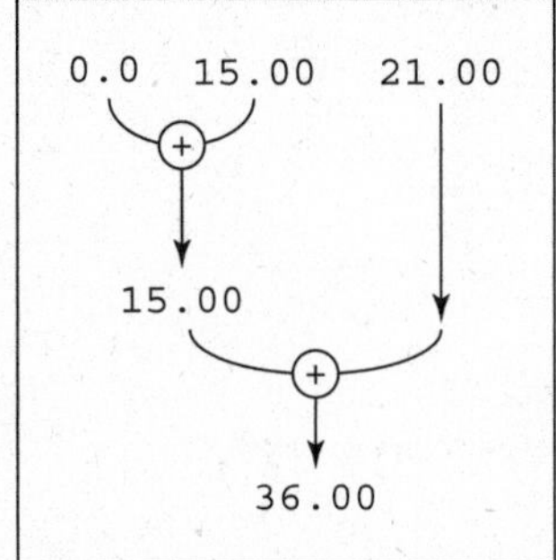

FIGURE 12-10: The reduce method adds two values from an incoming stream.

For comparison, imagine calling the method

```
reduce(10.0, (value1, value2) -> value1 * value2)
```

with the stream whose values include 3.0, 2.0, and 5.0. The resulting action is shown in Figure 12-11.

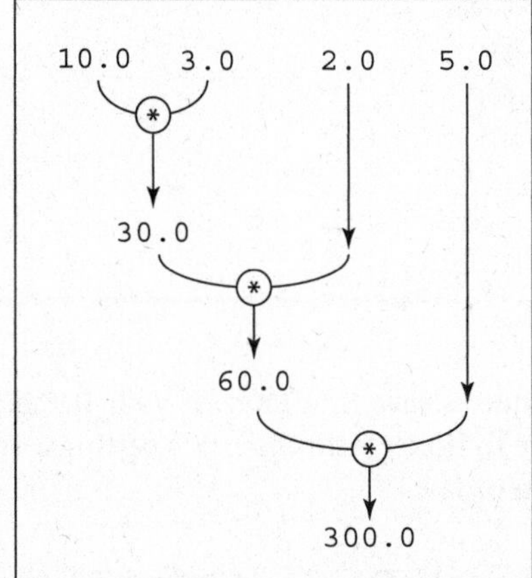

FIGURE 12-11: The reduce method multiplies values from an incoming stream.

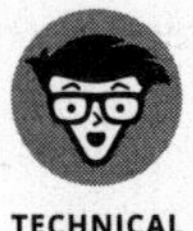

TECHNICAL STUFF

You might have heard of Google's MapReduce programming model. The similarity between the programming model's name and the Java method names map and reduce is not a coincidence.

Taken as a whole, the entire assembly line shown in Figure 12-9 adds up the prices of DVDs sold. Listing 12-5 contains a complete program using the streams and lambda expressions of Figure 12-9.

LISTING 12-5: Living the Functional Way of Life

```
import java.text.NumberFormat;
import java.util.ArrayList;

public class TallySales {

  public static void main(String[] args) {
    ArrayList<Sale> sales = new ArrayList<>();
    NumberFormat currency = NumberFormat.getCurrencyInstance();

    fillTheList(sales);

    double total = sales.stream()
                        .filter((sale) -> sale.getItem().equals("DVD"))
                        .map((sale) -> sale.getPrice())
                        .reduce(0.0, (price1, price2) -> price1 + price2);

    System.out.println(currency.format(total));
  }

  static void fillTheList(ArrayList<Sale> sales) {
    sales.add(new Sale("DVD", 15.00));
    sales.add(new Sale("Book", 12.00));
    sales.add(new Sale("DVD", 21.00));
    sales.add(new Sale("CD", 5.25));
  }
}
```

WARNING

The code in Listing 12-5 requires Java 8 or later. If your IDE is set for an earlier Java version, you might have to tinker with the IDE's settings. You may even have to download a newer version of Java.

The boldface code in Listing 12-5 is one big Java assignment statement. The right side of the statement contains a sequence of method calls. Each method call returns an object, and each such object is the thing before the dot in the next method call. That's how you form the assembly line.

For example, near the start of the boldface code, the name `sales` refers to an `ArrayList` object. Each `ArrayList` object has a `stream` method. In Listing 12-5, `sales.stream()` is a call to that `ArrayList` object's `stream` method.

The `stream` method returns an instance of Java's `Stream` class. (What a surprise!) So `sales.stream()` refers to a `Stream` object. (See Figure 12-12.)

Every `Stream` object has a `filter` method. So

```
sales.stream().filter((sale) -> sale.getItem().equals("DVD"))
```

is a call to the `Stream` object's `filter` method. (Refer to Figure 12-12.)

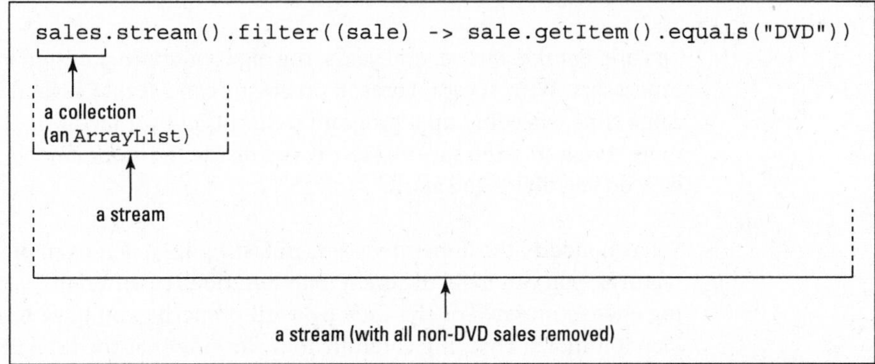

FIGURE 12-12: Getting all DVD sales.

The pattern continues. The `Stream` object's `map` method returns yet another `Stream` object — a `Stream` object containing prices. (See Figure 12-13.) To that `Stream` of prices you apply the `reduce` method, which yields one `double` value — the total of the DVD prices. (See Figure 12-14.)

sales.stream().filter((sale) -> sale.getItem().equals("DVD")).map((sale) -> sale.getPrice())

a stream (with all non-DVD sales removed)

a stream of prices

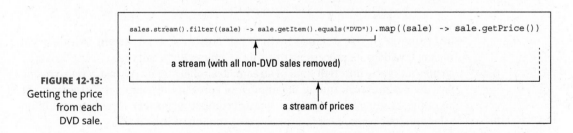

FIGURE 12-13: Getting the price from each DVD sale.

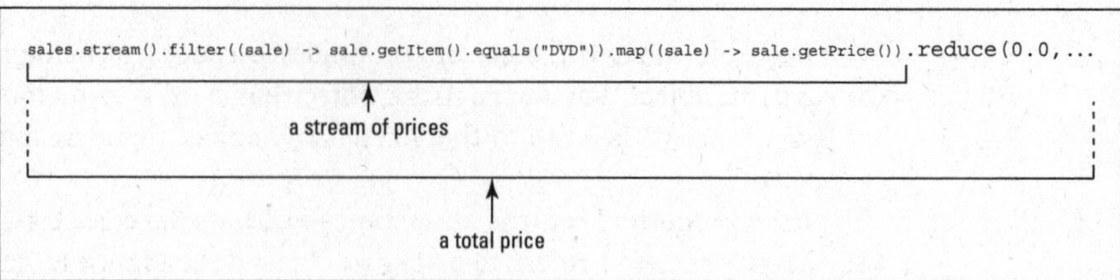

FIGURE 12-14: Getting the total price of all DVD sales.

Why bother?

The chain of method calls in Listing 12-5 accomplishes everything that the loop in Listing 12-4 accomplishes. But the code in Figure 12-14 uses concepts from functional programming. What's the big deal? Are you better off with Listing 12-5 than with Listing 12-4?

You are. For the past several years, the big trend in chip design has been multicore processors. With several cores, a processor can execute several statements at the same time, speeding up a program's execution by a factor of 2, or 4 or 8 or even more. Programs run much faster if you divide the work among several cores. But how do you divide the work?

You can modify the imperative code in Listing 12-4. For example, with some fancy features, you can hand different loop iterations to different cores. But the resulting code is messy. For the code to work properly, you have to micromanage the loop iterations, checking carefully to make sure that the final `total` is correct.

In contrast, the functional code is easy to modify. To take advantage of multicore processors, you change *only one word* in Listing 12-5!

```
sales.parallelStream()
     .filter((sale) -> sale.getItem().equals("DVD"))
     .map((sale) -> sale.getPrice())
     .reduce(0.0, (price1, price2) -> price1 + price2);
```

In Listing 12-5, the stream() method call creates a serial stream. With a *serial stream*, Java does its processing one sale at a time. But a call to `parallelStream()` creates a slightly different kind of stream: a parallel stream. With a *parallel stream*, Java divides the work among the number of cores in the computer's processor (or according to some other useful measure of computing power). If you have 4 million sales and four cores, each core processes 1 million of the sales.

Each core works independently of the others, and each core dumps its result into a final `reduce` method. The `reduce` method combines the cores' results into a final tally. In the best possible scenario, all the work gets done in one-fourth of the time it would take with an ordinary serial stream.

TECHNICAL STUFF

When you read the preceding paragraph, don't gloss over the phrase *best possible scenario.* Parallelism isn't magic. And sometimes, parallelism isn't your friend. Consider the situation in which you have only 20 sale amounts to tally. The time it takes to divide the problem into four groups of 5 sales each far exceeds the amount of time you save in using all four cores. In addition, some problems don't lend themselves to parallel processing. Imagine that the price of an item depends on the number of similar items being sold. In that case, you can't divide the problem among four independently operating cores. If you try, each core has to know what the other cores are doing. You lose the advantage of having four threads of execution.

NO VARIABLES? NO PROBLEM!

Consider the problems posed at the start of the earlier section "Functional Programming." Several clients try to update Oracle's stock price at the same time, or two visitors try to buy the same item on a website. The source of the problem is *shared data.* How many clients share access to Oracle's stock price? How many customers share access to a web page's Purchase button? How many of your processor's cores can modify the same variable's value? If you get rid of data sharing, your multicore processing problems go away.

In imperative programming, a variable is a place where statements share their values with one another. Can you avoid using variables in your code?

Compare the loop in Listing 12-4 with the functional programming code in Listing 12-5. In Listing 12-4, the `total` variable is shared among all loop iterations. Because each iteration can potentially change the value of `total`, you can't assign each iteration to a different processor core. If you did, you'd risk having two cores updating the total at the same time. (Chances are good that, because of the simultaneous updating, neither core would do its update correctly!) But the functional programming code in Listing 12-5 has no `total` variable. A running total plays no role in the functional version of the code. Instead, in Listing 12-5, the `reduce` method applies the sum operation to values coming from a stream. This incoming stream pops out of the previous method call (the `map` method), so the incoming stream has no name. That's nice. You don't even need a variable to store a stream of values.

In imperative programming, a variable is a place where statements share their values with one another. But functional programming shuns variables. So, when you do functional programming, you don't have a lot of data sharing. Many of the difficulties associated with multicore processors vanish into thin air. Your code can take advantage of many cores at the same time. When you write the code, you don't worry about data being shared among the cores. It's an elegant solution to an important computing problem.

Method references

Take a critical look at the last lambda expression in Listing 12-5:

```
(price1, price2) -> price1 + price2)
```

This expression does roughly the same work as a sum method. (In fact, you can find a sum method's declaration in the earlier section "Lambda expressions.") If your choice is between typing a 3-line sum method and typing a 1-line lambda expression, you'll probably choose the lambda expression. But what if you have a third alternative? Rather than type your own sum method, you can refer to an existing sum method. Using an existing method is the quickest and safest thing to do.

As luck would have it, Java's Double class contains a static sum method. You don't have to create your own sum method. If you run the following code:

```
double i = 5.0, j = 7.0;
System.out.println(Double.sum(i, j));
```

the computer displays 12.0. So, rather than type the price1 + price2 lambda expression in Listing 12-5, you can create a *method reference* — an expression that refers to an existing method.

```
sales.stream()
     .filter((sale) -> sale.getItem().equals("DVD"))
     .map((sale) -> sale.getPrice())
     .reduce(0.0, Double :: sum);
```

The expression Double::sum refers to the sum method belonging to Java's Double class. When you use this Double::sum method reference, you do the same thing that the last lambda expression does in Listing 12-5. Everybody is happy.

For information about static methods, see Chapter 10.

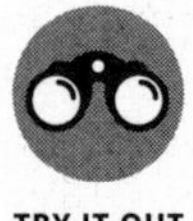

TRY IT OUT

You can always try the programming challenges that you dream up on your own. If you don't have any ideas to give you practice with functional programming, I have a couple of suggestions for you:

- Each employee has a name and a performance evaluation score. Find the total amount of money that you'll pay in bonuses if you give a $100 bonus to each employee whose score is 3 or higher.
- Each recipe has a name, a list of ingredients (some of which involve meat products), and an estimated preparation time. Find the average time estimate for cooking one of the vegetarian recipes.

» Making your code (more or less) crash proof

» Defining your own exception class

Chapter 13

Looking Good When Things Take Unexpected Turns

September 9, 1945: A moth flies into one of the relays of the Harvard Mark II computer and gums up the works. This becomes the first recorded case of a real computer bug.

April 19, 1957: Herbert Bright, manager of the data processing center at Westinghouse in Pittsburgh, receives an unmarked deck of computer punch cards in the mail (which is like getting an unlabeled CD-ROM in the mail today). Mr. Bright guesses that this deck comes from the development team for FORTRAN — the first computer programming language. He's been waiting a few years for this software. (No web downloads were available at the time.)

Armed with nothing but this good guess, Bright writes a small FORTRAN program and tries to compile it on his IBM 704. (The IBM 704 lives in its own, specially built, 2,000-square-foot room. With vacuum tubes instead of transistors, the machine has a whopping 32K of RAM. The operating system has to be loaded from tape before the running of each program, and a typical program takes between two and four hours to run.) After the usual waiting time, Bright's attempt to compile a FORTRAN program comes back with a single error: a missing comma in one of the statements. Bright corrects the error, and the program runs like a charm.

July 22, 1962: Mariner I, the first US spacecraft aimed at another planet, is destroyed when it behaves badly four minutes after launch. The bad behavior is attributed to a missing bar (like a hyphen) in the formula for the rocket's velocity.

Around the same time, orbit computation software at NASA is found to contain the incorrect statement `DO 10 I=1.10` (instead of the correct `DO 10 I=1,10`). In modern notation, this is like writing `do10i = 1.10` in place of `for (int i=1; i<=10; i++)`. The change from a comma to a period turns a loop into an assignment statement.

January 1, 2000: The Year 2000 Problem wreaks havoc on the modern world.

Any historically accurate facts in these notes were borrowed from the following sources: the Computer Folklore newsgroup (`https://groups.google.com/forum/#!forum/alt.folklore.computers`), the Free On-line Dictionary of Computing (`http://foldoc.org`), *Computer* magazine (`www.computer.org/computer-magazine/`), and other web pages of the IEEE (`www.computer.org`).

Handling Exceptions

You're taking inventory. This means counting item after item, box after box, and marking the numbers of such things on log sheets, in little handheld gizmos, and into forms on computer keyboards. A particular part of the project involves entering the number of boxes that you find on the Big Dusty Boxes That Haven't Been Opened Since Year One shelf. Rather than break the company's decades-old habit, you decide not to open any of these boxes. You arbitrarily assign the value $3.25 to each box.

Listing 13-1 shows the software to handle this bit of inventory. The software has a flaw, which is revealed in Figure 13-1. When the user enters a whole number value, things are okay. But when the user enters something else (like the number 3.5), the program comes crashing to the ground. Surely something can be done about this. Computers are stupid, but they're not so stupid that they should fail royally when a user enters an improper value.

LISTING 13-1: Counting Boxes

```
import static java.lang.System.out;
import java.util.Scanner;
import java.text.NumberFormat;

public class InventoryA {

   public static void main(String args[]) {
      final double boxPrice = 3.25;
      Scanner keyboard = new Scanner(System.in);
      NumberFormat currency = NumberFormat.getCurrencyInstance();

      out.print("How many boxes do we have? ");
      String numBoxesIn = keyboard.next();
      int numBoxes = Integer.parseInt(numBoxesIn);

      out.print("The value is ");
      out.println(currency.format(numBoxes * boxPrice));
      keyboard.close();
   }
}
```

```
How many boxes do we have? 3
The value is $9.75

How many boxes do we have? 3.5
Exception in thread "main" java.lang.NumberFormatException: For input string: "3.5"
        at java.lang.NumberFormatException.forInputString(Unknown Source)
        at java.lang.Integer.parseInt(Unknown Source)
        at java.lang.Integer.parseInt(Unknown Source)
        at InventoryA.main(InventoryA.java:15)

How many boxes do we have? three
Exception in thread "main" java.lang.NumberFormatException: For input string: "three"
        at java.lang.NumberFormatException.forInputString(Unknown Source)
        at java.lang.Integer.parseInt(Unknown Source)
        at java.lang.Integer.parseInt(Unknown Source)
        at InventoryA.main(InventoryA.java:15)
```

FIGURE 13-1: Three separate runs of the code in Listing 13-1.

The key to fixing a program bug is examining the message that appears when the program crashes. The inventory program's message says `java.lang.NumberFormatException`. That means a class named *NumberFormatException* is in the `java.lang` API package. Somehow, the call to `Integer.parseInt` brought this `NumberFormatException` class out of hiding.

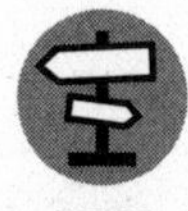

CROSS REFERENCE

For a brief explanation of the `Integer.parseInt` method, see Chapter 11.

Well, here's what's going on. The Java programming language has a mechanism called *exception handling.* With exception handling, a program can detect that things are about to go wrong and respond by creating a brand-new object. In the official terminology, the program is said to be *throwing* an exception. That new object, an instance of the Exception class, is passed like a hot potato from one piece of code to another until some piece of code decides to *catch* the exception. When the exception is caught, the program executes some recovery code, buries the exception, and moves on to the next normal statement as if nothing had ever happened. The process is illustrated in Figure 13-2.

The whole thing is done with the aid of several Java keywords. These keywords are described in this list:

- throw: Creates a new exception object.
- throws: Passes the buck from a method up to whatever code called the method.

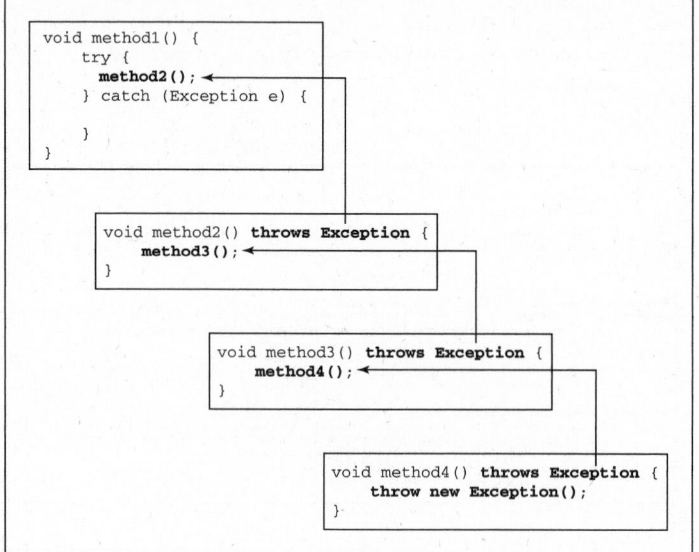

FIGURE 13-2: Throwing, passing, and catching an exception.

- try: Encloses code that has the potential to create a new exception object. In the usual scenario, the code inside a try clause contains calls to methods whose code can create one or more exceptions.
- catch: Deals with the exception, buries it, and then moves on.

So the truth is out. Through some chain of events like the one shown in Figure 13-2, the method Integer.parseInt can throw a NumberFormatException. When you call Integer.parseInt, this NumberFormatException is passed on to you.

TIP

The Java API (Application Programming Interface) documentation for the parseInt method says, "Throws: NumberFormatException — if the string does not contain a parsable integer." Once in a while, reading the documentation actually pays.

If you call yourself a hero, you'd better catch the exception so that all the other code can get on with its regular business. Listing 13-2 shows the catching of an exception.

LISTING 13-2: A Hero Counts Boxes

```
import static java.lang.System.out;
import java.util.Scanner;
import java.text.NumberFormat;

public class InventoryB {

   public static void main(String args[]) {
       final double boxPrice = 3.25;
       Scanner keyboard = new Scanner(System.in);
       NumberFormat currency = NumberFormat.getCurrencyInstance();

       out.print("How many boxes do we have? ");
       String numBoxesIn = keyboard.next();

       try {
           int numBoxes = Integer.parseInt(numBoxesIn);
           out.print("The value is ");
           out.println(currency.format(numBoxes * boxPrice));
       } catch (NumberFormatException e) {
           out.println("That's not a number.");
       }

       keyboard.close();
   }
}
```

Figure 13-3 shows three runs of the code from Listing 13-2. When a misguided user types **three** instead of **3**, the program maintains its cool by displaying `That's not a number`. The trick is to enclose the call to `Integer.parseInt` inside a `try` clause. If you do this, the computer watches for exceptions when any statement inside the `try` clause is executed. If an exception is thrown, the computer jumps from inside the `try` clause to a `catch` clause below it. In Listing 13-2, the computer jumps directly to the `catch (NumberFormatException e)` clause. The computer executes the `println` statement inside the clause and then marches on with normal processing. (If there were statements in Listing 13-2 after the end of the catch clause, the computer would go on and execute them.)

```
How many boxes do we have? 3
The value is $9.75

How many boxes do we have? three
That's not a number.


How many boxes do we have? -25
The value is ($81.25)
```

FIGURE 13-3: Three runs of the code in Listing 13-2.

An entire try-catch assembly — complete with a try clause, catch clause, and what-have-you — is called a *try statement*. Sometimes, for emphasis, I call it a *try-catch statement*.

The parameter in a catch clause

Take a look at the catch clause in Listing 13-2 and pay particular attention to the words (NumberFormatException e). This looks a lot like a method's parameter list, doesn't it? In fact, every catch clause is like a little mini-method with its own parameter list. The parameter list always has an exception type name and then a parameter.

In Listing 13-2, I don't do anything with the catch clause's e parameter, but I certainly could if I wanted to. ***Remember:*** The exception that's thrown is an object — an instance of the NumberFormatException class. When an exception is caught, the computer makes the catch clause's parameter refer to that exception object. In other words, the name *e* stores a bunch of information about the exception. To take advantage of this, you can call some of the exception object's methods.

```
} catch (NumberFormatException e) {
    out.println("Message: ***" + e.getMessage() + "***");
    e.printStackTrace();
}
```

With this new catch clause, a run of the inventory program may look like the run shown in Figure 13-4. When you call getMessage, you fetch some detail about the exception. (In Figure 13-4, the detail is Message: ***For input string: "three"***.) When you call printStackTrace, you get some additional information; namely, a display showing the methods that were running at the moment when the exception was thrown. (In Figure 13-4, the display includes Integer.parseInt and the main method.) Both getMessage and printStackTrace present information to help you find the source of the program's difficulties.

```
How many boxes do we have? three
Message: ***For input string: "three"***
java.lang.NumberFormatException: For input string: "three"
	at java.lang.NumberFormatException.forInputString(Unknown Source)
	at java.lang.Integer.parseInt(Unknown Source)
	at java.lang.Integer.parseInt(Unknown Source)
	at InventoryB.main(InventoryB.java:17)
```

FIGURE 13-4: Calling an exception object's methods.

TECHNICAL STUFF

When you mix `System.out.println` calls with `printStackTrace` calls, the order in which Java displays the information is not predictable. For example, in Figure 13-4, the text `Message: ***For input string: "three"***` may appear before or after the stack trace. If the ordering of this output matters to you, change `out.println("Message: ***"` to `System.err.println("Message: ***"`.

Exception types

What else can go wrong today? Are there other kinds of exceptions — things that don't come from the `NumberFormatException` class? Sure, plenty of different exception types are out there. You can even create one of your own. You wanna try? If so, look at Listings 13-3 and 13-4.

LISTING 13-3: Making Your Own Kind of Exception

```
@SuppressWarnings("serial")
class OutOfRangeException extends Exception {
}
```

LISTING 13-4: Using Your Custom-Made Exception

```
import static java.lang.System.out;
import java.util.Scanner;
import java.text.NumberFormat;

public class InventoryC {

   public static void main(String args[]) {
      final double boxPrice = 3.25;
      Scanner keyboard = new Scanner(System.in);
      NumberFormat currency = NumberFormat.getCurrencyInstance();

      out.print("How many boxes do we have? ");
      String numBoxesIn = keyboard.next();

      try {
         int numBoxes = Integer.parseInt(numBoxesIn);
```

(continued)

LISTING 13-4: (continued)

```
            if (numBoxes < 0) {
               throw new OutOfRangeException();
            }

            out.print("The value is ");
            out.println(currency.format(numBoxes * boxPrice));
         } catch (NumberFormatException e) {
            out.println("That's not a number.");
         } catch (OutOfRangeException e) {
            out.print(numBoxesIn);
            out.println("? That's impossible!");
         }

         keyboard.close();
      }
   }
```

Listings 13-3 and 13-4 remedy a problem that cropped up earlier, in Figure 13-3. Look at the last of the three runs in Figure 13-3. The user reports that the shelves have −25 boxes, and the computer takes this value without blinking an eye. The truth is that you would need a black hole (or some other exotic space-time warping phenomenon) to have a negative number of boxes on any shelf in your warehouse. So the program should get upset if the user enters a negative number of boxes, which is what the code in Listing 13-4 does. To see the upset code, look at Figure 13-5.

```
How many boxes do we have? 3
The value is $9.75


How many boxes do we have? three
That's not a number.


How many boxes do we have? -25
-25? That's impossible!
```

FIGURE 13-5: Three runs of the code from Listings 13-3 and 13-4.

The code in Listing 13-3 declares a new kind of exception class: `OutOfRangeException`. In many situations, typing a negative number would be just fine, so `OutOfRangeException` isn't built in to the Java API. However, in the inventory program, a negative number should be flagged as an anomaly.

The `OutOfRangeException` class in Listing 13-3 wins the award for the shortest self-contained piece of code in this book. The class's code is just a declaration line and an empty pair of braces. The code's operative phrase is `extends Exception`. Being a subclass of the Java API `Exception` class allows any instance of the `OutOfRangeException` class to be thrown.

Back in Listing 13-4, a new OutOfRangeException instance is thrown. When this happens, the catch clause (OutOfRangeException e) catches the instance. The clause echoes the user's input and displays the message That's impossible!

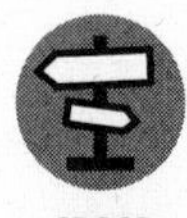

The text @SuppressWarnings("serial") in Listing 13-3 is a Java annotation. For an introduction to annotations, see Chapter 8. For a few words about the SuppressWarnings annotation, see Chapter 9.

If you use Eclipse, you might see a yellow warning marker next to the throw new OutOfRangeException() line in Listing 13-4. When you hover the pointer over the warning marker, Eclipse says, Resource leak: 'keyboard' is not closed at this location. Eclipse is being persnickety to make sure that your code eventually executes the keyboard.close() statement. (Yes, under certain circumstances, throwing the OutOfRangeException can cause the program to skip the keyboard.close() statement. But no, that can't happen when you run the code in Listing 13-4.) In my opinion, you can safely ignore this warning.

Who's going to catch the exception?

Take one more look at Listing 13-4. Notice that more than one catch clause can accompany a single try clause. When an exception is thrown inside a try clause, the computer starts going down the accompanying list of catch clauses. The computer starts at whatever catch clause comes immediately after the try clause and works its way down the program's text.

For each catch clause, the computer asks itself, "Is the exception that was just thrown an instance of the class in this clause's parameter list?"

- If not, the computer skips this catch clause and moves on to the next catch clause in line.
- If so, the computer executes this catch clause and then skips past all other catch clauses that come with this try clause. The computer goes on and executes whatever statements come after the whole try-catch statement.

For some concrete examples, see Listings 13-5 and 13-6.

LISTING 13-5: Yet Another Exception

```
@SuppressWarnings("serial")
class NumberTooLargeException extends OutOfRangeException {
}
```

LISTING 13-6: Where Does the Buck Stop?

```
import static java.lang.System.out;
import java.util.Scanner;
import java.text.NumberFormat;

public class InventoryD {

    public static void main(String args[]) {
        final double boxPrice = 3.25;
        Scanner keyboard = new Scanner(System.in);
        NumberFormat currency = NumberFormat.getCurrencyInstance();

        out.print("How many boxes do we have? ");
        String numBoxesIn = keyboard.next();

        try {
            int numBoxes = Integer.parseInt(numBoxesIn);

            if (numBoxes < 0) {
                throw new OutOfRangeException();
            }

            if (numBoxes > 1000) {
                throw new NumberTooLargeException();
            }

            out.print("The value is ");
            out.println(currency.format(numBoxes * boxPrice));
        }

        catch (NumberFormatException e) {
            out.println("That's not a number.");
        }

        catch (OutOfRangeException e) {
            out.print(numBoxesIn);
            out.println("? That's impossible!");
        }

        catch (Exception e) {
            out.print("Something went wrong, ");
            out.print("but I'm clueless about what ");
            out.println("it actually was.");
        }

        out.println("That's that.");

        keyboard.close();
    }
}
```

To run the code in Listings 13-5 and 13-6, you need one additional Java program file. You need the `OutOfRangeException` class in Listing 13-3.

Listing 13-6 addresses the scenario in which you have limited shelf space. You don't have room for more than 1,000 boxes, but once in a while the program asks how many boxes you have, and somebody enters the number *100000* by accident. In cases like this, Listing 13-6 does a quick reality check. Any number of boxes over 1,000 is tossed out as being unrealistic.

Listing 13-6 watches for a `NumberTooLargeException`, but to make life more interesting, Listing 13-6 doesn't have a `catch` clause for the `NumberTooLargeException`. In spite of this, everything still works out just fine. It's fine because `NumberTooLargeException` is declared to be a subclass of `OutOfRangeException`, and Listing 13-6 has a `catch` clause for the `OutOfRangeException`.

You see, because `NumberTooLargeException` is a subclass of `OutOfRangeException`, any instance of `NumberTooLargeException` is just a special kind of `OutOfRangeException`. So, in Listing 13-6, the computer may start looking for a clause to catch a `NumberTooLargeException`. When the computer stumbles upon the `OutOfRangeExceptioncatch` clause, the computer says, "Okay, I've found a match. I'll execute the statements in this `catch` clause."

To keep from having to write this whole story over and over again, I introduce some new terminology. I say that the `catch` clause with parameter `OutOfRangeException` *matches* the `NumberTooLargeException` that's been thrown. I call this `catch` clause a *matching catch clause.*

The following list describes different things that the user may do and how the computer responds. As you read, you can follow along by looking at the runs shown in Figure 13-6:

```
How many boxes do we have? 3
The value is $9.75
That's that.

How many boxes do we have? fish
That's not a number.
That's that.

How many boxes do we have? -25
-25? That's impossible!
That's that.

How many boxes do we have? 1001
1001? That's impossible!
That's that.
```

FIGURE 13-6: Four runs of the code from Listing 13-6.

» **The user enters an ordinary whole number, like the number *3*.** All statements in the `try` clause are executed. Then the computer skips past all the `catch` clauses and executes the code that comes immediately after all the `catch` clauses. (See Figure 13-7.)

» **The user enters something that's not a whole number, like the word *fish*.** The code throws a `NumberFormatException`. The computer skips past the remaining statements in the `try` clause. The computer executes the statements inside the first `catch` clause — the clause whose parameter is of type `NumberFormatException`. Then the computer skips past the second and third `catch` clauses and executes the code that comes immediately after all the `catch` clauses. (See Figure 13-8.)

```
try {
        //Normal processing (throw no exception)
}

catch (NumberFormatException e) {
        out.println("That's not a number.");
}

catch (OutOfRangeException e) {
        out.print(numBoxesIn);
        out.println("? That's impossible!");
}

catch (Exception e) {
        out.print("Something went wrong, ");
        out.print("but I'm clueless about what ");
        out.println("it actually was.");
}

out.println("That's that.");
```

FIGURE 13-7: No exception is thrown.

» **The user enters a negative number, like the number *–25*.** The code throws an `OutOfRangeException`. The computer skips past the remaining statements in the `try` clause. The computer even skips past the statements in the first `catch` clause. (After all, an `OutOfRangeException` isn't any kind of a `NumberFormatException`. The `catch` clause with parameter `NumberFormatException` isn't a match for this `OutOfRangeException`.) The computer executes the statements inside the second `catch` clause — the clause whose parameter is of type `OutOfRangeException`. Then the computer skips past the third `catch` clause and executes the code that comes immediately after all the `catch` clauses. (See Figure 13-9.)

```
try {

        throw new NumberFormatException ();

}

catch (NumberFormatException e) {
        out.println("That's not a number.");
}

catch (OutOfRangeException e) {
        out.print(numBoxesIn);
        out.println("? That's impossible!");
}

catch (Exception e) {
        out.print("Something went wrong, ");
        out.print("but I'm clueless about what ");
        out.println("it actually was.");
}

out.println("That's that.");
```

FIGURE 13-8: A `NumberFormatException` is thrown.

```
try {

        throw new OutOfRangeException ();

}

catch (NumberFormatException e) {
        out.println("That's not a number.");
}

catch (OutOfRangeException e) {
        out.print(numBoxesIn);
        out.println("? That's impossible!");
}

catch (Exception e) {
        out.print("Something went wrong, ");
        out.print("but I'm clueless about what ");
        out.println("it actually was.");
}

out.println("That's that.");
```

FIGURE 13-9: An `OutOfRangeException` is thrown.

» **The user enters an unrealistically large number, like the number *1001*.** The code throws a `NumberTooLargeException`. The computer skips past the remaining statements in the `try` clause. The computer even skips past the statements in the first `catch` clause. (After all, a `NumberTooLargeException` isn't any kind of `NumberFormatException`.)

But, according to the code in Listing 13-5, `NumberTooLargeException` is a subclass of `OutOfRangeException`. When the computer reaches the second `catch` clause, the computer says, "Hmm! A `NumberTooLargeException` is a kind of OutOfRangeException. I'll execute the statements in this catch clause — the clause with parameter of type OutOfRangeException." In other words, it's a match.

The computer executes the statements inside the second catch clause. Then the computer skips the third catch clause and executes the code that comes immediately after all the catch clauses. (See Figure 13-10.)

- **Something else, something quite unpredictable, happens. (I don't know what.)** With my unending urge to experiment, I reached into the try clause of Listing 13-6 and added a statement that throws an IOException. No reason — I just wanted to see what would happen.

```
try {

        throw new NumberTooLargeException ();

}

catch (NumberFormatException e) {
        out.println("That's not a number.");
}

catch (OutOfRangeException e) {
        out.print(numBoxesIn);
        out.println("? That's impossible!");
}

catch (Exception e) {
        out.print("Something went wrong, ");
        out.print("but I'm clueless about what ");
        out.println("it actually was.");
}

out.println("That's that.");
```

FIGURE 13-10: A NumberTooLargeException is thrown.

When the code threw an IOException, the computer skipped past the remaining statements in the try clause. Then the computer skipped past the statements in the first and second catch clauses. When the computer reached the third catch clause, I could hear the computer say, "Hmm! An IOException is a kind of Exception. I've found a matching catch clause — a clause with a parameter of type Exception. I'll execute the statements in this catch clause."

So the computer executed the statements inside the third catch clause. Then the computer executed the code that comes immediately after all the catch clauses. (See Figure 13-11.)

When the computer looks for a matching catch clause, the computer latches on to the topmost clause that fits one of the following descriptions:

» The clause's parameter type is the same as the type of the exception that was thrown.

» The clause's parameter type is a superclass of the exception's type.

If a better match appears farther down the list of catch clauses, that's just too bad. Imagine that you added a catch clause with a parameter of type NumberTooLargeException to the code in Listing 13-6. Imagine, also, that you put this new catch clause *after* the catch clause with parameter of type OutOfRangeException. Then, because NumberTooLargeException is a subclass of the OutOfRangeException class, the code in the new NumberTooLargeException clause would never be executed. That's just the way the cookie crumbles.

```
try {
    throw new IOException ();
}

catch (NumberFormatException e) {
    out.println("That's not a number.");
}

catch (OutOfRangeException e) {
    out.print(numBoxesIn);
    out.println("? That's impossible!");
}

catch (Exception e) {
    out.print("Something went wrong, ");
    out.print("but I'm clueless about what ");
    out.println("it actually was.");
}

out.println("That's that.");
```

FIGURE 13-11: An IOException is thrown.

Catching two or more exceptions at a time

Starting with Java 7, you can catch more than one kind of exception in a single catch clause. For example, in a particular inventory program, you might not want to distinguish between the throwing of a NumberFormatException and your own OutOfRangeException. In that case, you can rewrite part of Listing 13-6 this way:

```
try {
    int numBoxes = Integer.parseInt(numBoxesIn);
    if (numBoxes < 0) {
        throw new OutOfRangeException();
    }
    if (numBoxes > 1000) {
        throw new NumberTooLargeException();
    }
    out.print("The value is ");
    out.println(currency.format(numBoxes * boxPrice));
}
catch (NumberFormatException | OutOfRangeException e) {
    out.print(numBoxesIn);
    out.println("? That's impossible!");
}
catch (Exception e) {
    out.print("Something went wrong, ");
    out.print("but I'm clueless about what ");
    out.println("it actually was.");
}
```

The pipe symbol, `|`, tells Java to catch either a `NumberFormatException` or an `OutOfRangeException`. If you throw an exception of either type, the program displays the value of `numBoxesIn` followed by the text `? That's impossible!` If you throw an exception that is neither a `NumberFormatException` nor an `OutOfRangeException`, the program jumps to the last `catch` clause and displays `Something went wrong, but I'm clueless ....`

Throwing caution to the wind

Are you one of those obsessive-compulsive types? Do you like to catch every possible exception before the exception can possibly crash your program? Well, watch out. Java doesn't let you become paranoid. You can't catch an exception if the exception has no chance of being thrown.

Consider the following code. The code has an innocent `i++` statement inside a `try` clause. That's fair enough. But then the code's `catch` clause is pretending to catch an `IOException`:

```
// Bad code!
try {
    i++;
} catch (IOException e) {
    e.printStackTrace();
}
```

Who is this catch clause trying to impress? A statement like i++ doesn't do any input or output. The code inside the try clause can't possibly throw an IOException. So the compiler comes back and says, "Hey, catch clause. Get real. Get off your high horse." Well, to be a bit more precise, the compiler's reprimand reads as follows:

```
exception java.io.IOException is never thrown
in body of corresponding try statement
```

Doing useful things

So far, each example in this chapter catches an exception, prints a "bad input" message, and then closes up shop. Wouldn't it be nice to see a program that actually carries on after an exception has been caught? Well, it's time for something nice. Listing 13-7 has a try-catch statement inside a loop. The loop keeps running until the user types something sensible.

LISTING 13-7: Keep Pluggin' Along

```
import static java.lang.System.out;
import java.util.Scanner;
import java.text.NumberFormat;

public class InventoryLoop {

   public static void main(String args[]) {
      final double boxPrice = 3.25;
      boolean gotGoodInput = false;
      Scanner keyboard = new Scanner(System.in);
      NumberFormat currency = NumberFormat.getCurrencyInstance();

      do {
         out.print("How many boxes do we have? ");
         String numBoxesIn = keyboard.next();

         try {
            int numBoxes = Integer.parseInt(numBoxesIn);
            out.print("The value is ");
            out.println(currency.format(numBoxes * boxPrice));
            gotGoodInput = true;
         } catch (NumberFormatException e) {
            out.println();
            out.println("That's not a number.");
         }
      } while (!gotGoodInput);
```

(continued)

LISTING 13-7: *(continued)*

```
        out.println("That's that.");

        keyboard.close();
    }
}
```

Figure 13-12 shows a run of the code from Listing 13-7. In the first three attempts, the user types just about everything except a valid whole number. At last, the fourth attempt is a success. The user types **3**, and the computer leaves the loop.

```
How many boxes do we have? 3.5

That's not a number.
How many boxes do we have? three

That's not a number.
How many boxes do we have? fish

That's not a number.
How many boxes do we have? 3
The value is $9.75
That's that.
```

FIGURE 13-12: A run of the code in Listing 13-7.

Our friends, the good exceptions

A rumor is going around that Java exceptions always come from unwanted, erroneous situations. Although there's some truth to this rumor, the rumor isn't entirely accurate. Occasionally, an exception arises from a normal, expected occurrence. Take, for instance, the detection of the end of a file. The following code makes a copy of a file:

```
try {
    while (true) {
        dataOut.writeByte(dataIn.readByte());
    }
} catch (EOFException e) {
    numFilesCopied = 1;
}
```

To copy bytes from `dataIn` to `dataOut`, you just go into a `while` loop. With its `true` condition, the `while` loop is seemingly endless. But eventually, you reach the end of the `dataIn` file. When this happens, the `readByte` method throws an `EOFException` (an end-of-file exception). The throwing of this exception sends the computer out of the `try` clause and out of the `while` loop. From there, you do whatever you want to do in the `catch` clause and then proceed with normal processing.

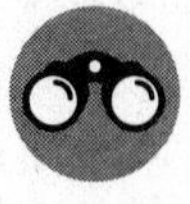

TRY IT OUT

Try your hand at these coding tasks:

- Add `try-catch` statements to keep the following code from crashing:

```
import java.util.Scanner;

public class Main {

  public static void main(String[] args) {
    Scanner keyboard = new Scanner(System.in);
    String[] words = new String[5];

    int i = 0;
    do {
      words[i] = keyboard.next();
    } while (!words[i++].equals("Quit"));

    for (int j = 0; j < 5; j++) {
      System.out.println(words[j].length());
    }

    keyboard.close();
  }
}
```

- In Listing 13-6, the price of each box and the number of boxes that are too large are fixed values. Make improvements to the code so that the user enters both of those values. Remember that some values for these quantities don't make sense. For example, a negative number of boxes is never too many boxes. Use `try-catch` statements to handle inappropriate user input.

Handle an Exception or Pass the Buck

So you're getting to know Java, hey? What? You say you're all the way up to Chapter 13? I'm impressed. You must be a hard worker. But remember, all work and no play . . .

So, how about taking a break? A little nap could do you a world of good. Is ten seconds okay? Or is that too long? Better make it five seconds.

Listing 13-8 has a program that's supposed to pause its execution for five seconds. The problem is that the program in Listing 13-8 is incorrect. Take a look at Listing 13-8 for a minute, and then I'll tell you what's wrong with it.

LISTING 13-8: An Incorrect Program

```
/*
 * This code does not compile.
 */

import static java.lang.System.out;

public class NoSleepForTheWeary {

    public static void main(String args[]) {
        out.print("Excuse me while I nap ");
        out.println("for just five seconds...");

        takeANap();

        out.println("Ah, that was refreshing.");
    }

    static void takeANap() {
        Thread.sleep(5000);
    }
}
```

The strategy in Listing 13-8 isn't bad. The idea is to call the `sleep` method, which is defined in the Java API. This `sleep` method belongs to the API `Thread` class. When you call the `sleep` method, the number that you feed it is a number of milliseconds. So `Thread.sleep(5000)` means pause for five seconds.

The problem is that the code inside the `sleep` method can throw an exception. This kind of exception is an instance of the `InterruptedException` class. When you try to compile the code in Listing 13-8, you get a message such as

```
unreported exception java.lang.InterruptedException;
must be caught or declared to be thrown
```

Maybe the message reads

```
Unhandled exception type InterruptedException
```

One way or another, the message is unwelcome.

TECHNICAL STUFF

For the purpose of understanding exceptions in general, you don't need to know exactly what an `InterruptedException` is. All you really have to know is that a call to `Thread.sleep` can throw one of these `InterruptedException` objects. But if you're really curious, an `InterruptedException` is thrown when some code interrupts some other code's sleep. Imagine that you have two pieces of code running at the same time. One piece of code calls the `Thread.sleep` method. At the same time, another piece of code calls the `interrupt` method. By calling the `interrupt` method, the second piece of code brings the first code's `Thread.sleep` method to a screeching halt. The `Thread.sleep` method responds by spitting out an `InterruptedException`.

Now, the Java programming language has two kinds of exceptions. They're called *checked* and *unchecked* exceptions:

- The potential throwing of a checked exception must be acknowledged in the code.
- The potential throwing of an unchecked exception doesn't need to be acknowledged in the code.

An `InterruptedException` is one of Java's checked exception types. When you call a method that has the potential to throw an `InterruptedException`, you need to acknowledge that exception in the code.

Now, when I say that an exception is *acknowledged in the code*, what do I really mean?

```
// The author wishes to thank that InterruptedException,
// without which this code could not have been written.
```

No, that's not what it means to be acknowledged in the code. Acknowledging an exception in the code means one of two things:

- The statements (including method calls) that can throw the exception are inside a `try` clause. That `try` clause has a `catch` clause with a matching exception type in its parameter list.
- The statements (including method calls) that can throw the exception are inside a method that has a `throws` clause in its header. The `throws` clause contains a matching exception type.

If you're confused by the wording of these two bullets, don't worry. The next two listings illustrate the points made in the bullets.

In Listing 13-9, the method call that can throw an InterruptedException is inside a try clause. That try clause has a catch clause with exception type InterruptedException.

LISTING 13-9: Acknowledging with a try-catch Statement

```
import static java.lang.System.out;

public class GoodNightsSleepA {

    public static void main(String args[]) {
        out.print("Excuse me while I nap ");
        out.println("for just five seconds...");

        takeANap();

        out.println("Ah, that was refreshing.");
    }

    static void takeANap() {
        try {
            Thread.sleep(5000);
        } catch (InterruptedException e) {
            out.println("Hey, who woke me up?");
        }
    }
}
```

It's my custom, at this point in a section, to remind you that a run of Listing Such-and-Such is shown in Figure So-and-So. But the problem here is that Figure 13-13 doesn't do justice to the code in Listing 13-9. When you run the program in Listing 13-9, the computer displays Excuse me while I nap for just five seconds, pauses for five seconds, and then displays Ah, that was refreshing. The code works because the call to the sleep method, which can throw an InterruptedException, is inside a try clause. That try clause has a catch clause whose exception is of type InterruptedException.

```
Excuse me while I nap for just five seconds...
Ah, that was refreshing.
```

FIGURE 13-13: A 5-second pause before the "Ah" line.

So much for acknowledging an exception with a try-catch statement. You can acknowledge an exception another way, shown in Listing 13-10.

LISTING 13-10: Acknowledging with throws

```
import static java.lang.System.out;

public class GoodNightsSleepB {

    public static void main(String args[]) {
        out.print("Excuse me while I nap ");
        out.println("for just five seconds...");

        try {
            takeANap();
        } catch (InterruptedException e) {
            out.println("Hey, who woke me up?");
        }

        out.println("Ah, that was refreshing.");
    }

    static void takeANap() throws InterruptedException {
        Thread.sleep(5000);
    }
}
```

To see a run of the code in Listing 13-10, refer to Figure 13-13. Once again, Figure 13-13 fails to capture the true essence of the run, but that's okay. Just remember that in Figure 13-13, the computer pauses for five seconds before it displays `Ah, that was refreshing.`

The important part of Listing 13-10 is in the `takeANap` method's header. That header ends with `throws InterruptedException`. By announcing that it throws an `InterruptedException`, method `takeANap` passes the buck. What this `throws` clause really says is, "I realize that a statement inside this method has the potential to throw an `InterruptedException`, but I'm not acknowledging the exception in a `try-catch` statement. Java compiler, please don't bug me about this. Instead of having a `try-catch` statement, I'm passing the responsibility for acknowledging the exception to the `main` method (the method that called the `takeANap` method)."

Indeed, in the `main` method, the call to `takeANap` is inside a `try` clause. That `try` clause has a `catch` clause with a parameter of type `InterruptedException`. So everything is okay. Method `takeANap` passes the responsibility to the `main` method, and the `main` method accepts the responsibility with an appropriate `try-catch` statement. Everybody's happy. Even the Java compiler is happy.

To better understand the throws clause, imagine a volleyball game in which the volleyball is an exception. When a player on the other team serves, that player is throwing the exception. The ball crosses the net and comes right to you. If you pound the ball back across the net, you're catching the exception. But if you pass the ball to another player, you're using the throws clause. In essence, you're saying, "Here, other player. You deal with this exception."

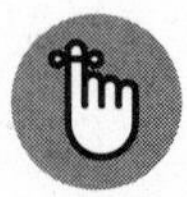
REMEMBER

A statement in a method can throw an exception that's not matched by a catch clause. This includes situations in which the statement throwing the exception isn't even inside a try block. When this happens, execution of the program jumps out of the method that contains the offending statement. Execution jumps back to whatever code called the method in the first place.

TIP

A method can name more than one exception type in its throws clause. Just use commas to separate the names of the exception types, as in the following example:

```
throws InterruptedException, IOException, ArithmeticException
```

The Java API has hundreds of exception types. Several of them are subclasses of the RuntimeException class. Anything that's a subclass of RuntimeException (or a sub-subclass, sub-sub-subclass, and so on) is unchecked. Any exception that's not a descendent of RuntimeException is checked. The unchecked exceptions include things that would be hard for the computer to predict. Such things include the NumberFormatException (of Listings 13-2, 13-4, and others), the ArithmeticException, the IndexOutOfBoundsException, the infamous NullPointerException, and many others. When you write Java code, much of your code is susceptible to these exceptions, but enclosing the code in try clauses (or passing the buck with throws clauses) is completely optional.

The Java API also has its share of checked exceptions. The computer can readily detect exceptions of this kind. So Java insists that, for an exception of this kind, any potential exception-throwing statement is acknowledged with either a try statement or a throws clause. Java's checked exceptions include the InterruptedException (Listings 13-9 and 13-10), the IOException, the SQLException, and a gang of other interesting exceptions.

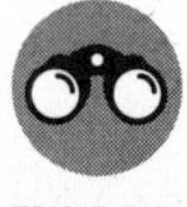
TRY IT OUT

I can't think of a clever way to connect the "Try" in "TryItOut" with the try in try-catch statements. If you think of something, scribble it in the margin on this page. Then try these little challenges:

» The following code doesn't compile because the code throws an unacknowledged `FileNotFoundException`:

```
// BAD CODE:
import java.io.File;
import java.util.Scanner;

public class Main {

  public static void main(String[] args) {
    Scanner diskScanner = new Scanner(new File("numbers.txt"));

    int[] numerators = new int[5];
    int[] denominators = new int[5];

    int i = 0;
    while (diskScanner.hasNextInt()) {
      numerators[i] = diskScanner.nextInt();
      denominators[i] = diskScanner.nextInt();
      i++;
    }

    for (int j = 0; j < numerators.length; j++) {
      System.out.println(numerators[j] / denominators[j]);
    }

    diskScanner.close();
  }
}
```

Fix the unacknowledged `FileNotFoundException` so that the code compiles. Then notice that, depending on the values in the `numbers.txt` file, some other exceptions may be thrown during a run of the program. Add one or more `try-catch` statements to display messages about these exceptions without letting the program crash.

» Add `try-catch` statements or `throws` clauses (or a mixture of these two things) to fix the following broken code:

```
// BAD CODE:
import java.io.DataInputStream;
import java.io.DataOutputStream;
import java.io.EOFException;
import java.io.File;
import java.io.FileInputStream;
import java.io.FileOutputStream;
```

```
public class Main {

  public static void main(String[] args) {
    File fileIn = new File("input");
    FileInputStream fileInStrm = new FileInputStream(fileIn);
    DataInputStream dataInStrm = new DataInputStream(fileInStrm);

    File fileOut = new File("output");
    FileOutputStream fileOutStrm = new FileOutputStream(fileOut);
    DataOutputStream dataOutStrm = new DataOutputStream(fileOutStrm);

    int numFilesCopied = 0;

    try {
      while (true) {
        dataOutStrm.writeByte(dataInStrm.readByte());
      }
    } catch (EOFException e) {
      numFilesCopied = 1;
    }
  }
}
```

When you've gotten the code to compile, create a file named `input` and run the code to see whether it creates the file named `output`.

Finishing the Job with a finally Clause

Once upon a time, I was a young fellow, living with my parents in Philadelphia, just starting to drive a car. I was heading toward a friend's house and thinking about who-knows-what when another car came from nowhere and bashed my car's passenger door. This kind of thing is called a *RunARedLightException.*

Anyway, both cars were still drivable, and we were right in the middle of a busy intersection. To avoid causing a traffic jam, we both pulled over to the nearest curb. I fumbled for my driver's license (which had a very young picture of me on it) and opened the door to get out of my car.

And that's when the second accident happened. As I was getting out of my car, a city bus was coming by. The bus hit me and rolled me against my car a few times. This kind of thing is called a *DealWithLawyersException.*

The truth is that everything came out just fine. I was bruised but not battered. My parents paid for the damage to the car, so I never suffered any financial consequences. (I managed to pass on the financial burden by putting the RunARedLightException into my throws clause.)

This incident helps to explain why I think the way I do about exception handling. In particular, I wonder, "What happens if, while the computer is recovering from one exception, a second exception is thrown?" After all, the statements inside a catch clause aren't immune to calamities.

Well, the answer to this question is anything but simple. For starters, you can put a try statement inside a catch clause. This protects you against unexpected, potentially embarrassing incidents that can crop up during the execution of the catch clause. But when you start worrying about cascading exceptions, you open up a very slimy can of worms. The number of scenarios is large, and things can become complicated very quickly.

One not-too-complicated thing that you can do is to create a finally clause. Like a catch clause, a finally clause comes after a try clause. The big difference is that the statements in a finally clause are executed whether or not an exception is thrown. The idea is, "No matter what happens, good or bad, execute the statements inside this finally clause." Listing 13-11 has an example.

LISTING 13-11: Jumping Around

```
import static java.lang.System.out;

public class DemoFinally {

    public static void main(String args[]) {
        try {
            doSomething();
        } catch (Exception e) {
            out.println("Exception caught in main.");
        }
    }

    static void doSomething() {
        try {
            out.println(0 / 0);
        } catch (Exception e) {
            out.println("Exception caught in doSomething.");
            out.println(0 / 0);
```

(continued)

LISTING 13-11: (continued)

```
            } finally {
                out.println("I'll get printed.");
            }

            out.println("I won't get printed.");
        }
    }
```

Normally, when I think about a `try` statement, I think about the computer recovering from an unpleasant situation. The recovery takes place inside a `catch` clause, and then the computer marches on to whatever statements come after the `try` statement. Well, if something goes wrong during execution of a `catch` clause, this picture can start looking different.

Listing 13-11 gets a workout in Figure 13-14. First, the `main` method calls `doSomething`. Then the stupid `doSomething` method goes out of its way to cause trouble. The `doSomething` method divides 0 by 0, which is illegal and undoable in anyone's programming language. This foolish action by the `doSomething` method throws an `ArithmeticException`, which is caught by the `try` statement's one and only `catch` clause.

```
Exception caught in doSomething.
I'll get printed.
Exception caught in main.
```

FIGURE 13-14: Running the code from Listing 13-11.

Inside the `catch` clause, that lowlife `doSomething` method divides 0 by 0 again. This time, the statement that does the division isn't inside a protective `try` clause. That's okay, because an `ArithmeticException` isn't checked. (It's one of those `RuntimeException` subclasses. It's an exception that doesn't have to be acknowledged in a `try` or a `throws` clause. For details, see the preceding section.)

Well, checked or not, the throwing of another `ArithmeticException` causes control to jump out of the `doSomething` method. But, before leaving the `doSomething` method, the computer executes the `try` statement's last will and testament: the statements inside the `finally` clause. That's why in Figure 13-14 you see the words `I'll get printed.`

Interestingly enough, you don't see the words `I won't get printed` in Figure 13-14. Because the `catch` clause's execution throws its own, uncaught exception, the computer never makes it down past the `try-catch-finally` statement.

So the computer goes back to where it left off in the `main` method. Back in the `main` method, word of the `doSomething` method's `ArithmeticException` mishaps causes execution to jump into a `catch` clause. The computer prints `Exception caught in main`, and then this terrible nightmare of a run is finished.

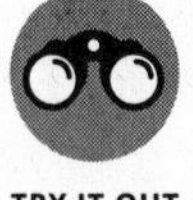

TRY IT OUT

At the end of the earlier section "Handle an Exception or Pass the Buck," you add exception-handling code to a program that makes a copy of a file. Along with your code, you may see warnings telling you that you've forgotten to close `dataInStrm` and `dataOutStrm`. Fix this by adding `dataInStrm.close()` and `dataOutStrm.close()` calls inside `finally` clauses.

A try Statement with Resources

Imagine a program that gets input from two different files or from a `Scanner` and a disk file. To make sure that you clean up properly, you put `close` method calls in a `finally` clause. (See Listing 13-12.)

LISTING 13-12: Using Two Files

```
import java.io.File;
import java.io.IOException;
import java.util.Scanner;

public class Main {

    public static void main(String args[]) {
        Scanner scan1 = null;
        Scanner scan2 = null;
        try {
            scan1 = new Scanner(new File("File1.txt"));
            scan2 = new Scanner(new File("File2.txt"));
            // Do useful stuff
        } catch (IOException e) {
            // Oops!
        } finally {
            scan1.close();
            scan2.close();
            System.out.println("Done!");
        }
    }
}
```

In theory, the computer always executes `scan1.close()` and `scan2.close()` no matter what goes wrong during execution of the `try` clause. But that's theory. In reality, another programmer (not you, of course) might modify the code by closing `scan1` in the middle of the `try` clause:

```
try {
    scan1 = new Scanner(new File("File1.txt"));
    scan2 = new Scanner(new File("File2.txt"));
    // Do useful stuff but also ...
    scan1.close();
    scan1 = null;
} catch (IOException e) {
    // Oops!
} finally {
    scan1.close();
    scan2.close();
    System.out.println("Done!");
}
```

Now you have a real predicament. Inside the `finally` clause, the value of `scan1` is `null`. The call to `scan1.close()` fails, so the program throws a `NullPointerException` and stops running before reaching the call to `scan2.close()`. In the worst of circumstances, `scan2` isn't closed and your program has `File2.txt` locked up so that no other program can use the file.

When a program uses several resources (many files, a database and a file, or whatever) the buildup of `try` statements becomes quite complicated. You can make `try` statements within `catch` clauses and all kinds of crazy combinations. But Java has a better way to solve the problem: In Java 7 (and later versions of Java), you can create a *try-with-resources statement.* Listing 13-13 shows you how.

LISTING 13-13: Making Sure to Close Resources

```
import java.io.File;
import java.io.IOException;
import java.util.Scanner;

public class NewMain {

    public static void main(String args[]) {
        try (Scanner scan1 = new Scanner(new File("File1.txt"));
             Scanner scan2 = new Scanner(new File("File2.txt"))) {
            // Do useful stuff
        } catch (IOException e) {
```

```
            // Oops!
        }
        System.out.println("Done!");
    }
}
```

In Listing 13-13, the declarations of `scan1` and `scan2` are in parentheses after the word `try`. The parenthesized declarations tell Java to close `scan1` and `scan2` automatically after execution of the statements in the `try` clause. You can declare several resources inside one `try` statement's parentheses. When you do, Java closes all the resources automatically after execution of the `try` clause's statements. You can add `catch` clauses and a `finally` clause, if you want. You can access all kinds of resources (files, databases, connections to servers, and others) and have peace of mind knowing that Java will sever the connections automatically.

Life is good.

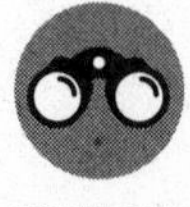

TRY IT OUT

At the end of the earlier section "Handle an Exception or Pass the Buck," you add exception-handling code to a program that makes a copy of a file. Along with your code, you may see warnings telling you that you've forgotten to close `dataInStrm` and `dataOutStrm`. In a subsequent section ("Finishing the Job with a finally Clause"), you got rid of the warnings by adding `dataInStrm.close()` and `dataOutStrm.close()` calls inside `finally` clauses. Instead of adding calls to the `close` method, fix the problem using a `try`-with-resources statement.

» Exposing names to other classes

» Tweaking your code to find the right middle ground

Chapter 14

Sharing Names among the Parts of a Java Program

Speaking of private fields and methods (and I do speak about these things in this chapter) . . .

I'm eating lunch with some friends at work. "They can read your email," says one fellow. Another chimes in, "They know every single website that you visit. They know what products you buy, what you eat for dinner, what you wear, what you think. They even know your deepest, darkest secrets. Why, I wouldn't be surprised if they know when you're going to die."

A third voice enters the fray. "It's getting to the point where you can't blow your nose without someone taking a record of it. I visited a website a few weeks ago, and the page wished me Happy Birthday. How did they know it was me, and how did they remember that it was my birthday?"

"Yeah," says the first guy. "I have a tag on my car that lets me sail through toll booths. It senses that I'm going through and puts the charge on my credit card automatically. Every month, I get a list from the company showing where I've been and when I was there. I'm amazed it doesn't say whom I was visiting and what I did when I got there."

I think quietly to myself. I think about saying, "That's just a bunch of baloney. Personally, I'd be flattered if my employer, the government, or some big company thought so much of me that they tracked my every move. I have enough trouble getting people's attention when I really want it. And most agencies that keep logs of all my purchasing and viewing habits can't even spell my name right when they send me junk mail. 'Hello, this is a courtesy call for Larry Burg. Is Mr. Burg at home?' Spying on people is really boring. I can just see the headline on the front page of *The Times:* 'Author of *Java For Dummies* Wears His Undershirt Inside Out!' Big deal!"

I think for a few seconds, and then I say, "They're out to get us. TV cameras! That's the next big thing — TV cameras everywhere."

Access Modifiers

If you've read this far into *Java For Dummies*, 7th Edition, you probably know one thing: Object-oriented programming is big on hiding details. Programmers who write one piece of code shouldn't tinker with the details inside another programmer's code. It's not a matter of security and secrecy. It's a matter of modularity. When you hide details, you keep the intricacies inside one piece of code from being twisted and broken by another piece of code. Your code comes in nice, discrete, manageable lumps. You keep complexity to a minimum. You make fewer mistakes. You save money. You help promote world peace.

Other chapters have plenty of examples of the use of private fields. When a field is declared private, it's hidden from all outside meddling. This hiding enhances modularity, minimizes complexity, and so on.

Elsewhere in the annals of *Java For Dummies*, 7th Edition, are examples of things that are declared public. Just like a public celebrity, a field that's declared public is left wide open. Plenty of people probably know what kind of toothpaste Elvis used, and any programmer can reference a public field, even a field that's not named *Elvis.*

In Java, the words *public* and *private* are called *access modifiers.* No doubt you've seen fields and methods without access modifiers in their declarations. A method or field of this kind is said to have *default access.* Many examples in this book use default access without making a big fuss about it. That's okay in some chapters, but not in this chapter. In this chapter, I describe the nitty-gritty details about default access.

And you can find out about yet another access modifier that isn't used in any example before this chapter. (At least, I don't remember using it in any earlier examples.) It's the `protected` access modifier. Yes, this chapter covers some of the slimy, grimy facts about protected access.

Classes, Access, and Multipart Programs

With this topic, you can become all tangled up in terminology, so you need to get some basics out of the way. (Most of the terminology that you need comes from Chapter 10, but it's worth reviewing at the start of this chapter.) Here's a fake piece of Java code:

```
class MyClass {
    int myField;              //a field (a member)

    void myMethod() {         //a method (another member)
        int myOtherField;     //a method-local variable (NOT a member)
    }
}
```

The comments on the right side of the code tell the whole story. Two kinds of variables exist here: fields and method-local variables. This chapter isn't about method-local variables. It's about methods and fields.

Believe me, carrying around the phrase *methods and fields* wherever you go isn't easy. It's much better to give these things one name and be done with it. That's why both methods and fields are called *members* of a class.

Members versus classes

At this point, you make an important distinction. Think about Java's `public` keyword. As you may already know from earlier chapters, you can put `public` in front of a member. For example, you can write

```
public static void main(String args[]) {
```

or

```
public amountInAccount = 50.22;
```

These uses of the public keyword come as no big surprise. What you may not already know is that you can put the public keyword in front of a class. For example, you can write

```
public class Drawing {
    // Your code goes here
}
```

In Java, the public keyword has two slightly different meanings — one meaning for members and another meaning for classes. Most of this chapter deals with the meaning of public (and other such keywords) for members. The last part of this chapter (appropriately titled "Access Modifiers for Java Classes") deals with the meaning for classes.

Access modifiers for members

Sure, this section is about members. But that doesn't mean that you can ignore Java classes. Members or not, the Java class is still where all the action takes place. Each field is declared in a particular class, belongs to that class, and is a member of that class. The same is true of methods. Each method is declared in a particular class, belongs to that class, and is a member of that class. Can you use a certain member name in a particular place in your code? To begin answering the question, check whether that place is inside or outside of the member's class:

- If the member is private, only code that's inside the member's class can refer directly to that member's name:

```
class SomeClass {
    private int myField = 10;
}

class SomeOtherClass {

    public static void main(String args[]) {
        SomeClass someObject = new SomeClass();

        //This doesn't work:
        System.out.println(someObject.myField);
    }
}
```

» If the member is public, any code running in the same Java Virtual Machine can refer directly to that member's name.

```
class SomeClass {
    public int myField = 10;
}

class SomeOtherClass {

    public static void main(String args[]) {
        SomeClass someObject = new SomeClass();

        //This works:
        System.out.println(someObject.myField);
    }
}
```

Figures 14-1 through 14-3 illustrate the ideas in a slightly different way.

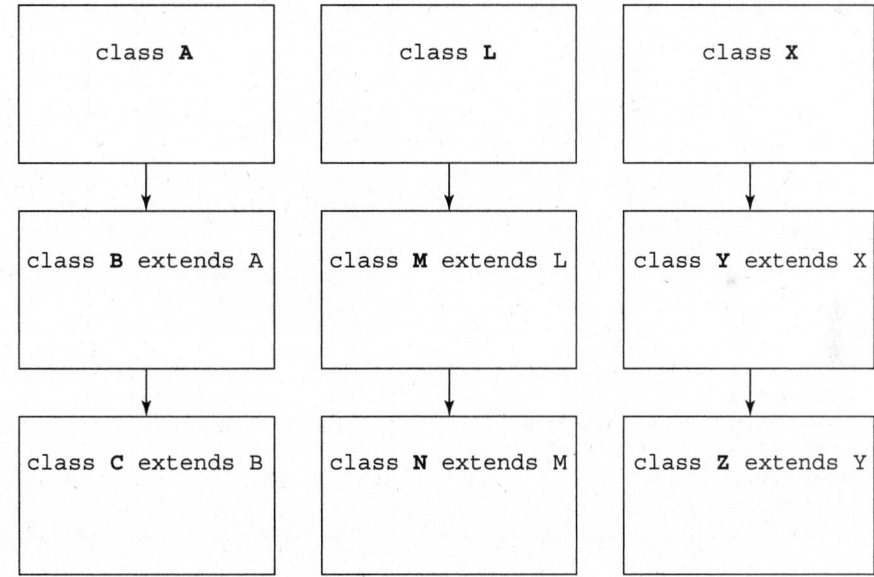

FIGURE 14-1: Several classes and their subclasses.

WARNING

When you see this section's examples, you may come to the wrong conclusion. You may have this little conversation with yourself: "In the example with `private int myField`, the code doesn't work. But in the example with `public int myField`, the code works. So, to have a better chance of getting my code to work, I should make my fields `public` and avoid making them `private`. Right?"

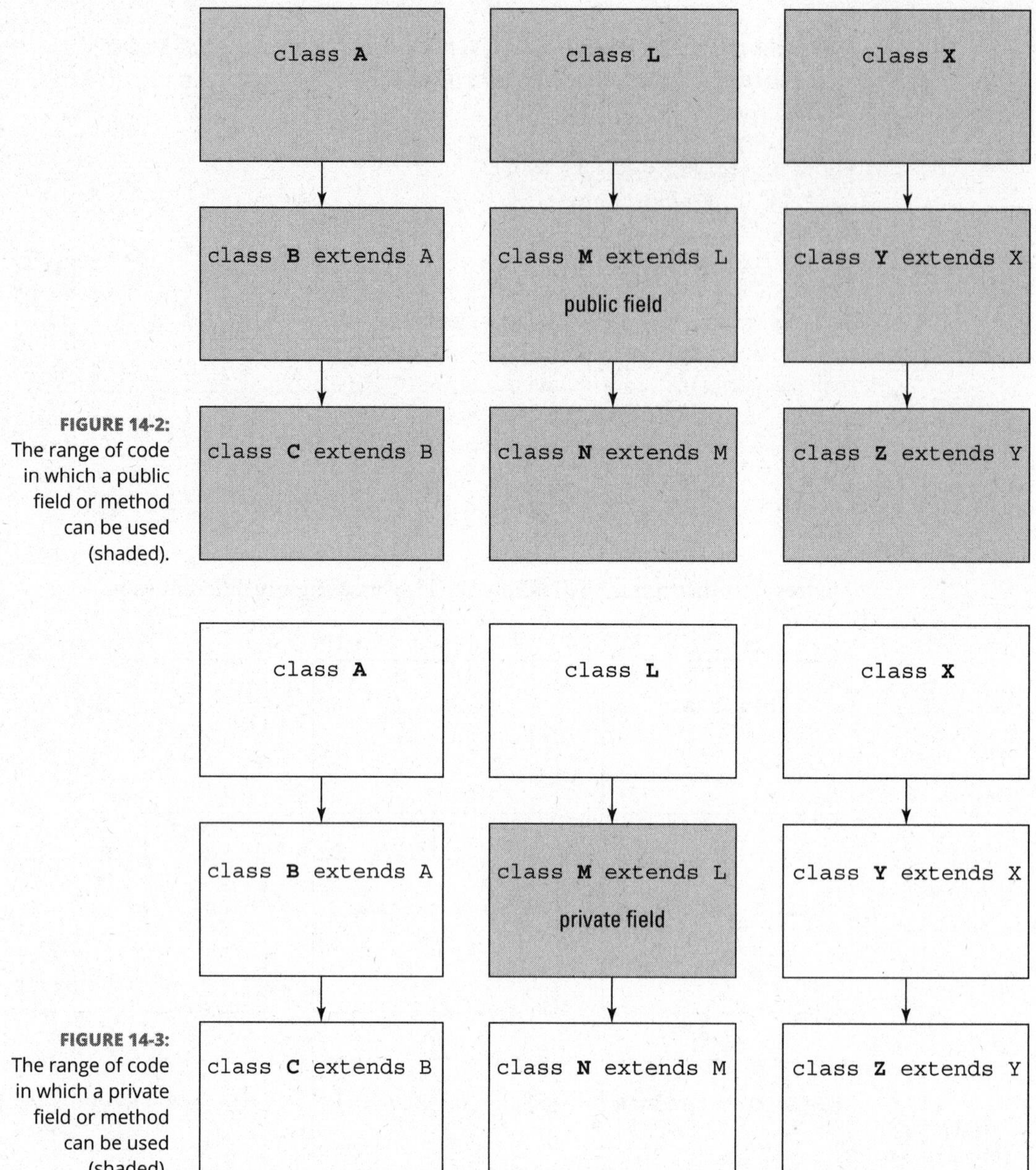

FIGURE 14-2: The range of code in which a public field or method can be used (shaded).

FIGURE 14-3: The range of code in which a private field or method can be used (shaded).

No, dear reader. That's not right!

Public fields are easy to use and even easier to misuse. The best way to engineer your code is to make access to each field as restrictive as possible. If a field doesn't absolutely need to be public, try making it private. If other classes have to get or set the field's values, provide public getter and setter methods. And that leads nicely into the next paragraph . . . .

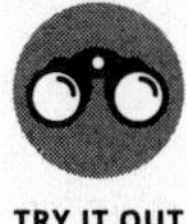

TRY IT OUT

In one of this section's examples, you can't write `someObject.myField` because, in `SomeClass`, the variable `myField` is declared to be private. Fix this by adding getters and setters, and modify the `someObject.myField` reference appropriately.

Putting a drawing on a frame

To make this business about access modifiers clear, you need an example or two. In this chapter's first example, almost everything is public. With public access, you don't have to worry about who can use what.

The code for this first example comes in several parts. The first part, which is in Listing 14-1, displays an `ArtFrame`. On the face of the `ArtFrame` is a `Drawing`. If all the right pieces are in place, running the code of Listing 14-1 displays a window like the one shown in Figure 14-4.

LISTING 14-1: Displaying a Frame

```
import com.burdbrain.drawings.Drawing;
import com.burdbrain.frames.ArtFrame;

class ShowFrame {

    public static void main(String args[]) {
        ArtFrame artFrame = new ArtFrame(new Drawing());

        artFrame.setSize(200, 100);
        artFrame.setVisible(true);
    }
}
```

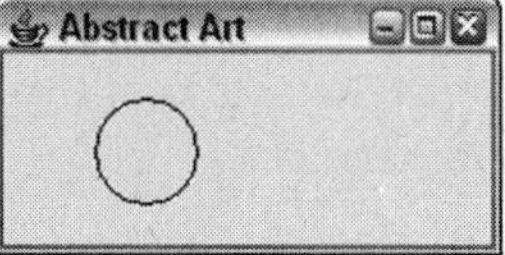

FIGURE 14-4: An ArtFrame.

The code in Listing 14-1 creates a new `ArtFrame` instance. You may suspect that `ArtFrame` is a subclass of a Java `frame` class, and that's certainly the case. Chapter 9 says that Java frames are, by default, invisible. So, in Listing 14-1, to make the `ArtFrame` instance visible, you call the `setVisible` method.

Now notice that Listing 14-1 starts with two `import` declarations. The first `import` declaration allows you to abbreviate the name `Drawing` from the `com.burdbrain.drawings` package. The second import declaration allows you to abbreviate the name `ArtFrame` from `com.burdbrain.frames`.

CROSS REFERENCE

For a review of `import` declarations, see Chapter 4.

The detective in you may be thinking, "He must have written more code (code that I don't see here) and put that code in packages that he named *com.burdbrain.drawings* and *com.burdbrain.frames*." And, indeed, you are correct. To make Listing 14-1 work, I create something called a *Drawing*, and I'm putting all my drawings in the `com.burdbrain.drawings` package. I also need an `ArtFrame` class, and I'm putting all such classes in my `com.burdbrain.frames` package.

So, really, what's a `Drawing`? Well, if you're so eager to know, look at Listing 14-2.

LISTING 14-2: The Drawing Class

```
package com.burdbrain.drawings;

import java.awt.Graphics;

public class Drawing {
    public int x = 40, y = 40, width = 40, height = 40;

    public void paint(Graphics g) {
        g.drawOval(x, y, width, height);
    }
}
```

The code for the `Drawing` class is pretty slim — it contains a few `int` fields and a `paint` method. That's all. Well, when I create my classes, I try to keep 'em lean. Anyway, here are some notes about my `Drawing` class:

- **At the top of the code is a *package declaration*.** Lo and behold! I've made my `Drawing` class belong to a package — the `com.burdbrain.drawings` package. I didn't pull this package name out of the air. The convention (handed down by the people who created Java) says that you start a package name by reversing the parts of your domain name, so I reversed `burdbrain.com`. Then you add one or more descriptive names, separated by dots. I added the name *drawings* because I intend to put all my drawing goodies in this package.

- **The `Drawing` class is *public*.** A public class is vulnerable to intrusion from the outside. In general, I avoid plastering the `public` keyword in front of any old class. But in Listing 14-2, I have to declare my `Drawing` class to be public. If I don't, classes that aren't in the `com.burdbrain.drawings` package can't use the goodies in Listing 14-2. In particular, the line

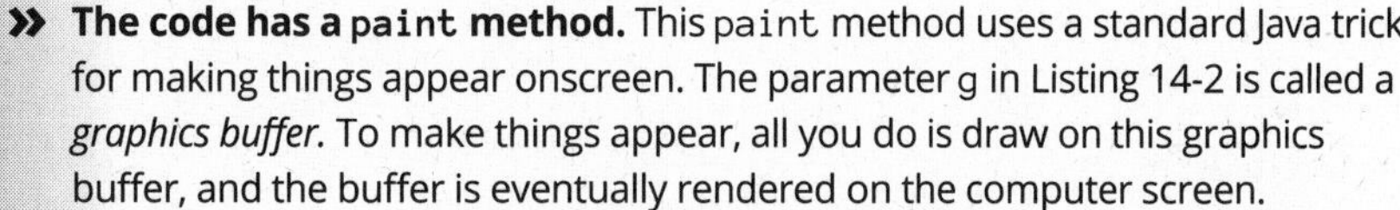

```
ArtFrame artFrame = new ArtFrame(new Drawing());
```

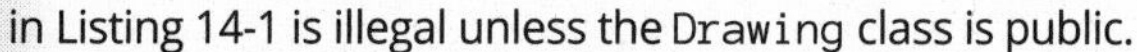

in Listing 14-1 is illegal unless the `Drawing` class is public.

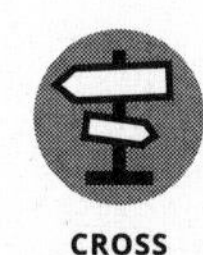

CROSS REFERENCE

For more information on public and nonpublic classes, see the section "Access Modifiers for Java Classes," later in this chapter.

- **The code has a `paint` method.** This `paint` method uses a standard Java trick for making things appear onscreen. The parameter `g` in Listing 14-2 is called a *graphics buffer.* To make things appear, all you do is draw on this graphics buffer, and the buffer is eventually rendered on the computer screen.

  Here's a little more detail: In Listing 14-2, the `paint` method takes a `g` parameter. This `g` parameter refers to an instance of the `java.awt.Graphics` class. Because a `Graphics` instance is a buffer, the things that you put onto this buffer are eventually displayed on the screen. Like all instances of the `java.awt.Graphics` class, this buffer has several drawing methods — and one of them is `drawOval`. When you call `drawOval`, you specify a starting position (`x` pixels from the left edge of the frame and `y` pixels from the top of the frame). You also specify an oval size by putting numbers of pixels in the `width` and `height` parameters. Calling the `drawOval` method puts a little round thing into the `Graphics` buffer. That `Graphics` buffer, round thing and all, is displayed onscreen.

Directory structure

The code in Listing 14-2 belongs to the `com.burdbrain.drawings` package. When you put a class into a package, you have to create a directory structure that mirrors the name of the package.

To house code that's in the `com.burdbrain.drawings` package, you have to have three directories: a `com` directory, a subdirectory of `com` named `burdbrain`, and a subdirectory of `burdbrain` named `drawings`. The overall directory structure is shown in Figure 14-5.

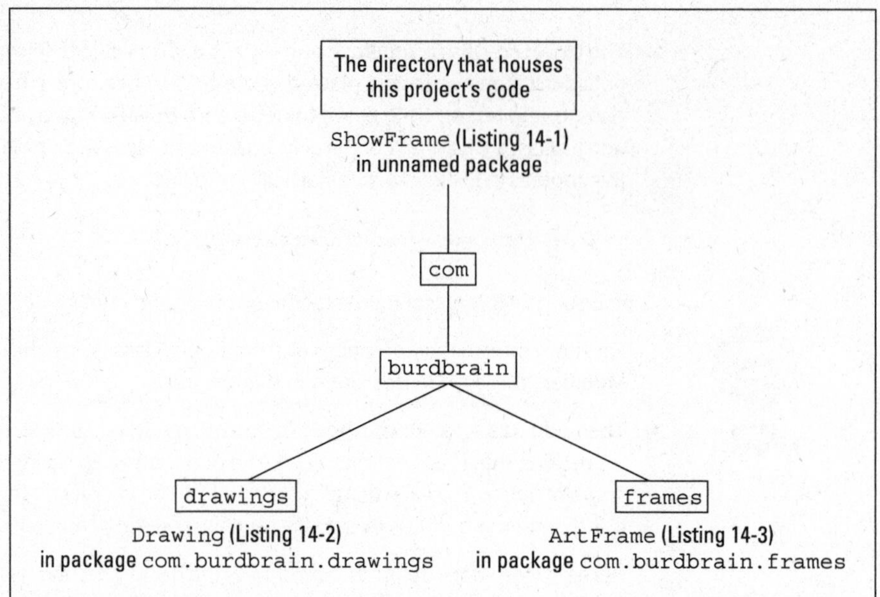

FIGURE 14-5: The files and directories in your project.

WARNING

If you don't have your code in the appropriate directories, you get a repulsive and disgusting `NoClassDefFoundError`. Believe me, this error is never fun to get. When you see this error, you don't have any clues to help you figure out where the missing class is or where the compiler expects to find it. If you stay calm, you can figure out all this stuff on your own. If you panic, you'll be poking around for hours. As a seasoned Java programmer, I can remember plenty of scraped knuckles that came from this heinous `NoClassDefFoundError`.

Making a frame

This chapter's first three listings develop one multipart example. This section has the last of three pieces in that example. This last piece isn't crucial for the understanding of access modifiers, which is the main topic of this chapter. So, if you want to skip past the explanation of Listing 14-3, you can do so without losing the chapter's thread. On the other hand, if you want to know more about the Java `Swing` classes, read on.

LISTING 14-3: The ArtFrame Class

```
package com.burdbrain.frames;

import java.awt.Graphics;
import javax.swing.JFrame;
import com.burdbrain.drawings.Drawing;
```

```
public class ArtFrame extends JFrame {
    private static final long serialVersionUID = 1L;

    Drawing;

    public ArtFrame(Drawing drawing) {
        this.drawing = drawing;
        setTitle("Abstract Art");
        setDefaultCloseOperation(EXIT_ON_CLOSE);
    }

    public void paint(Graphics g) {
        drawing.paint(g);
    }
}
```

LOOKING FOR FILES IN ALL THE RIGHT PLACES

You try to compile the program in Listing 14-1. The Java compiler pokes through the code and stumbles upon some missing pieces. First there's this thing called an `ArtFrame`. Then you have this `Drawing` business. Listing 14-1 defines a class named `ShowFrame`, not `ArtFrame` or `Drawing`. So where does the compiler go for information about the `ArtFrame` and `Drawing` classes?

If you stop to think about it, the problem can be daunting. Should the compiler go searching all over your hard drive for files named `ArtFrame.java` or `Drawing.class`? How large is your new hard drive? 500GB? 750GB? 6,000,000GB? And what about references to files on network drives? The search space is potentially unlimited. What if the compiler eventually resolves all these issues? Then you try to run your code, and the Java Virtual Machine (JVM) starts searching all over again. (For info on the Java Virtual Machine, see Chapter 2.)

To tame this problem, Java defines something called a *CLASSPATH.* The *CLASSPATH* is a list of places where the compiler and the JVM look for code. There are several ways to set a CLASSPATH. Some programmers create a new CLASSPATH each time they run a Java program. Others create a system-wide CLASSPATH variable. (If you're familiar with the PATH variable on Windows and Unix computers, you may already know how this stuff works.) One way or another, the compiler and the JVM need a list of places to look for code. Without such a list, these Java tools don't look anywhere. They don't find classes like `ArtFrame` or `Drawing`. You get a `cannot find symbol` message or a `NoClassDefFoundError` message, and you're very unhappy.

Listing 14-3 has all the gadgetry that you need for putting a drawing on a Java frame. The code uses several names from the Java API (Application Programming Interface). I explain most of these names in Chapters 9 and 10.

The only new name in Listing 14-3 is the word *paint*. The `paint` method in Listing 14-3 defers to another `paint` method — the `paint` method belonging to a `Drawing` object. The `ArtFrame` object creates a floating window on your computer screen. What's drawn in that floating window depends on whatever `Drawing` object was passed to the `ArtFrame` constructor.

If you trace the flow of Listings 14-1 through 14-3, you may notice something peculiar: The `paint` method in Listing 14-3 never seems to be called. Well, for many of Java's window-making components, you just declare a `paint` method and let the method sit there quietly in the code. When the program runs, the computer calls the `paint` method automatically.

That's what happens with `javax.swing.JFrame` objects. In Listing 14-3, the frame's `paint` method is called from behind the scenes. Then the frame's `paint` method calls the `Drawing` object's `paint` method, which in turn draws an oval on the frame. That's how you get the stuff you see in Figure 14-4.

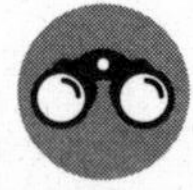
TRY IT OUT

In your computer's File Explorer or Finder, navigate to this book's `14-01` project folder. In that folder, poke around and find the `ShowFrame.java`, `Drawing.java`, and `ArtFrame.java` files. Notice how these Java files are nested inside a few different folders.

Sneaking Away from the Original Code

Your preferred software vendor, Burd Brain Consulting, has sold you two files: `Drawing.class` and `ArtFrame.class`. As a customer, you can't see the code inside the files `Drawing.java` and `ArtFrame.java`. So you have to live with whatever happens to be inside these two files. (If only you'd purchased a copy of *Java For Dummies*, 6th Edition, which has the code for these files in Listings 14-2 and 14-3!) Anyway, you want to tweak the way the oval looks in Figure 14-4 so that it's a bit wider. To do this, you create a subclass of the `Drawing` class — `DrawingWide` — and put it in Listing 14-4.

LISTING 14-4: A Subclass of the Drawing Class

```
import java.awt.Graphics;
import com.burdbrain.drawings.Drawing;

public class DrawingWide extends Drawing {
    int width = 100, height = 30;

    public void paint(Graphics g) {
        g.drawOval(x, y, width, height);
    }
}
```

To make use of the code in Listing 14-4, you remember to change one of the lines in Listing 14-1. You change the line to

```
ArtFrame = new ArtFrame(new DrawingWide());
```

In Listing 14-1 you can also remove the `com.burdbrain.drawings.Drawing` import declaration because you no longer need it.

Listing 14-4 defines a subclass of the original `Drawing` class. In that subclass, you override the original class's `width` and `height` fields and the original class's `paint` method. The frame that you get is shown in Figure 14-6.

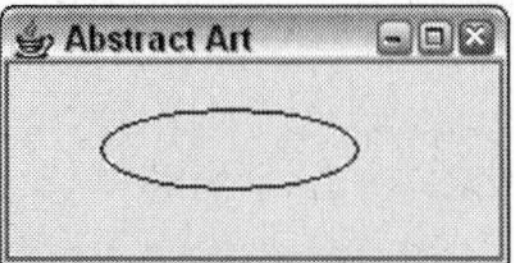

FIGURE 14-6: Another art frame.

In passing, you may notice that the code in Listing 14-4 doesn't start with a package declaration. This means that your whole collection of files comes from the following three packages:

- **The `com.burdbrain.drawings` package:** The original `Drawing` class from Listing 14-2 is in this package.
- **The `com.burdbrain.frames` package:** The `ArtFrame` class from Listing 14-3 is in this package.

» **An ever-present, unnamed package:** In Java, when you don't start a file with a package declaration, all the code in that file goes into one big, unnamed package. Listings 14-1 and 14-4 are in the same unnamed package. In fact, most of the listings from the first 13 chapters of this book are in Java's unnamed package.

At this point, your project has two drawing classes: the original `Drawing` class and your new `DrawingWide` class. Similar as these classes may be, they live in two separate packages. That's not surprising. The `Drawing` class, developed by your friends at Burd Brain Consulting, lives in a package whose name starts with *com.burdbrain.* But you developed `DrawingWide` on your own, so you shouldn't put it in a `com.burdbrain` package.

The most sensible thing to do is to put it in one of your own packages, such as `com.myhomedomain.drawings`; but putting your class in the unnamed package will do for now.

One way or another, your `DrawingWide` subclass compiles and runs as planned. You go home, beaming with the confidence of having written useful, working code.

Default access

If you're reading these paragraphs in order, you know that the last example ends happily. The code in Listing 14-4 runs like a charm. Everyone, including my wonderful editor, Paul Levesque, is happy.

But, wait! Do you ever wonder what life would be like if you hadn't chosen that particular career, dated that certain someone, or read that certain *For Dummies* book? In this section, I roll back the clock a bit to show you what would have happened if one word had been omitted from the code in Listing 14-2.

Dealing with different versions of a program can give you vertigo, so I start this discussion by describing what you have. First, you have a `Drawing` class. In this class, the fields aren't declared to be public and have the default access. The `Drawing` class lives in the `com.burdbrain.drawings` package. (See Listing 14-5.)

LISTING 14-5: Fields with Default Access

```
package com.burdbrain.drawings;

import java.awt.Graphics;
```

```
public class Drawing {
    int x = 40, y = 40, width = 40, height = 40;

    public void paint(Graphics g) {
        g.drawOval(x, y, width, height);
    }
}
```

Next, you have a `DrawingWide` subclass (copied, for your convenience, in Listing 14-6). The `DrawingWide` class is in Java's unnamed package.

LISTING 14-6: A Failed Attempt to Create a Subclass

```
import com.burdbrain.drawings.*;
import java.awt.Graphics;

public class DrawingWide extends Drawing {
    int width = 100, height = 30;

    public void paint(Graphics g) {
        g.drawOval(x, y, width, height);
    }
}
```

The trouble is that the whole thing falls apart at the seams. The code in Listing 14-6 doesn't compile. Instead, you get the following error messages:

```
x is not public in com.burdbrain.drawings.Drawing;
cannot be accessed from outside package
y is not public in com.burdbrain.drawings.Drawing;
cannot be accessed from outside package
```

The code doesn't compile, because a field that has default access can't be directly referenced outside its package — not even by a subclass of the class containing the field. The same holds true for any methods that have default access.

A class's fields and methods are called *members* of the class. The rules for access — default and otherwise — apply to all members of classes.

REMEMBER

The access rules that I describe in this chapter don't apply to method-local variables. A method-local variable can be accessed only within its own method.

For the rundown on method-local variables, see Chapter 10.

In Java, the default access for a member of a class is package-wide access. A member declared without the word *public, private,* or *protected* in front of it is accessible in the package in which its class resides. Figures 14-7 and 14-8 illustrate the point.

WARNING

The names of packages, with all their dots and subparts, can be slightly misleading. For instance, when you write a program that responds to button clicks, you normally import classes from two separate packages. On one line, you may have `import java.awt.*;`. On another line, you may have `import java.awt.event.*;`. Importing all classes from the `java.awt` package doesn't automatically import classes from the `java.awt.event` package.

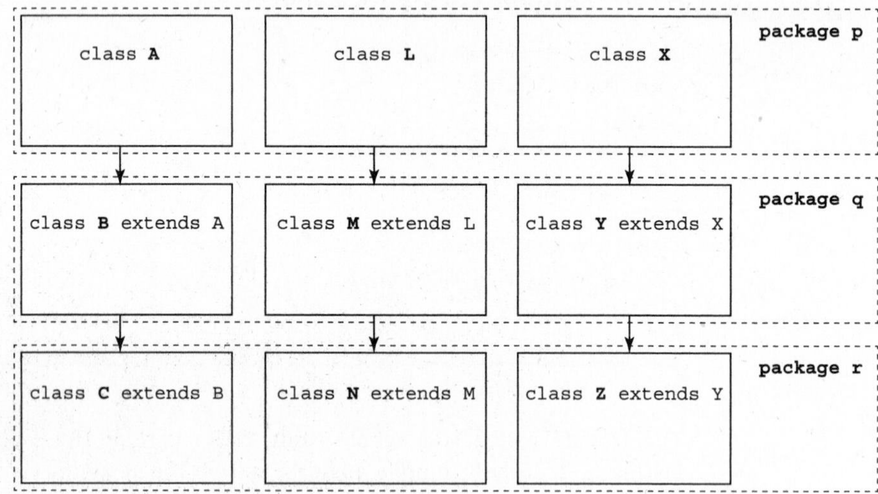

FIGURE 14-7: Packages cut across subclass hierarchies.

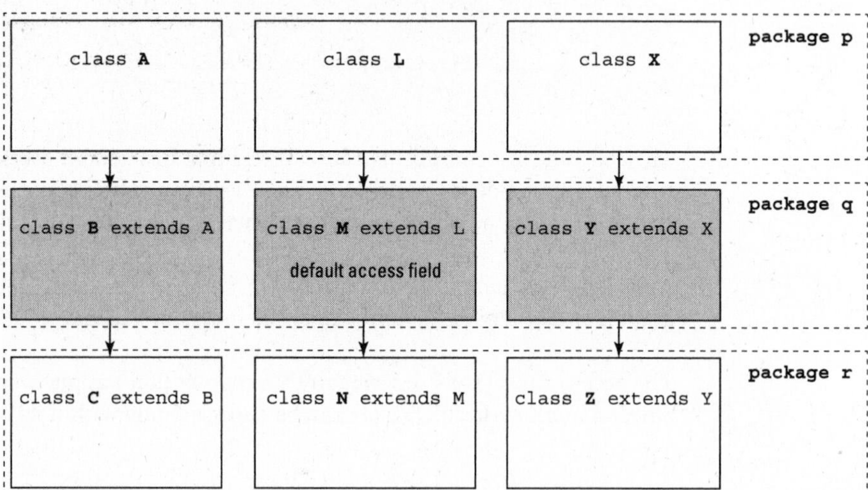

FIGURE 14-8: The range of code in which a default field or method can be used (shaded).

Crawling back into the package

I love getting things in the mail. At worst, it's junk mail that I can throw right into the trash. At best, it's something I can use, a new toy, or something somebody sent especially for me.

Well, today is my lucky day. Somebody from Burd Brain Consulting sent a subclass of the `Drawing` class. It's essentially the same as the code in Listing 14-6. The only difference is that this new `DrawingWideBB` class lives inside the `com.burdbrain.drawings` package. The code is shown in Listing 14-7. To run this code, I have to modify Listing 14-1 with the line

```
ArtFrame artFrame = new ArtFrame(new DrawingWideBB());
```

LISTING 14-7: Yes, Virginia, This Is a Subclass

```
package com.burdbrain.drawings;

import java.awt.Graphics;

public class DrawingWideBB extends Drawing {
    int width = 100, height = 30;

    public void paint(Graphics g) {
        g.drawOval(x, y, width, height);
    }
}
```

When you run Listing 14-7 alongside the `Drawing` class in Listing 14-5, everything works just fine. The reason? It's because `Drawing` and `DrawingWideBB` are in the same package. Look back at Figure 14-8 and notice the shaded region that spans across an entire package. The code in the `DrawingWideBB` class has every right to use the `x` and `y` fields, which are defined with default access in the `Drawing` class because `Drawing` and `DrawingWideBB` are in the same package.

REMEMBER

To use the `DrawingWideBB` class in Listing 14-7, you make two changes in the original Listing 14-1. Change the first import declaration to

```
import com.burdbrain.drawings.DrawingWideBB;
```

Also, change the `ArtFrame` object's constructor call to `new ArtFrame(new DrawingWideBB())`.

WARNING

This section explains default access, the kind of access that I use in most of the book's examples. I use default access a lot because, with default access, you don't have to make sense of the words `public` or `private`. So, in many examples, you have fewer words to worry about.

But in real life, programmers shun the use of default access. With default access, all the other classes in your package can view and change the values of your fields. Other programmers can set `daysInThisMonth` to 32 or `chaptersInThisBook` to −7.

By far, the best policy is to use default access only when such access is absolutely necessary. In most situations, if other classes have to get or set your field's values, you should use private access and provide public getter and setter methods.

Protected Access

When I was first getting to know Java, I thought the word *protected* meant *nice and secure* or something like that. "Wow, that field is protected. It must be hard to get at." Well, this notion turned out to be wrong. In Java, a member that's protected is less hidden, less secure, and available for use in more classes than one that has default access. In other words, protected access is more permissive than default access. For me, the terminology is misleading. But that's the way it is.

Subclasses that aren't in the same package

Think of protected access this way. You start with a field that has default access (a field without the word `public`, `private`, or `protected` in its declaration). That field can be accessed only inside the package in which it lives. Now add the word `protected` to the front of the field's declaration. Suddenly, classes outside that field's package have some access to the field. You can now reference the field from a subclass (of the class in which the field is declared). You can also reference the field from a sub-subclass, a sub-sub-subclass, and so on. Any descendent class will do. For an example, see Listings 14-8 and 14-9.

LISTING 14-8: Protected Fields

```
package com.burdbrain.drawings;

import java.awt.Graphics;

public class Drawing {
    protected int x = 40, y = 40, width = 40, height = 40;
```

```
    public void paint(Graphics g) {
        g.drawOval(x, y, width, height);
    }
}
```

LISTING 14-9: The Subclass from the Blue Lagoon, Part II

```
import java.awt.Graphics;
import com.burdbrain.drawings.Drawing;

public class DrawingWide extends Drawing {
    int width = 100, height = 30;

    public void paint(Graphics g) {
        g.drawOval(x, y, width, height);
    }
}
```

Listing 14-8 defines the `Drawing` class. Listing 14-9 defines `DrawingWide`, which is a subclass of the `Drawing` class.

In the `Drawing` class, the `x`, `y`, `width`, and `height` fields are `protected`. The `DrawingWide` class has its own `width` and `height` fields, but `DrawingWide` references the `x` and `y` fields that are defined in the parent `Drawing` class. That's okay, even though `DrawingWide` isn't in the same package as its parent `Drawing` class. (The `Drawing` class is in the `com.burdbrain.drawings` package; the `DrawingWide` class is in Java's great, unnamed package.) It's okay because the `x` and `y` fields are protected in the `Drawing` class.

Compare Figures 14-8 and 14-9. Notice the extra bit of shading in Figure 14-9. A subclass can access a protected member of a class, even if that subclass belongs to some other package.

TIP

Do you work with a team of programmers? Do people from outside your team use their own team's package names? If so, when they use your code, they may make subclasses of the classes that you've defined. This is where protected access comes in handy. Use protected access when you want people from outside your team to make direct references to your code's fields or methods.

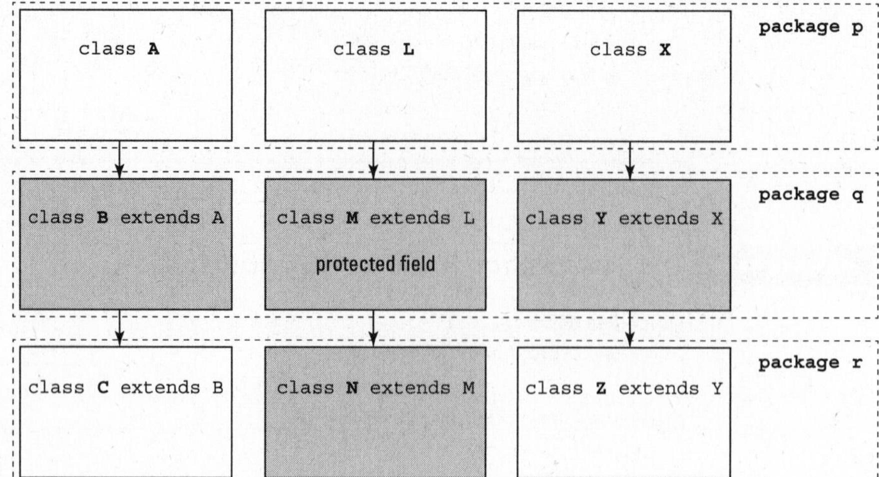

FIGURE 14-9: The range of code in which a protected field or method can be used (shaded).

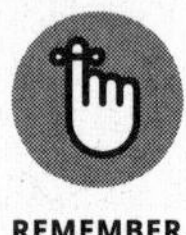

REMEMBER

For the members of a class, private access is the most restrictive, then comes default access, then protected access, and finally, public access.

Classes that aren't subclasses (but are in the same package)

Those people from Burd Brain Consulting are sending you one piece of software after another. This time, they've sent an alternative to the ShowFrame class — the class in Listing 14-1. This new ShowFrameWideBB class displays a wider oval (how exciting!), but it does this without creating a subclass of the old Drawing class. Instead, the new ShowFrameWideBB code creates a Drawing instance and then changes the value of the instance's width and height fields. The code is shown in Listing 14-10.

LISTING 14-10: Drawing a Wider Oval

```
package com.burdbrain.drawings;

import com.burdbrain.frames.ArtFrame;

class ShowFrameWideBB {

    public static void main(String args[]) {
        Drawing drawing = new Drawing();
        drawing.width = 100;
        drawing.height = 30;
```

```
        ArtFrame artFrame = new ArtFrame(drawing);
        artFrame.setSize(200, 100);
        artFrame.setVisible(true);
    }
}
```

Here's the story. This ShowFrameWideBB class in Listing 14-10 is in the same package as the Drawing class (the com.burdbrain.drawings package). But ShowFrameWideBB isn't a subclass of the Drawing class.

Now imagine compiling ShowFrameWideBB with the Drawing class that's shown in Listing 14-8 — the class with all those protected fields. What happens? Well, everything goes smoothly because a protected member is available in two (somewhat unrelated) places. Look again at Figure 14-9. A protected member is available to subclasses outside the package, but the member is also available to code (subclasses or not) within the member's package.

Listing 14-10 has a main method, which is inside a class, which is in turn inside the com.burdbrain.drawings package. With most Integrated Development Environments (IDEs), you don't think twice about running a main method that's in a named package. But if you run programs from the command line, you may need to type a fully qualified class name. For example, to run the code in Listing 14-10, you type java com.burdbrain.drawings.ShowFrameWideBB.

TECHNICAL STUFF

The real story about protected access is one step more complicated than the story that I describe in this section. The Java Language Specification (https://docs.oracle.com/javase/specs) mentions a hair-splitting point about code being responsible for an object's implementation. When you're first figuring out how to program in Java, don't worry about this point. Wait until you've written many Java programs. Then when you stumble upon a variable has protected access error message, you can start worrying. Better yet, skip the worrying and take a careful look at the protected access section in the Java Language Specification.

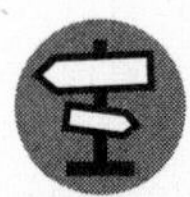
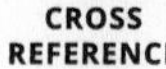
CROSS REFERENCE

For info about the Java Language Specification, visit Chapter 3.

Here are some things for you to try:

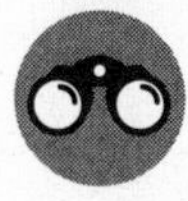
TRY IT OUT

» In Listing 14-2, I draw a circle on a frame. To fill the circle with green color, use the Graphics class's setColor and fillOval methods, like this:

```
g.setColor(Color.GREEN)
g.fillOval(x, y, width, height);
```

Values such as Color.GREEN belong to Color class in the java.awt package.

Create a frame that displays a traffic signal with its green, yellow, and red lights.

- A Book has a title (a String) and an author (an instance of the Author class). An Author has a name (a String) and an ArrayList of Book instances. A separate class contains a main method that creates several books and several authors. The main method also displays information about the books and authors.

  Put each class in its own package. Wherever possible, make your fields private, and provide public getters and setters.

- An Item has a name (a String) and an artist (an instance of the Artist class). Each Artist instance has a name (a String) and an ArrayList of items.

  The Song and Album classes are subclasses of the Item class. Each Song instance has a genre (a value from an enum named Genre). The values of Genre are ROCK, POP, BLUES, and CLASSICAL. Each Album instance has an ArrayList of songs.

  Finally, a Playlist has an ArrayList of items.

  Create these classes. In a separate class, construct instances of each class, and display information about these instances on the screen.

- The following four classes live in four different .java files. Without typing these classes in an IDE's editor, decide which statements will cause the IDE to display error messages. For each such statement, decide on the least permissive access change that would eliminate the error message:

```
// THIS CODE DOES NOT COMPILE:

package com.allmycode.things;

import com.allyourcode.stuff.Stuff;
import com.allyourcode.stuff.morestuff.MoreStuff;

public class Things {
  protected int i = 0;
  private int j = 0;
  int k = 0;

  public static void main(String[] args) {
    Stuff stuff = new Stuff();
    System.out.println(stuff.i);
```

```
    MoreStuff moreStuff = new MoreStuff();
    System.out.println(moreStuff.i);
  }
}

package com.allyourcode.stuff;

import com.allyourcode.stuff.morestuff.MoreStuff;

public class Stuff {
  protected int i = 0;

  void aMethod() {
    new MoreStuff().myMethod();
  }
}

package com.allyourcode.stuff.morestuff;

import com.allmycode.things.Things;

public class MoreStuff extends Things {

  protected void myMethod() {
    System.out.println(i);
  }
}

package com.allmycode.things;

public class MoreThings extends Things {

  public void anotherMethod() {
    System.out.println(i);
    System.out.println(j);
    System.out.println(k);
  }
}
```

Access Modifiers for Java Classes

Maybe the things that you read about access modifiers for members make you a tad dizzy. After all, member access in Java is a complicated subject with lots of plot twists and cliffhangers. Well, the dizziness is over. Compared with the saga for fields and methods, the access story for classes is rather simple.

A class can be either public or nonpublic. If you see something like

```
public class Drawing
```

you're looking at the declaration of a public class. But, if you see plain old

```
class ShowFrame
```

the class that's being declared isn't public.

Public classes

If a class is public, you can refer to the class from anywhere in your code. Of course, some restrictions apply. You must obey all the rules in this chapter's "Directory structure" section. You must also refer to a packaged class properly. For example, in Listing 14-1, you can write

```
import com.burdbrain.drawings.Drawing;
import com.burdbrain.frames.ArtFrame;
...
ArtFrame artFrame = new ArtFrame(new Drawing());
```

or you can do without the import declarations and write

```
com.burdbrain.frames.ArtFrame artFrame =
    new com.burdbrain.frames.ArtFrame(new com.burdbrain.drawings.Drawing());
```

One way or another, your code must acknowledge that the `ArtFrame` and `Drawing` classes are in named packages.

Nonpublic classes

If a class isn't public, you can refer to the class only from code within the class's package.

I tried it. First, I went back to Listing 14-2 and deleted the word *public*. I turned `public class Drawing` into plain old `class Drawing`, like this:

```
package com.burdbrain.drawings;

import java.awt.Graphics;

class Drawing {
    public int x = 40, y = 40, width = 40, height = 40;

    public void paint(Graphics g) {
        g.drawOval(x, y, width, height);
    }
}
```

Then I compiled the code in Listing 14-7. Everything was peachy because Listing 14-7 contains the following lines:

```
package com.burdbrain.drawings;

public class DrawingWideBB extends Drawing
```

Because both pieces of code are in the same `com.burdbrain.drawings` package, access from `DrawingWideBB` back to the nonpublic `Drawing` class was no problem at all.

But then I tried to compile the code in Listing 14-3. The code in Listing 14-3 begins with

```
package com.burdbrain.frames;
```

That code isn't in the `com.burdbrain.drawings` package. So when the computer reached the line

```
Drawing drawing;
```

from Listing 14-3, the computer went *poof!* To be more precise, the computer displayed this message:

```
com.burdbrain.drawings.Drawing is not public in com.burdbrain.drawings;
cannot be accessed from outside package
```

Well, I guess I got what was coming to me.

Things are never as simple as they seem. The rules that I describe in this section apply to almost every class in this book. But Java has fancy things called *inner classes*, and inner classes follow a different set of rules. Fortunately, a typical novice programmer has little contact with inner classes. The only inner classes in this book are in Chapter 15 (and a few inner classes disguised as `enum` types). So for now, you can live quite happily with the rules that I describe in this section.

» Working with abstract classes

Chapter 15
Fancy Reference Types

In previous chapters, you may have read about the things that full-time and part-time employees have in common. In particular, both the FullTimeEmployee and PartTimeEmployee classes can extend the Employee class. That's nice to know if you're running a small business, but what if you're not running a business? What if you're taking care of house pets?

This chapter explores the care of house pets and other burning issues.

Java's Types

Chapter 4 explains that Java has these two kinds of types:

» **Java has eight primitive types.**

The four that you use most often are int, double, boolean, and char.

» **Java's API has thousands of reference types. And, when you write a Java program, you define new reference types.**

Java's String type is a reference type. So are Java's Scanner, JFrame, ArrayList, and File types. My DummiesFrame is a reference type. In Chapter 7, you create your own Employee, FullTimeEmployee, and PartTimeEmployee reference types. Your first *You'll love Java!* program has a main method inside of a class, and that class is a reference type. You may not realize it, but every array belongs to a reference type.

In Java, reference types are everywhere. But until this point in the book, the only reference types that you see are classes and arrays. Java has other kinds of reference types, and this chapter explores the possibilities.

The Java Interface

Think about a class (such as an `Employee` class) and a subclass (such as a `FullTimeEmployee` class). The relationship between a class and its subclass is one of inheritance. In many real-life families, a child inherits assets from a parent. And in Chapter 8, the `FullTimeEmployee` class inherits `name` and `jobTitle` fields from the `Employee` class. That's the way it works.

But consider the relationship between an editor and an author. The editor says, "By signing this contract, you agree to submit a completed manuscript by the ninth of January." Despite any excuses that the author gives before the deadline date (and, believe me, authors make plenty of excuses), the relationship between the editor and the author is one of obligation. The author agrees to take on certain responsibilities; and, in order to continue being an author, the author must fulfill those responsibilities. (By the way, there's no subtext in this paragraph — none at all.)

Now consider Barry Burd. Who? Barry Burd — that guy who writes *Java For Dummies* and certain other *For Dummies* books (all from Wiley Publishing). He's a college professor, and he's also an author. You want to mirror this situation in a Java program, but Java doesn't support multiple inheritance. You can't make Barry extend both a `Professor` class and an `Author` class at the same time.

Fortunately for Barry, Java has interfaces. An interface is a kind of reference type. In fact, the code to create an interface looks a lot like the code to create a class:

```
public interface MyInterfaceName {
  // blah, blah, blah
}
```

An interface is a lot like a class, but an interface is different. (So, what else is new? A cow is like a planet, but it's quite a bit different. Cows moo; planets hang in space.)

Anyway, when you read the word *interface*, you can start by thinking of a class. Then, in your head, note that

- A class can extend only one parent class, but a class can implement many interfaces.

- A parent class is a bunch of stuff that a class inherits. But an *interface* is a bunch of stuff that an implementing class is *obliged to provide*.

What about poor Barry? He can be an instance of a `Person` class with all the fields that any person has — `name`, `address`, `age`, `height`, `weight`, and so on. He can also implement more than one interface:

- Because Barry implements a `Professor` interface, he must have methods named `teachStudents`, `adviseStudents`, and `gradePapers`.
- Because he implements an `Author` interface, he must have methods named `writeChapters`, `reviewChapters`, `answerEmail`, and so on.

Two interfaces

Imagine two different kinds of data. One is a column of numbers that comes from an array. Another is a table (with rows and columns) that comes from a disk file. What might these two things have in common?

I don't know about you, but I may want to display both kinds of data. So I can write code to create a contract. The contract says, "Whoever signs this contract agrees to have a `display` method." In Listing 15-1, I declare a `Displayable` interface.

LISTING 15-1: Behold! An Interface!

```
public interface Displayable {

    public void display();

}
```

Wait just a darn minute! The `display` method declaration in Listing 15-1 has a header but no body. There are no curly braces after `display()` — only a lonely-looking semicolon. What's going on here?

To answer the question, I'll let the code in Listing 15-1 speak for itself. If the code in the listing could talk, here's what the code would say:

> "As an interface, my `display` method has a header but no body. A class that claims to implement me (the `Displayable` interface) must provide (either directly or indirectly) a body for the `display` method. That is, a class that claims to

implement `Displayable` must, in one way or another, provide its own code of the following kind:

```
public void display() {
    // Some statements go here
}
```

In order to implement me (the interface in Listing 15-1), the new code's `display` method must take no parameters and return nothing (also known as `void`)."

The `Displayable` interface is like a legal contract. The `Displayable` interface doesn't tell you what an implementing class already has. Instead, the `Displayable` interface tells you what an implementing class must declare in its own code.

In addition to displaying columns of numbers and tables, I may also want to summarize both kinds of data. How do you summarize a column of numbers? I don't know. Maybe you display the total of all the numbers. And how do you summarize a table? Maybe you display the table's column headings. How you summarize the data isn't my concern. All I care about is that you have some way to summarize the data.

So I create code containing a second Java contract. The second contract says, "Whoever signs this contract agrees to have a `summarize` method." In Listing 15-2, I declare a `Summarizable` interface.

LISTING 15-2: Another Interface

```
public interface Summarizable {

    public String summarize();

}
```

Any class claiming to implement the `Summarizable` interface must, by hook or by crook, provide an implementation of a `summarize` method — a method with no parameters that returns a `String` value.

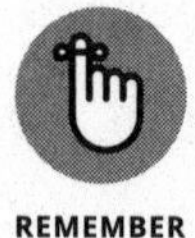

REMEMBER

In the declaration of an interface, a particular method might have no body of its own. A method with no body is called an *abstract method.*

Implementing interfaces

Listing 15-3 implements the `Displayable` and `Summarizable` interfaces, and provides bodies for the `display` and `summarize` methods.

LISTING 15-3: Implementing Two Interfaces

```
public class ColumnOfNumbers implements Displayable, Summarizable {
    double numbers[];

    public ColumnOfNumbers(double[] numbers) {
        this.numbers = numbers;
    }

    @Override
    public void display() {
        for (double d : numbers) {
            System.out.println(d);
        }
    }

    @Override
    public String summarize() {
        double total = 0.0;
        for (double d : numbers) {
            total += d;
        }
        return Double.toString(total);
    }
}
```

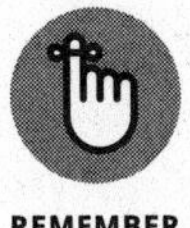

REMEMBER

When you implement an interface, you provide bodies for the interface's abstract methods.

Java's compiler is serious about the use of the `implements` keyword. If you remove either of the two method declarations from Listing 15-3 without removing the `implements` clause, you see some frightening error messages in your IDE's editor. Java expects you to honor the contract that the `implements` keyboard implies. If you don't honor the contract, Java refuses to compile your code. So there!

TIP

You can use Java's error messages to your advantage. Start by typing some code containing the clause `implements Displayable, Summarizable`. Because of the `implements` clause, the editor displays an error mark and lists the names of the methods that you should have declared but didn't. In this section's example, those method names are `display` and `summarize`. After a few more mouse clicks, the IDE generates simple `display` and `summarize` methods for you.

Listing 15-4 contains another class that implements the `Displayable` and `Summarizable` interfaces.

LISTING 15-4: Another Class Implements the Interfaces

```
import java.io.File;
import java.io.FileNotFoundException;
import java.util.ArrayList;
import java.util.Scanner;

public class Table implements Displayable, Summarizable {
    Scanner diskFile;
    ArrayList<String> lines = new ArrayList<>();

    public Table(String fileName) {
        try {
            diskFile = new Scanner(new File(fileName));

        } catch (FileNotFoundException e) {
            e.printStackTrace();
        }
        while (diskFile.hasNextLine()) {
            lines.add(diskFile.nextLine());
        }
    }

    @Override
    public void display() {
        for (String line : lines) {
            System.out.println(line);
        }
    }

    @Override
    public String summarize() {
        return lines.get(0);
    }
}
```

In Listings 15-3 and 15-4, notice several uses of the @Override annotation. Chapter 8 introduces the use of the @Override annotation. Normally, you use @Override to signal the replacement of a method that's already been declared in a superclass. But from Java 6 onward, you can also use @Override to signal an interface method's implementation. That's what I do in Listings 15-3 and 15-4.

Putting the pieces together

The code in Listing 15-5 makes use of all the stuff in Listings 15-1 to 15-4.

LISTING 15-5: Getting the Most out of Your Interfaces

```
public class Main {

    public static void main(String[] args) {
        double numbers[] = { 21.7, 68.3, 5.5 };
        ColumnOfNumbers column = new ColumnOfNumbers(numbers);

        displayMe(column);
        summarizeMe(column);

        Table table = new Table("MyTable.txt");

        displayMe(table);
        summarizeMe(table);
    }

    static void displayMe(Displayable displayable) {
        displayable.display();
        System.out.println();
    }

    static void summarizeMe(Summarizable summarizable) {
        System.out.println(summarizable.summarize());
        System.out.println();
    }
}
```

With the `MyTable.txt` file shown in Figure 15-1, the output from Listing 15-5 is shown in Figure 15-2.

```
Name  ID Balance
Barry 01 19.51
Carol 02 100.35
Myrna 03 10.07
```

FIGURE 15-1: The `MyTable.txt` file.

```
21.7
68.3
5.5

95.5

Name   ID Balance
Barry 01 19.51
Carol 02 100.35
Myrna 03 10.07

Name   ID Balance
```

FIGURE 15-2: Running the code in Listing 15-5.

Feast your eyes on the `displayMe` method in Listing 15-5. What kind of parameter does the `displayMe` method take? Is it a `ColumnOfNumbers`? No. Is it a `Table`? No.

The `displayMe` method doesn't know anything about `ColumnOfNumbers` instances or `Table` instances. All the `displayMe` method knows about is things that implement `Displayable`. That's what the `displayMe` method's parameter list says. When you hand something that implements the `Displayable` interface to the `displayMe` method, the `displayMe` method knows what it can do. The `displayMe` method can call the parameter's `display` method, because that parameter object is guaranteed to have a `display` method.

The same kind of thing is true about the `summarizeMe` method in Listing 15-5. How do you know that you can call `summarizable.summarize()` inside the body of the `summarizeMe` method? You can make this call because `summarizable` has to have a `summarize()` method. The rules about Java interfaces guarantee it.

That's the real power behind Java's interfaces.

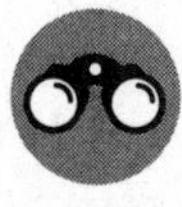

TRY IT OUT

In this section, the `ColumnOfNumbers` and `Table` classes implement the `Displayable` and `Summarizable` interfaces. What about a `Deletable` interface? Any class implementing the `Deletable` interface must have its own `delete` method.

Create the `DeletableColumnOfNumbers` class — a subclass of the `ColumnOfNumbers` class. In addition to all the things `ColumnOfNumbers` does, the `DeletableColumnOfNumbers` class also implements the `Deletable` interface. When you `delete` a column of numbers, you set the values of each of its entries to 0.0.

Create the `DeletableTable` class — a subclass of the `Table` class. In addition to all the things `Table` does, the `DeletableTable` class also implements the `Deletable` interface. When you `delete` a table, you remove all rows except the first (table heading) row. (*Hint:* If you call the `lines` list's `remove` method starting from the `1` row and going to the `lines.size()` row, you won't be happy with the results. A call to the `remove` method modifies the list immediately, and that can mess up your loop.)

TWO KINDS OF METHODS

Inside an interface declaration, any method without a body is called an abstract method. If you run Java 8 or later, you can also put methods with bodies inside an interface declaration. A method with a body is called a *default method*. In an interface's code, each default method declaration starts with the `default` keyword.

```
public interface MyInterface {

    void method1();

    default void method2() {
        System.out.println("Hello!");
    }
}
```

In `MyInterface`, `method1` is an abstract method, and `method2` is a default method. If you create a class that implements `MyInterface`, like so

```
class MyClass implements MyInterface
```

then your newly declared `MyClass` must declare its own `method1` and provide a body for `method1`. Optionally, your `MyClass` may declare its own `method2`. If `MyClass` doesn't declare its own `method2`, then `MyClass` inherits a `method2` body from `MyInterface`.

Abstract Classes

Is there anything you can say that applies to animals of every kind? If you're a biologist, maybe there is. But if you're a programmer, you can say very little. If you don't believe me, consider the wondrous variety of life on the planet Earth:*

» A gelada monkey spends the day on a grassy plateau. But at night the gelada goes for a snooze on the rocky, perilous edge of a mountain cliff. With any luck, the sleeping monkey doesn't toss and turn much.

---

*See `smithsonianmag.com/science-nature/ethiopias-exotic-monkeys-147893502`, `http://news.nationalgeographic.com/news/2004/12/1208_041208_pompeii_worms.html`, `psychologytoday.com/blog/choke/201207/how-humans-learn-lessons-the-sea-squirt`, and `esa.int/Our_Activities/Human_Spaceflight/Research/Tiny_animals_survive_exposure_to_space`.

- A Pompeii worm lives in an underwater tube. The temperature by the worm's head is about 72 degrees Fahrenheit (22 degrees Celsius). But at the other end of the worm, the water temperature is normally 176 degrees Fahrenheit (80 degrees Celsius). If you know one of these worms personally, don't buy any warm socks for it.
- A sea squirt lives part of its life as an animal. At a certain point in its life cycle, the sea squirt attaches itself permanently to a rock and then digests its own brain, effectively turning itself into a plant.
- A tiny water bear can survive 12 days (and maybe more) with no atmosphere in the vacuum of outer space. Even the cosmic radiation in outer space doesn't harm a water bear. That's what I want to be in my next life — a water bear.

With so much biological diversity on our planet, the only thing I can say that applies to every animal is that every animal has a certain weight (measured in pounds or kilograms) and every animal makes (or, possibly, doesn't make) a characteristic sound. Listing 15-6 has the complete scoop.

LISTING 15-6: What a Programmer Knows about Animals

```
public class Animal {
    double weight;
    String sound;

    public Animal(double weight, String sound) {
        this.weight = weight;
        this.sound = sound;
    }
}
```

While I typed the code for the `Animal` class, I had to stop and correct several typing mistakes. The mistakes weren't really my fault. My cat was walking back and forth across my computer keyboard. And that brings me from the subject of all animals to the topic of house pets.

A house pet is an animal. But every house pet has a name — like Fluffy, Blacky, or Princess. And every house pet has a recommended routine for taking care of the pet.

Of course, the care routines differ greatly from one kind of pet to another. If I had a dog, I'd have to walk the dog. But I'd never try to walk a cat. In fact, I don't even let our cat out of the house. So when I define my `HousePet` class, I want to be vague about pet care instructions. And in Java, a class that's somewhat vague is called an *abstract class*. Listing 15-7 has an example.

LISTING 15-7: What It Means to Be a House Pet

```
public abstract class HousePet extends Animal {
    String name;

    public HousePet(String name, double weight, String sound) {
        super(weight, sound);
        this.name = name;
    }

    abstract public void howToCareFor();

    public void about() {
        System.out.print(name + " weighs " + weight + " pounds");
        System.out.print(sound != null ? (" and says '" + sound + "'") : "");
        System.out.println(".");
    }
}
```

On the first line of Listing 15-7, the keyword `abstract` tells Java that `HousePet` is an abstract class. Because `HousePet` is an abstract class, `HousePet` can have an abstract method. And in Listing 15-7, `howToCareFor` is an abstract method. An abstract method has a header but no body. In an abstract method's declaration, there are no curly braces — only a semicolon where curly braces would normally appear.

So, when you try to execute the `howToCareFor` method, what happens? Well, you can't really execute the `howToCareFor` method in Listing 15-7. In fact, you can't even create an instance of the abstract class declared in Listing 15-7. The following code is illegal:

```
// VERY BAD CODE:
HousePet myPet = new HousePet("Boop", 12.0, "Meow");
```

An abstract class has no life of its own. In order to use an abstract class, you have to create an ordinary (non-abstract) class that extends the abstract class. In the ordinary class, all methods have bodies. So everything works out.

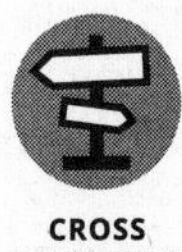
CROSS REFERENCE

Before you walk away from Listing 15-7, notice the `super(weight, sound)` call in that listing. As in Chapter 9, the keyword `super` triggers a call to the superclass's constructor. In Listing 15-7, calling `super(weight, sound)` is like calling the `Animal(double weight, String sound)` constructor from Listing 15-6. The constructor assigns values to the new object's `weight` and `sound` fields.

Caring for your pet

Here's a quotation from the book *Java For Dummies*, 7th Edition:

> "In order to use an abstract class, you have to create an ordinary (non-abstract) class that extends the abstract class."

So, to use the HousePet class in Listing 15-7, you have to create a class that extends the HousePet class. The code in Listing 15-8 extends the abstract HousePet class and provides a body for the method named howToCareFor.

LISTING 15-8: It's a Dog's Life

```
public class Dog extends HousePet {
    int walksPerDay;

    public Dog(String name, double weight, int walksPerDay) {
        super(name, weight, "Woof");
        this.walksPerDay = walksPerDay;
    }

    @Override
    public void howToCareFor() {
        System.out.print("Walk " + name);
        System.out.println(" " + walksPerDay + " times each day.");
    }
}
```

In addition to having a name, a weight, and a sound, every dog gets walked a certain number of times per day. And now, because of the howToCareFor method's body, you know what caring for a dog means: It means walking the dog a certain number of times each day. It's a good thing that the howToCareFor method is abstract in the HousePet class. You wouldn't necessarily want to walk some other kind of pet.

Take, for example, a domestic cat. "Caring" for a cat may mean not bothering it too often. And cats have other characteristics — characteristics that don't apply to dogs. For example, some cats go outdoors; others don't. You can make walksPerDay be 0 for an indoor cat, but that feels like cheating. Instead, each cat can have a boolean value representing the cat's outdoor indoor/outdoor status. Listing 15-9 has the code.

LISTING 15-9: How to Be a Cat

```
public class Cat extends HousePet {
    boolean isOutdoor;

    public Cat(String name, double weight, boolean isOutdoor) {
        super(name, weight, "Meow");
        this.isOutdoor = isOutdoor;
    }

    @Override
    public void howToCareFor() {
        System.out.println(
          isOutdoor ? "Let " : "Do not let " + name + " outdoors.");
    }
}
```

Both the `Dog` and `Cat` classes are subclasses of the `HousePet` class. And, because of the abstract method declaration in Listing 15-7, both the `Dog` and `Cat` classes must have `howToCareFor` methods. But the `howToCareFor` methods in the two classes are quite different. One method refers to a `walksPerDay` field; the other method refers to an `isOutdoor` field. And because the `HousePet` class's `howToCareFor` method is abstract, there's no default behavior. Either the `Dog` and `Cat` classes implement their own `howToCareFor` methods or the `Dog` and `Cat` classes can't claim to extend `HousePet`.

TECHNICAL STUFF

This paragraph describes a picky detail, and you should ignore it if you have any inclination to do so: The `Dog` and `Cat` classes must implement the `howToCareFor` method because the `Dog` and `Cat` classes aren't abstract. If the `Dog` and `Cat` classes were abstract (that is, if they were abstract classes extending the abstract `HousePet` class), then the `Dog` and `Cat` classes would not have to implement the `howToCareFor` method. The `Dog` and `Cat` classes could pass the implementation buck to their own subclasses. For that matter, an abstract class that implements an interface doesn't have to provide bodies for all the interfaces abstract methods. Abstract classes can take advantage of many little loopholes. But in order to use these loopholes, you have to create some exotic programming examples. So, in this chapter I simplify the story and write that (a) a class that extends an abstract class must provide bodies for the abstract class's abstract methods, and (b) a class that implements an interface must provide bodies for the interface's abstract methods. It's not exactly true, but it's good enough for now.

If you live in a very small apartment, you may not have room for a dog or a cat. In that case, Listing 15-10 is for you.

LISTING 15-10: You May Grow Up to Be a Fish

```
public class Fish extends HousePet {

    public Fish(String name, double weight) {
        super(name, weight, null);
    }

    @Override
    public void howToCareFor() {
        System.out.println("Feed " + name + " daily.");

    }
}
```

I could go on and on creating subclasses of the HousePet class. Many years ago, our daughter had some pet mice. Caring for the mice meant keeping the cat away from them.

In Java, subclasses multiply like rabbits.

Using all your classes

Your work isn't finished until you've tested your code. Most programs require hours, days, and even months of testing. But for this chapter's HousePet example, I'll do only one test. The test is in Listing 15-11.

LISTING 15-11: The Class Menagerie

```
public class Main {

    public static void main(String[] args) {
        Dog dog1 = new Dog("Fido", 54.7, 3);

        Dog dog2 = new Dog("Rover", 15.2, 2);

        Cat cat1 = new Cat("Felix", 10.0, false);

        Fish fish1 = new Fish("Bubbles", 0.1);

        dog1.howToCareFor();
        dog2.howToCareFor();
        cat1.howToCareFor();
        fish1.howToCareFor();

        dog1.about();
        dog2.about();
```

```
        cat1.about();
        fish1.about();
    }
}
```

When you run the code in Listing 15-11, you get the output shown in Figure 15-3.

```
Walk Fido 3 times each day.
Walk Rover 2 times each day.
Do not let Felix outdoors.
Feed Bubbles daily.
Fido weighs 54.7 pounds and says 'Woof'.
Rover weighs 15.2 pounds and says 'Woof'.
Felix weighs 10.0 pounds and says 'Meow'.
Bubbles weighs 0.1 pounds.
```

FIGURE 15-3: Please don't pet the Pompeii worm.

Notice how the code in Listing 15-11 seamlessly and effortlessly calls many versions of the howToCareFor method. With the dog1.howToCareFor() and dog2.howToCareFor() calls, Java executes the method in Listing 15-8. With the cat1.howToCareFor() call, Java executes the method in Listing 15-9. And, with the fish1.howToCareFor() call, Java executes the method in Listing 15-10 — it's like having a big if statement without writing the if statement's code. When you add a new class for a pet mouse, you don't have to enlarge an existing if statement. There's no if statement to enlarge.

Notice also how the about method in the abstract HousePet class keeps track of the object that called it. For example, when you call dog1.about() in Listing 15-11, the HousePet class's nonspecific about method knows that the sound dog1 makes is Woof. Everything falls into place very nicely.

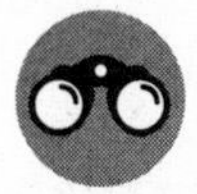

TRY IT OUT

Do you like abstract art? You can use abstract classes to create abstract art!

- Create an abstract class named Shape. The Shape class has a size field (of type int) and an abstract show method. Extend the abstract Shape class with two other classes: a Square class and a Triangle class. In the bodies of the Square and Triangle classes' show methods, place the code that creates a text-based rendering of the shape in question. For example, a Square of size 5 looks like this:

```
--------
|      |
|      |
|      |
--------
```

A `Triangle` of size 2 looks like this:

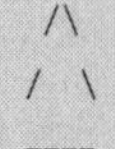

```
 /\
/  \
----
```

- For an extra-special challenge, create an abstract `Shape` class with an abstract `paint` method. The `Shape` class also has `size`, `color`, and `isFilled` fields. The `size` field has type `int`, the `color` field has type `java.awt.Color`, and the `isFilled` field has type `boolean`. Extend the abstract `Shape` class with two other classes: a `Square` class and a `Circle` class. In the bodies of the `Square` and `Circle` classes' `paint` methods, place the code that draws the shape in question on a Java `JFrame`.

Relax! You're Not Seeing Double!

If you've read this chapter's earlier sections on interfaces and abstract methods, your head might be spinning. Both interfaces and abstract classes have abstract methods. But the abstract methods play slightly different roles in these two kinds of reference types. How can you keep it all straight in your mind?

The first thing to do is to remember that no one learns about object-oriented programming concepts without getting lots of practice in writing code. If you've read this chapter and you're confused, that may be a good thing. It means you've understood enough to know how complicated this stuff is. The more code you write, the more comfortable you'll become with classes, interfaces, and all these other ideas.

The next thing to do is to sort out the differences in the way you declare abstract methods. Table 15-1 has the story.

Both interfaces and abstract classes have abstract methods. So you may be wondering how you should choose between declaring an interface and declaring an abstract class. In fact, you might ask three professional programmers how interfaces and abstract classes differ from one another. If you do, you may get five different answers. (Yes, five answers; not three answers.)

Interfaces and abstract classes are similar beasts, and the new features in Java 8 made them even more similar than in previous Java versions. But the basic idea is about the relationships among things.

TABLE 15-1: Using (or Not Using) Abstract Methods

	In an Ordinary (Non-Abstract) Class	In an Interface	In an Abstract Class
Are abstract methods allowed?	No	Yes	Yes
Can a method declaration contain the `abstract` keyword?	No	Yes	Yes
Can a method declaration contain the `default` keyword (meaning "not abstract")?	No	Yes	No
With neither the `abstract` nor the `default` keyword, a method is:	Not abstract	Abstract	Not abstract

- **Extending a subclass represents an *is a* relationship.**

  Think about the relationships in this chapter's earlier section "Abstract Classes." A house pet is an animal. A dog is a house pet. A cat is a house pet. A fish is a house pet.

- **Implementing an interface represents a *can do* relationship.**

  Think about the relationships in this chapter's earlier section "The Java Interface." The first line in Listing 15-3 says `implements Displayable`. With these words, the code promises that each `ColumnOfNumbers` object can be displayed. Later in same listing, you make good on the promise by declaring a `display` method.

  Think about the relationships in this chapter's earlier section "The Java Interface." A column of numbers isn't always a summarizable thing. But in Listing 15-3, you promise that the `ColumnOfNumbers` objects will be summarizable, and you make good on the promise by declaring a `summarize` method.

If you want more tangible evidence of the difference between an interface and an abstract class, consider this: A class can implement many interfaces, but a class can extend only one other class, even if that one class is an abstract class. So, after you've declared

```
public class Dog extends HousePet
```

you can't also make `Dog` extend a `Friend` class. But you can make `Dog` implement a `Befriendable` interface. And then you can make the same `Dog` class implement a `Trainable` interface. (By the way, I've tried making my `Cat` class implement a `Trainable` interface but, for some reason, it never works.)

And, if you want an even *more* tangible difference between an interface and an abstract class, I have one for you: An interface can't contain any non-static, non-final fields. For example, if the `HousePet` class in Listing 15-7 were an interface, it couldn't have a `name` field. That simply wouldn't be allowed.

So there. Interfaces and abstract classes are different from one another. But if you're new at the game, you shouldn't worry about the difference. Just read as much code as you can, and don't get scared when you see an abstract method. That's all there is to it.

» Responding when the user presses a key or selects a drop down box item

» Putting classes inside of other classes

Chapter 16
Responding to Keystrokes and Mouse Clicks

In the late 1980s, I bought my first mouse. I paid $100 and, because I didn't really need a mouse, I checked with my wife before buying it. (At the time, my computer ran a hybrid text/windowed environment. Anything that I could do with a mouse, I could just as easily do with the Alt key.)

Now it's the 21st century. The last ten mice that I got were free. Ordinary ones just fall into my lap somehow. A few exotic mice were on sale at the local computer superstore. One cost $10 and came with a $10 rebate.

As I write this chapter, I'm using the most recent addition to my collection: an official *For Dummies* mouse. This yellow-and-white beauty has a little compartment filled with water. Instead of a snowy Atlantic City scene, the water surrounds a tiny Dummies Man charm. It's so cute. It was a present from the folks at Wiley Publishing.

Go On . . . Click That Button

In previous chapters, I create windows that don't do much. A typical window displays some information but doesn't have any interactive elements. Well, the time has come to change all that. This chapter's first example is a window with a button on it. When the user clicks the button, darn it, something happens. The code is shown in Listing 16-1, and the `main` method that calls the code in Listing 16-1 is in Listing 16-2.

LISTING 16-1: A Guessing Game

```
import java.awt.FlowLayout;
import java.awt.event.ActionEvent;
import java.awt.event.ActionListener;
import java.util.Random;

import javax.swing.JButton;
import javax.swing.JFrame;
import javax.swing.JLabel;
import javax.swing.JTextField;

class GameFrame extends JFrame implements ActionListener {
   private static final long serialVersionUID = 1L;

   int randomNumber = new Random().nextInt(10) + 1;
   int numGuesses = 0;

   JTextField textField = new JTextField(5);
   JButton button = new JButton("Guess");
   JLabel label = new JLabel(numGuesses + " guesses");

   public GameFrame() {
      setDefaultCloseOperation(JFrame.EXIT_ON_CLOSE);
      setLayout(new FlowLayout());
      add(textField);
      add(button);
      add(label);
      button.addActionListener(this);
      pack();
      setVisible(true);
   }

   @Override
   public void actionPerformed(ActionEvent e) {
      String textFieldText = textField.getText();
```

```
      if (Integer.parseInt(textFieldText)==randomNumber) {
         button.setEnabled(false);
         textField.setText(textField.getText() + " Yes!");
         textField.setEnabled(false);
      } else {
         textField.setText("");
         textField.requestFocus();
      }

      numGuesses++;
      String guessWord = (numGuesses == 1) ? " guess" : " guesses";
      label.setText(numGuesses + guessWord);
   }
}
```

LISTING 16-2: Starting the Guessing Game

```
public class ShowGameFrame {

   public static void main(String args[]) {
      new GameFrame();
   }
}
```

Some snapshots from a run of this section's code are shown in Figures 16-1 and 16-2. In a window, the user plays a guessing game. Behind the scenes, the program chooses a secret number (a number from 1 to 10). Then the program displays a text field and a button. The user types a number in the text field and clicks the button. One of two things happens next:

- **If the number that the user types isn't the same as the secret number,** the computer posts the number of guesses made so far. The user gets to make another guess.
- **If the number that the user types is the same as the secret number,** the text field displays Yes!. Meanwhile, the game is over, so both the text field and the button become disabled. Both components have that gray, washed-out look, and neither component responds to keystrokes or mouse clicks.

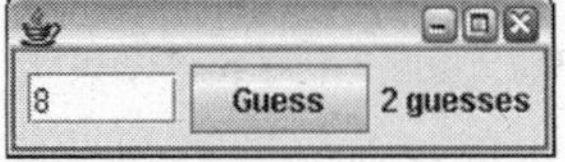

FIGURE 16-1: An incorrect guess.

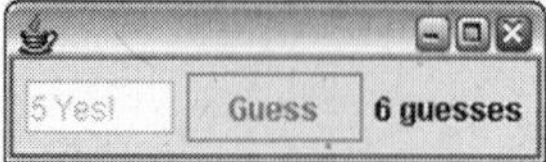

FIGURE 16-2: The correct guess.

In Listing 16-1, the code to create the frame, the button, and the text field isn't earth-shattering. I did similar things in Chapters 9 and 10. The `JTextField` class is new in this chapter, but a text field isn't much different from a button or a label. Like so many other components, the `JTextField` class is defined in the `javax.swing` package. When you create a new `JTextField` instance, you can specify a number of columns. In Listing 16-1, I create a text field that's five columns wide.

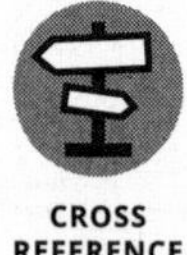

CROSS REFERENCE

Listing 16-1 uses a fancy operator to decide between the singular *guess* and the plural *guesses*. If you're not familiar with this use of the question mark and colon, see Chapter 11.

Events and event handling

The big news in Listing 16-1, shown in the preceding section, is the handling of the user's button click. When you're working in a graphical user interface (GUI), anything the user does (like pressing a key, moving the mouse, clicking the mouse, or whatever) is called an *event*. The code that responds to the user's press, movement, or click is called *event-handling code*.

Listing 16-1 deals with the button-click event with three parts of its code:

- The top of the `GameFrame` class declaration says that this class implements `ActionListener`.

  By announcing that it will implement the `ActionListener` interface, the code in Listing 16-1 agrees that it will give meaning to the interface's abstract `actionPerformed` method. In this situation, *giving meaning* means declaring an `actionPerformed` method with curly braces, a body, and maybe some statements to execute.

- Sure enough, the code for the `GameFrame` class has an `actionPerformed` method, and that `actionPerformed` method has a body.
- Finally, the constructor for the `GameFrame` class adds `this` to the button's list of action listeners.

  Java will call *this* code's `actionPerformed` method when the user clicks the button. Hooray!

Taken together, all three of these tricks make the `GameFrame` class handle button clicks.

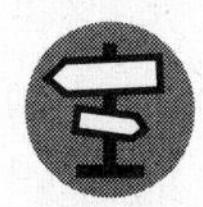

CROSS REFERENCE

For the full story about Java interfaces, refer to Chapter 15.

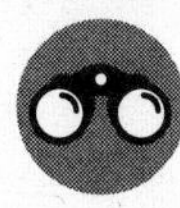

TRY IT OUT

You can learn a lot about the code in Listing 16-1 by removing certain statements and observing the results. For each suggested removal, see whether your IDE displays any error messages. If not, try to run the program. After observing the results, put the element back and try the next suggested removal:

- Remove the entire `actionPerformed` method declaration — header and all.
- Remove the call to `setVisible(true)`.
- Remove the call to `pack()`.
- Remove the call to `button.addActionListener()`.

Threads of execution

Here's a well-kept secret: Java programs are *multithreaded,* which means that several things are going on at once whenever you run a Java program. Sure, the computer is executing the code that you've written, but it's executing other code as well (code that you didn't write and don't see). All this code is being executed at the same time. While the computer executes your `main` method's statements, one after another, the computer takes time out, sneaks away briefly, and executes statements from other, unseen methods. For most simple Java programs, these other methods are ones that are defined as part of the Java Virtual Machine (JVM).

For instance, Java has an event-handling thread. While your code runs, the event-handling thread's code runs in the background. The event-handling thread's code listens for mouse clicks and takes appropriate action whenever a user clicks the mouse. Figure 16-3 illustrates how this works.

Your code's thread	The event handling thread
`setLayout(new FlowLayout());`	Did the user click the mouse?
`add(textField);`	.
`add(button);`	.
`add(label);`	Did the user click the mouse?
	.
`button.addActionListener(this);`	.
`pack();`	Did the user click the mouse?
`setVisible(true);`	Yes? Okay, then. I'll call the `actionPerformed` method.

FIGURE 16-3: Two Java threads.

When the user clicks the button, the event-handling thread says, "Okay, the button was clicked. What should I do about that?" And the answer is, "Call some actionPerformed methods." It's as if the event-handling thread has code that looks like this:

```
if (buttonJustGotClicked()) {
    object1.actionPerformed(infoAboutTheClick);
    object2.actionPerformed(infoAboutTheClick);
    object3.actionPerformed(infoAboutTheClick);
}
```

Of course, behind every answer is yet another question. In this situation, the follow-up question is, "Where does the event-handling thread find actionPerformed methods to call?" And there's another question: "What if you don't want the event-handling thread to call certain actionPerformed methods that are lurking in your code?"

Well, that's why you call the addActionListener method. In Listing 16-1, the call

```
button.addActionListener(this);
```

tells the event-handling thread, "Put this code's actionPerformed method on your list of methods to be called. Call this code's actionPerformed method whenever the button is clicked."

So that's how it works. To have the computer call an actionPerformed method, you register the method with Java's event-handling thread. You do this registration by calling addActionListener. The addActionListener method belongs to the object whose clicks (and other events) you're waiting for. In Listing 16-1, you're waiting for the button object to be clicked, and the addActionListener method belongs to that button object.

The keyword this

In Chapters 9 and 10, the keyword this gives you access to instance variables from the code inside a method. What does the this keyword really mean? Well, compare it with the English phrase *state your name:*

> *I, (state your name), do solemnly swear, to uphold the constitution of the Philadelphia Central High School Photography Society. . . .*

The phrase *state your name* is a placeholder. It's a space in which each person puts his or her own name:

> *I, Bob, do solemnly swear . . .*
>
> *I, Fred, do solemnly swear . . .*

Think of the pledge ("I . . . do solemnly swear . . .") as a piece of code in a Java class. In that piece of code is the placeholder phrase *state your name.* Whenever an instance of the class (a person) executes the code (that is, takes the pledge), the instance fills in its own name in place of the phrase *state your name.*

The `this` keyword works the same way. It sits inside the code that defines the `GameFrame` class. Whenever an instance of `GameFrame` is constructed, the instance calls `addActionListener(this)`. In that call, the `this` keyword stands for the instance itself.

```
button.addActionListener(thisGameFrameInstance);
```

By calling `button.addActionListener(this)`, the `GameFrame` instance is saying, "Add my `actionPerformed` method to the list of methods that are called whenever the button is clicked." And indeed, the `GameFrame` instance has an `actionPerformed` method. The `GameFrame` has to have an `actionPerformed` method because the `GameFrame` class implements the `ActionListener` interface. It's funny how that all fits together.

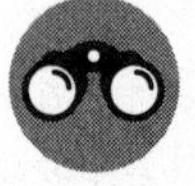

TRY IT OUT

In your own words, describe the uses of the keyword `this` in the following code:

```
public class Main {

  public static void main(String[] args) {
    new IntegerHolder(42).displayMyN();
    new IntegerHolder(7).displayMyN();
  }
}

class IntegerHolder {
  private int n;

  IntegerHolder(int n) {
    this.n = n;
  }

  void displayMyN() {
    Displayer.display(this);
  }
```

```
  public int getN() {
    return n;
  }
}

class Displayer {

  public static void display(IntegerHolder holder) {
    System.out.println(holder.getN());
  }
}
```

Inside the actionPerformed method

The `actionPerformed` method in Listing 16-1 uses a bunch of tricks from the Java API. Here's a brief list of those tricks:

- Every instance of `JTextField` (and of `JLabel`) has its own getter and setter methods, including `getText` and `setText`. Calling `getText` fetches whatever string of characters is in the component. Calling `setText` changes the characters that are in the component. In Listing 16-1, judicious use of `getText` and `setText` pulls a number out of the text field and replaces the number with either nothing (the empty string `""`) or the number, followed by the word *Yes!*
- Every component in the `javax.swing` package (`JTextField`, `JButton`, or whatever) has a `setEnabled` method. When you call `setEnabled(false)`, the component gets that limp, gray, washed-out look and can no longer receive button clicks or keystrokes.
- Every component in the `javax.swing` package has a `requestFocus` method. When you call `requestFocus`, the component gets the privilege of receiving the user's next input. For example, in Listing 16-1, the call `textField.requestFocus()` says, "Even though the user may have just clicked the button, put a cursor in the text field. That way, the user can type another guess in the text field without clicking the text field first."

TIP

You can perform a test to make sure that the object referred to by the button variable is really the thing that was clicked. Just write `if (e.getSource() == button)`. If your code has two buttons, `button1` and `button2`, you can test to find out which button was clicked. You can write `if (e.getSource() == button1)` and `if (e.getSource() == button2)`.

The serialVersionUID

Chapter 9 introduces the `SuppressWarnings` annotation to avoid dealing with something called a `serialVersionUID`. A `serialVersionUID` is a number that helps Java avoid version conflicts when you send an object from one place to another. For example, you can send the state of your `JFrame` object to another computer's screen. Then the other computer can check the frame's version number to make sure that no funny business is taking place.

In Chapter 9, I side-step the `serialVersionUID` issue by telling Java to ignore any warnings about missing serial version numbers. But in Listing 16-1, I take a bolder approach. I give my `JFrame` object a real `serialVersionUID`. This is my first version of `GameFrame`, so I give this `GameFrame` the version number 1. (Actually, I give this `GameFrame` the number `1L`, meaning the `long` value 1. See Chapter 4.)

So, when would you bother to change a class's `serialVersionUID` number? If version number 1 is nice, is version number 2 even better? The answer is complicated, but the bottom line is, don't change the `serialVersionUID` number unless you make incompatible changes to the class's code. By "incompatible changes," I mean changes that make it impossible for the receiving computer's existing code to handle your newly created objects.

CROSS REFERENCE

For more details about the `serialVersionUID` and what constitutes an incompatible code change, check out this site:

```
http://docs.oracle.com/javase/8/docs/platform/serialization/spec/version.
  html
```

Every major Java IDE has visual tools to help you design a GUI interface.

- **Eclipse has WindowBuilder:** `www.eclipse.org/windowbuilder`
- **IntelliJ IDEA has GUI Designer:** `www.jetbrains.com/help/idea/2016.3/gui-designer-basics.html`
- **NetBeans has GUI Builder:** `http://netbeans.org/kb/docs/java/quickstart-gui.html`

With any of these tools, you drag components from a palette onto a frame. (The components include buttons, text fields, and other goodies.) Using the mouse, you can move and resize each component. As you design the frame visually, the tools creates the frame's code automatically. Each component on the frame has a little spreadsheet showing the component's properties. For example, you can change the text on a button's face by changing the *text* entry in the button's spreadsheet. When you right-click or control-click the picture of a component, you get the option of jumping to the component's `actionPerformed` method. In the actionPerformed method, you add Java code, such as button.setText("You clicked me!"). Tools like WindowBuilder, GUI Designer, and GUI Builder make the design of GUI interfaces quicker, more natural, and more intuitive.

This chapter describes features of Java's Swing framework. Since 1998, Swing has been Java's primary framework for developing GUI applications. But late in 2011, Oracle added a newer framework — JavaFX — to Java's core. JavaFX provides a richer set of components than Swing. But for simple applications, JavaFX is more difficult to use. If you're interested in reading more about JavaFX, visit Oracle's Getting Started with JavaFX page. It's at http://docs.oracle.com/javafx/2/get_started/jfxpub-get_started.htm.

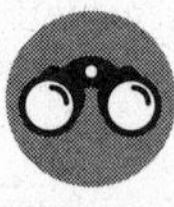

Using the techniques shown in this chapter, create a program that displays a frame containing three components: a text field (JTextField), a button (JButton), and a label (JLabel). The user types text into the text field. Then, when the user clicks the button, the program copies any text that's in the text field onto the label.

Responding to Things Other Than Button Clicks

When you know how to respond to one kind of event, responding to other kinds of events is easy. Listings 16-3 and 16-4 display a window that converts between US and UK currencies. The code in these listings responds to many kinds of events. Figures 16-4, 16-5, and 16-6 show some pictures of the code in action.

LISTING 16-3: Displaying the Local Currency

```
import java.awt.Color;
import java.awt.FlowLayout;
import java.awt.event.ItemEvent;
import java.awt.event.ItemListener;
import java.awt.event.KeyEvent;
import java.awt.event.KeyListener;
import java.awt.event.MouseEvent;
import java.awt.event.MouseListener;
import java.text.NumberFormat;
import java.util.Locale;

import javax.swing.JComboBox;
import javax.swing.JFrame;
import javax.swing.JLabel;
import javax.swing.JTextField;
```

```
class MoneyFrame extends JFrame implements
                                KeyListener, ItemListener, MouseListener {
    private static final long serialVersionUID = 1L;

    JLabel fromCurrencyLabel = new JLabel(" ");
    JTextField textField = new JTextField(5);
    JLabel label = new JLabel("           ");
    JComboBox<String> combo = new JComboBox<>();
    NumberFormat currencyUS = NumberFormat.getCurrencyInstance();
    NumberFormat currencyUK = NumberFormat.getCurrencyInstance(Locale.UK);

    public MoneyFrame() {
        setLayout(new FlowLayout());

        add(fromCurrencyLabel);
        add(textField);
        combo.addItem("US to UK");
        combo.addItem("UK to US");
        add(label);
        add(combo);

        textField.addKeyListener(this);
        combo.addItemListener(this);
        label.addMouseListener(this);
        setDefaultCloseOperation(JFrame.EXIT_ON_CLOSE);

        setSize(300, 100);
        setVisible(true);
    }

    void setTextOnLabel() {
        String amountString = "";
        String fromCurrency = "";

        try {
            double amount = Double.parseDouble(textField.getText());

            if(combo.getSelectedItem().equals("US to UK")) {
                amountString = " = " + currencyUK.format(amount * 0.61214);
                fromCurrency = "$";
            }

            if(combo.getSelectedItem().equals("UK to US")) {
                amountString = " = " + currencyUS.format(amount * 1.63361);
                fromCurrency = "\u00A3";
            }
```

(continued)

LISTING 16-3: *(continued)*

```
        } catch (NumberFormatException e) {
        }

        label.setText(amountString);
        fromCurrencyLabel.setText(fromCurrency);
    }

    @Override
    public void keyReleased(KeyEvent k) {
        setTextOnLabel();
    }

    @Override
    public void keyPressed(KeyEvent k) {
    }

    @Override
    public void keyTyped(KeyEvent k) {
    }

    @Override
    public void itemStateChanged(ItemEvent i) {
        setTextOnLabel();
    }

    @Override
    public void mouseEntered(MouseEvent m) {
        label.setForeground(Color.red);
    }

    @Override
    public void mouseExited(MouseEvent m) {
        label.setForeground(Color.black);
    }

    @Override
    public void mouseClicked(MouseEvent m) {
    }

    @Override
    public void mousePressed(MouseEvent m) {
    }

    @Override
    public void mouseReleased(MouseEvent m) {
    }
}
```

LISTING 16-4: Calling the Code in Listing 16-3

```
public class ShowMoneyFrame {

    public static void main(String args[]) {
        new MoneyFrame();
    }
}
```

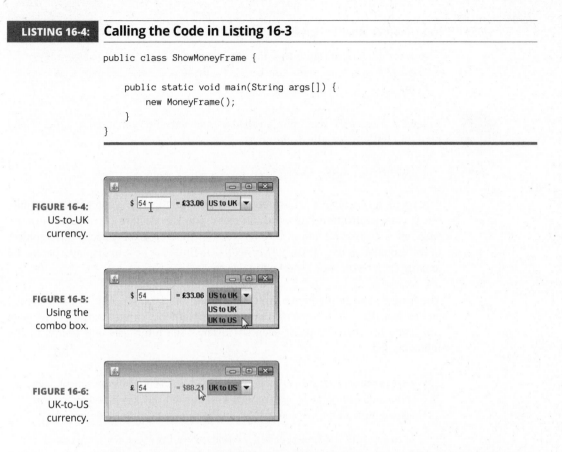

FIGURE 16-4: US-to-UK currency.

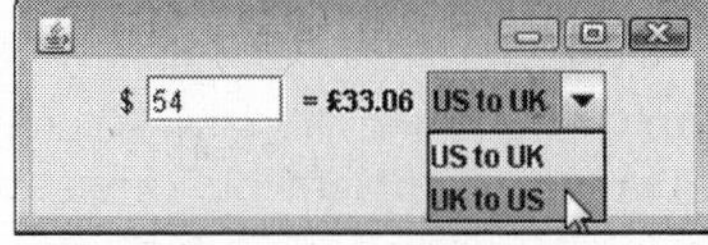

FIGURE 16-5: Using the combo box.

FIGURE 16-6: UK-to-US currency.

Okay, so Listing 16-3 is a little long. Even so, the outline of the code in Listing 16-3 isn't too bad. Here's what the outline looks like:

```
class MoneyFrame extends JFrame implements
                                KeyListener, ItemListener, MouseListener {
    Variable declarations
    Constructor for the MoneyFrame class
    Declaration of a method named setTextOnLabel
    Methods that are required because the class implements three interfaces
}
```

The constructor in Listing 16-3 adds the following four components to the new `MoneyFrame` window:

- **A label:** In Figure 16-4, the label displays a dollar sign.
- **A text field:** In Figure 16-4, the user types **54** in the text field.

» **Another label:** In Figure 16-4, the label displays £33.06.

» **A combo box:** In Figure 16-4, the combo box displays *US to UK*. In Figure 16-5, the user selects an item in the box. In Figure 16-6, the selected item is *UK to US*.

TECHNICAL STUFF

In Java, a JComboBox (commonly called a *drop-down list*) can display items of any kind. In Listing 16-3, the declaration

```
JComboBox<String> combo = new JComboBox<>();
```

constructs a JComboBox whose entries have type String. That seems sensible, but if your application has a Person class, you can declare JComboBox<Person> peopleBox. In that situation, Java has to know how to display each Person object in the drop-down list. (It isn't a big deal. Java finds out how to display a person by looking for a toString() method inside the Person class.)

The MoneyFrame implements three interfaces: the KeyListener, ItemListener, and MouseListener interfaces. Because it implements three interfaces, the code can listen for three kinds of events. I discuss the interfaces and events in the following list:

» **KeyListener:** A class that implements the KeyListener interface must have three methods named keyReleased, keyPressed, and keyTyped. When you lift your finger off a key, the event-handling thread calls keyReleased.

In Listing 16-3, the keyReleased method calls setTextOnLabel. My setTextOnLabel method checks to see what's currently selected in the combo box. If the user selects the US-to-UK option, the setTextOnLabel method converts dollars to pounds. If the user selects the UK-to-US option, the setTextOnLabel method converts pounds to dollars.

TECHNICAL STUFF

In the setTextOnLabel method, I use the string "\u00A3". The funny-looking \u00A3 code is Java's UK pound sign. (The u in \u00A3 stands for *Unicode* — an international standard for representing characters in the world's alphabets.) If my operating system's settings defaulted to UK currency, in the runs of Java programs the pound sign would appear on its own. For information about all of this, check out the Locale class in 's API documentation (https://docs.oracle.com/javase/8/docs/api/java/util/Locale.html).

By the way, if you're thinking in terms of real currency conversion, forget about it. This program uses rates that may or may not have been accurate at one time. Sure, a program can reach out on the Internet for the most up-to-date currency rates, but at the moment, you have other Javafish to fry.

- **ItemListener:** A class that implements the ItemListener interface must have an itemStateChanged method. When you select an item in a combo box, the event-handling thread calls itemStateChanged.

  In Listing 16-3, when the user selects US-to-UK or UK-to-US in the combo box, the event-handling thread calls the itemStateChanged method. In turn, the itemStateChanged method calls setTextOnLabel, and so on.

- **MouseListener:** A class that implements the MouseListener interface must have mouseEntered, mouseExited, mouseClicked, mousePressed, and mouseReleased methods. Implementing MouseListener is different from implementing ActionListener. When you implement ActionListener, as in Listing 16-1, the event-handling thread responds only to mouse clicks. But with MouseListener, the thread responds to the user pressing the mouse, releasing the mouse, and more.

  In Listing 16-3, the mouseEntered and mouseExited methods are called whenever you move over or away from the label. How do you know that the label is involved? Just look at the code in the MoneyFrame constructor. The label variable's addMouseListener method is the one that's called.

  Look at the mouseEntered and mouseExited methods in Listing 16-3. When mouseEntered or mouseExited is called, the computer forges ahead and calls setForeground. This setForeground method changes the color of the label's text.

  Isn't modern life wonderful? The Java API even has a Color class with names like Color.red and Color.black.

Listing 16-3 has several methods that aren't really used. For instance, when you implement MouseListener, your code has to have its own mouseReleased method. You need the mouseReleased method not because you're going to do anything special when the user releases the mouse button, but because you made a promise to the Java compiler and have to keep that promise.

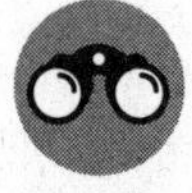

TRY IT OUT

In a previous section, you create a program that copies text from a text field to a label whenever the user clicks a button. Modify the program so that the user doesn't have to click a button. The program automatically updates the label's text whenever the user modifies the text field's content.

Creating Inner Classes

Here's big news! You can define a class inside of another class! For the user, Listing 16-5 behaves the same way as Listing 16-1. But in Listing 16-5, the GameFrame class contains a class named MyActionListener.

LISTING 16-5: A Class within a Class

```
import java.awt.FlowLayout;
import java.awt.event.ActionEvent;
import java.awt.event.ActionListener;
import java.util.Random;

import javax.swing.JButton;
import javax.swing.JFrame;
import javax.swing.JLabel;
import javax.swing.JTextField;

class GameFrame extends JFrame {
   private static final long serialVersionUID = 1L;

   int randomNumber = new Random().nextInt(10) + 1;
   int numGuesses = 0;

   JTextField textField = new JTextField(5);
   JButton button = new JButton("Guess");
   JLabel label = new JLabel(numGuesses + " guesses");

   public GameFrame() {
      setDefaultCloseOperation(JFrame.EXIT_ON_CLOSE);
      setLayout(new FlowLayout());
      add(textField);
      add(button);
      add(label);
      button.addActionListener(new MyActionListener());
      pack();
      setVisible(true);
   }

   class MyActionListener implements ActionListener {

      @Override
      public void actionPerformed(ActionEvent e) {
         String textFieldText = textField.getText();

         if (Integer.parseInt(textFieldText) == randomNumber) {
            button.setEnabled(false);
            textField.setText(textField.getText() + " Yes!");
            textField.setEnabled(false);
         } else {
            textField.setText("");
            textField.requestFocus();
         }
```

```
            numGuesses++;
            String guessWord = (numGuesses == 1) ? " guess" : " guesses";
            label.setText(numGuesses + guessWord);
        }
    }
}
```

The `MyActionListener` class in Listing 16-5 is an *inner class*. An inner class is a lot like any other class. But within an inner class's code, you can refer to the enclosing class's fields. For example, several statements inside `MyActionListener` use the name `textField`, and `textField` is defined in the enclosing `GameFrame` class.

Notice that the code in Listing 16-5 uses the `MyActionListener` class only once. (The only use is in a call to `button.addActionListener`.) So I ask, do you really need a name for something that's used only once? No, you don't. You can substitute the entire definition of the inner class inside the call to `button.addActionListener`. When you do this, you have an *anonymous inner class*. Listing 16-6 shows you how it works.

LISTING 16-6: **A Class with No Name (Inside a Class with a Name)**

```
import java.awt.FlowLayout;
import java.awt.event.ActionEvent;
import java.awt.event.ActionListener;
import java.util.Random;

import javax.swing.JButton;
import javax.swing.JFrame;
import javax.swing.JLabel;
import javax.swing.JTextField;

class GameFrame extends JFrame {
    private static final long serialVersionUID = 1L;

    int randomNumber = new Random().nextInt(10) + 1;
    int numGuesses = 0;

    JTextField textField = new JTextField(5);
    JButton button = new JButton("Guess");
    JLabel label = new JLabel(numGuesses + " guesses");

    public GameFrame() {
        setDefaultCloseOperation(JFrame.EXIT_ON_CLOSE);
        setLayout(new FlowLayout());
```

(continued)

LISTING 16-6: *(continued)*

```
        add(textField);
        add(button);
        add(label);

        button.addActionListener(new ActionListener() {

            @Override
            public void actionPerformed(ActionEvent e) {
                String textFieldText = textField.getText();

                if (Integer.parseInt(textFieldText) == randomNumber) {
                    button.setEnabled(false);
                    textField.setText(textField.getText() + " Yes!");
                    textField.setEnabled(false);
                } else {
                    textField.setText("");
                    textField.requestFocus();
                }

                numGuesses++;
                String guessWord = (numGuesses == 1) ? " guess" : " guesses";
                label.setText(numGuesses + guessWord);
            }
        });
        pack();
        setVisible(true);
    }
}
```

Inner classes are good for things like event handlers, such as the `actionPerformed` method in this chapter's examples. The most difficult thing about an *anonymous* inner class is keeping track of the parentheses, the curly braces, and the indentation. My humble advice is, start by writing code without any inner classes, as in the code from Listing 16-1. Later, when you become bored with ordinary Java classes, experiment by changing some of your ordinary classes into inner classes.

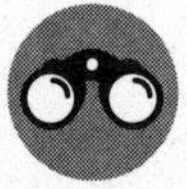

TRY IT OUT

In a previous section, you create a program that copies text from a text field to a label whenever the user clicks a button. Modify the code so that it has an inner class. Then if you're really ambitious, modify the code so that it has an anonymous inner class.

» **Inserting values into a database**

» **Making queries to a database**

Chapter 17
Using Java Database Connectivity

Whenever I teach Java to professional programmers, I always hear the same old thing: "We don't need to make attractive-looking layouts. No glitzy GUIs for us. We need to access databases. Yup, just [shut up and] show us how to write Java programs that talk to databases."

So here it is, folks — the real deal!

The *Java Database Connectivity** (JDBC) classes provide common access to most database management systems. Just get a driver for your favorite vendor's system, customize one line of code in each of this chapter's examples, and you're ready to go.

*Apparently, there's no evidence in any of Oracle's literature that the acronym *JDBC* actually stands for *Java Database Connectivity.* But that's okay. If *Java Database Connectivity* isn't the correct terminology, it's close enough. In the Java world, *JDBC* certainly doesn't stand for *John Digests Bleu Cheese.*

Creating a Database and a Table

The crux of JDBC is contained in two packages: `java.sql` and `javax.sql`, which are both in the Java API. This chapter's examples use the classes in `java.sql`. The first example is shown in Listing 17-1.

LISTING 17-1: Creating a Database and a Table

```
import java.sql.Connection;
import java.sql.DriverManager;
import java.sql.SQLException;
import java.sql.Statement;

public class CreateTable {

  public static void main(String args[]) {

    final String CONNECTION = "jdbc:derby:AccountDatabase;create=true";

    try (Connection conn = DriverManager.getConnection(CONNECTION);
         Statement statement = conn.createStatement()) {

      statement.executeUpdate("create table ACCOUNTS                   " +
                              "  (NAME VARCHAR(32) NOT NULL PRIMARY KEY, " +
                              "   ADDRESS VARCHAR(32),                 " +
                              "   BALANCE FLOAT                       )");
      System.out.println("ACCOUNTS table created.");

    } catch (SQLException e) {
      e.printStackTrace();
    }
  }
}
```

Running the examples in this chapter is a bit trickier than running other chapters' examples. To talk to a database, you need an intermediary piece of software known as a *database driver*. Database drivers come in all shapes and sizes, and many of them are quite expensive. But Listing 17-1 points to a small, freebie driver: the Derby JDBC driver. The code for the Derby JDBC driver is kept in the `EmbeddedDriver` class (which is a Java class). This class lives inside the `org.apache.derby.jdbc` package.

When you install Java 9, you don't get this `org.apache.derby.jdbc` package. You need a separate file named `derby.jar`, which you can download from `http://db.apache.org/derby/derby_downloads.html`.

Even after you've downloaded a copy of `derby.jar`, your IDE might not know where you've put the file on your computer's hard drive. It's usually not enough to put `derby.jar` in a well-known directory. Instead, you have to tell Eclipse, IntelliJ IDEA, or NetBeans exactly where to find your `derby.jar` file. Here's what you do:

- **Eclipse:** Select Project ⇨ Properties. In the resulting dialog box, select Java Build Path, and then select the Libraries tab. Click the Add External JARs button, and then navigate to the `derby.jar` file on your computer's hard drive.
- **IntelliJ IDEA:** Select File ⇨ Project Structure. In the resulting dialog box, select Libraries. Click the plus sign (+) icon and, in the resulting drop-down box, select Java. Navigate to the `derby.jar` file on your computer's hard drive.
- **NetBeans:** Select File ⇨ Project Properties. In the resulting dialog box, select Libraries and then select the Run tab. Click the Add JAR/Folder button, and navigate to the `derby.jar` file on your computer's hard drive.

What happens when you run the code

During a successful run of the code in Listing 17-1, you see an `ACCOUNTS table created` message. That's about it. The code has no other visible output because most of the output goes to a database.

If you poke around a bit, you can find direct evidence of the new database's existence. Using your computer's File Explorer or Finder, you can navigate to the project folder containing the code in Listing 17-1. (If you've downloaded the code from this book's website, look in your IDE's *17-01* project folder.) Inside that folder, you'll see a brand-new *AccountDatabase* subfolder. That's where the newly created database lives.

Unfortunately, you can't see what's inside the database unless you run a couple more programs. Read on!

Using SQL commands

In Listing 17-1, the heart of the code lies in the call to `executeUpdate`. The `executeUpdate` call contains a string — a normal, Java, double-quoted string of characters. To keep the code readable, I've chopped the string into four parts, and separate the parts with plus signs (Java's string concatenation operator).

WHOSE DATABASE IS IT ANYWAY?

Databases come in many shapes and sizes from many different vendors. In 2017, the top database vendors include Oracle, Microsoft, IBM, and SAP. Some popular open-source databases include PostgreSQL and Oracle's MySQL. The code in Listing 17-1 (and this chapter's other listings) uses an open-source database from The Apache Software Foundation known as Apache Derby.

If you don't want to use Apache Derby, you have to replace the `CONNECTION` string in this chapter's examples. What other string you use depends on the kind of database software you have, and on other factors. Check your database vendor's documentation.

By the way, database drivers are like people: some are quite old and others aren't so old. As of January 2017, the latest version of JDBC is version 4.2. A "quite old" JDBC database driver is one that was created for a version of JDBC before Version 4.0 (circa December 2006). If your database driver doesn't meet the JDBC 4.0 standards, you have to add a few extra statements to each of this chapter's examples, as follows:

```
final public String DRIVER = "com.databasevendorname.databasebrandname.maybe
   otherstuff";
try {
  Class.forName(DRIVER).newInstance();
} catch (InstantiationException |
        IllegalAccessException |
        ClassNotFoundException e) {
  e.printStackTrace();
}
```

Again, check your database vendor's documentation.

If you're familiar with Structured Query Language, or SQL, the command strings in the calls to `executeUpdate` make sense to you. If not, pick up a copy of *SQL For Dummies*, 8th Edition, by Allen G. Taylor (Wiley). One way or another, don't go fishing around this chapter for an explanation of the `create table` command. You won't find an explanation, because the big `create table` string in Listing 17-1 isn't part of Java. This command is just a string of characters that you feed to Java's `executeUpdate` method. This string, which is written in SQL, creates a new database table with three columns (columns for a customer's `NAME`, the customer's `ADDRESS`, and the account's `BALANCE`). When you write a Java database program, that's what you do. You write ordinary SQL commands and surround those commands with calls to Java methods.

Connecting and disconnecting

Aside from the call to the executeUpdate method, the code in Listing 17-1 is copy-and-paste stuff. Here's a rundown on what each part of the code means:

- **DriverManager.getConnection:** Establish a session with a particular database.

  The getConnection method lives in a Java class named DriverManager. In Listing 17-1, the call to getConnection creates an AccountDatabase and opens a connection to that database. Of course, you may already have an AccountDatabase before you start running the code in Listing 17-1. If you do, the text ;create=true in the CONNECTION string has no effect.

  In the CONNECTION string, notice the colons. The code doesn't simply name the AccountDatabase — it tells the DriverManager class what protocols to use to connect with the database. The code jdbc:derby: — which is a lot like the http: in a web address — tells the computer to use the jdbc protocol to talk to the derby protocol, which in turn talks directly to your AccountDatabase.

- **conn.createStatement:** Make a statement.

  It seems strange, but in Java Database Connectivity, you create a single statement object. After you've created a statement object, you can use that object many times, with many different SQL strings, to issue many different commands to the database. So, before you start calling the statement.executeUpdate method, you have to create an actual statement object. The call to conn.createStatement creates that statement object for you.

- **try-with-resources:** Release resources, come what may!

  As Ritter always says, you're not being considerate of others if you don't clean up your own messes. Every connection and every database statement lock up some system resources. When you're finished using these resources, you release them.

  In Listing 17-1, Java's try-with-resources block automatically closes and releases your resources at the end of the block's execution. In addition, try-with-resources takes care of all the messy details associated with failed attempts to catch exceptions gracefully.

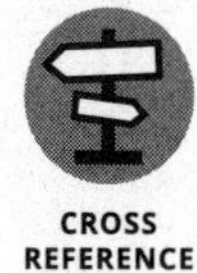
CROSS REFERENCE

For the scoop about try-with-resources, see Chapter 13.

Putting Data in the Table

Like any other tabular configuration, a database table has columns and rows. When you run the code in Listing 17-1, you get an empty table. The table has three columns (NAME, ADDRESS, and BALANCE) but no rows. To add rows to the table, run the code in Listing 17-2.

LISTING 17-2: Inserting Data

```
import java.sql.Connection;
import java.sql.DriverManager;
import java.sql.SQLException;
import java.sql.Statement;

public class AddData {

  public static void main(String args[]) {

    final String CONNECTION = "jdbc:derby:AccountDatabase";

    try (Connection conn = DriverManager.getConnection(CONNECTION);
         Statement statement = conn.createStatement()) {

      statement.executeUpdate("insert into ACCOUNTS values          " +
                              "  ('Barry Burd', '222 Cyber Lane', 24.02) ");

      statement.executeUpdate("insert into ACCOUNTS values          " +
                              "  ('Joe Dow', '111 Luddite Street', 55.63)");

      System.out.println("Rows added.");

    } catch (SQLException e) {
      e.printStackTrace();
    }
  }
}
```

Listing 17-2 uses the same strategy as the code in Listing 17-1: Create Java strings containing SQL commands, and make those strings be arguments to Java's executeUpdate method. In Listing 17-2, I put two rows in the ACCOUNTS table — one for me and another for Joe Dow. (Joe, I hope you appreciate this.)

TIP

For the best results, put all this chapter's listings in the same project. That way, you don't have to add the `derby.jar` file to more than one project. You can also count on the *AccountDatabase* folder being readily available to all four of this chapter's code listings. If you download this book's examples for Eclipse, IntelliJ IDEA, or NetBeans, you'll find all the code from this chapter in the project named *17-01*.

Retrieving Data

What good is a database if you can't get data from it? In this section, you query the database that you created in the previous sections. The code to issue the query is shown in Listing 17-3.

LISTING 17-3: Making a Query

```
import static java.lang.System.out;

import java.sql.Connection;
import java.sql.DriverManager;
import java.sql.ResultSet;
import java.sql.SQLException;
import java.sql.Statement;
import java.text.NumberFormat;

public class GetData {

  public static void main(String args[]) {
    NumberFormat currency = NumberFormat.getCurrencyInstance();
    final String CONNECTION = "jdbc:derby:AccountDatabase";

    try (Connection conn = DriverManager.getConnection(CONNECTION);
         Statement statement = conn.createStatement();
         ResultSet resultset = statement.executeQuery("select * from ACCOUNTS"))
    {

      while (resultset.next()) {
        out.print(resultset.getString("NAME"));
        out.print(", ");
        out.print(resultset.getString("ADDRESS"));
        out.print(" ");
        out.println(currency.format(resultset.getFloat("BALANCE")));
      }
```

(continued)

LISTING 17-3: *(continued)*

```
      } catch (SQLException e) {
        e.printStackTrace();
      }
    }
  }
```

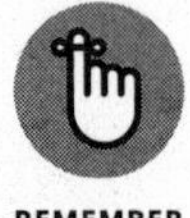

REMEMBER

To use a database other than Apache Derby, change the value of CONNECTION in each of this chapter's examples.

A run of the code from Listing 17-3 is shown in Figure 17-1. The code queries the database and then steps through the rows of the database, printing the data from each of the rows.

FIGURE 17-1: Getting data from the database.

```
Barry Burd, 222 Cyber Lane $24.02
Joe Dow, 111 Luddite Street $55.63
```

Listing 17-3 calls executeQuery and supplies the call with an SQL command. For those who know SQL commands, this particular command gets all data from the ACCOUNTS table (the table that you create in Listing 17-1).

The thing returned from calling executeQuery is of type java.sql.ResultSet. (That's one of the differences between the executeUpdate and executeQuery methods: executeQuery returns a result set, and executeUpdate doesn't.) A *result set* is much like a database table. Like the original table, the result set has rows and columns. Each row contains the data for one account. In this example, each row has a name, an address, and a balance amount.

After you call executeQuery and get your result set, you can step through the result set one row at a time. To do this, you go into a little loop and test the condition resultset.next() at the top of each loop iteration. Each time around, the call to resultset.next() does two things:

- It moves you to the next row of the result set (the next account) if another row exists.
- It tells you whether another row exists by returning a boolean value — true or false.

If the condition resultset.next() is true, the result set has another row. The computer moves to that other row, so you can march into the body of the loop and scoop data from that row. On the other hand, if resultset.next() is false, the result set doesn't have any more rows. You jump out of the loop and start closing everything.

Now, imagine that the computer is pointing to a row of the result set, and you're inside the loop in Listing 17-3. Then you're retrieving data from the result set's row by calling the result set's `getString` and `getFloat` methods. Back in Listing 17-1, you set up the `ACCOUNTS` table with the columns `NAME`, `ADDRESS`, and `BALANCE`. Here in Listing 17-3, you're getting data from these columns by calling your `get`*`SomeTypeOrOther`* methods and feeding the original column names to these methods. After you have the data, you display the data on the computer screen.

TIP

Each Java `ResultSet` instance has several nice `get`*`SomeTypeOrOther`* methods. Depending on the type of data you put into a column, you can call methods `getArray`, `getBigDecimal`, `getBlob`, `getInt`, `getObject`, `getTimestamp`, and several others.

Destroying Data

It's true. All good things must come to an end. By writing this, I'm referring both to this book's content and to the information in this chapter's `AccountDatabase`.

To get rid of the database table that you create in Listing 17-1, run the code in Listing 17-4.

LISTING 17-4: Arrivederci, Database Table

```
import java.sql.Connection;
import java.sql.DriverManager;
import java.sql.SQLException;
import java.sql.Statement;

public class DropTable {

  public static void main(String[] args) {
    final String CONNECTION = "jdbc:derby:AccountDatabase";

    try (Connection conn = DriverManager.getConnection(CONNECTION);
         Statement statement = conn.createStatement()) {

      statement.executeUpdate("drop table ACCOUNTS");
```

(continued)

LISTING 17-4: (continued)

```
      System.out.println("ACCOUNTS table dropped.");
    } catch (SQLException e) {
      e.printStackTrace();
    }
  }
}
```

When you run this code, you wipe the slate clean. Your AccountDatabase no longer contains an ACCOUNTS table. So, if you want to run Listing 17-1 again (perhaps with a change or two), you can.

Who knows? You may even create a table to store your favorite *Java For Dummies* jokes.

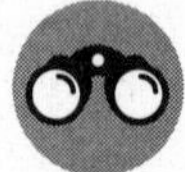

TRY IT OUT

Naturally, I have some things for you to try:

» Rerun the code in Listing 17-3. This time, use the following string in the executeQuery call:

```
"select * from ACCOUNTS where BALANCE > 30"
```

» Run the AddData program (from Listing 17-2) two times in a row without modifying any of the program's code. What error messages do you see? Why?

» Create a table containing three columns: an item name, a price, and a tax rate. Store data in several rows of the table.

Retrieve the data from the table and display a row of output for each row in the table. Each row of output contains the item name followed by the price with tax added. For example, if an item's price is $10 and the item's tax rate is 0.05 (meaning 5 percent), the item's output row contains the number $10.50.

On the last line of the program's output, display the total of all items' tax-added prices.

5

The Part of Tens

IN THIS PART . . .

Catch common mistakes before you make them.

Explore the best resources for Java on the web.

» **Watching out for fall-through**

» **Putting methods, listeners, and constructors where they belong**

» **Using static and non-static references**

» **Avoiding other heinous errors**

Chapter 18
Ten Ways to Avoid Mistakes

"The only people who never make mistakes are the people who never do anything at all." One of my college professors said that. I don't remember the professor's name, so I can't give him proper credit. I guess that's my mistake.

Putting Capital Letters Where They Belong

Java is a case-sensitive language, so you really have to mind your p's and q's — along with every other letter of the alphabet. Here are some details to keep in mind as you create Java programs:

» Java's keywords are all completely lowercase. For instance, in a Java `if` statement, the word *if* can't be *If* or *IF*.

» When you use names from the Java API (Application Programming Interface), the case of the names has to match what appears in the API.

» You also need to make sure that the names you make up yourself are capitalized the same way throughout your entire program. If you declare a `myAccount` variable, you can't refer to it as `MyAccount`, `myaccount`, or `Myaccount`. If you capitalize the variable name two different ways, Java thinks you're referring to two completely different variables.

For more info on Java's case-sensitivity, see Chapter 3.

Breaking Out of a switch Statement

If you don't break out of a `switch` statement, you get fall-through. For instance, if the value of `verse` is 3, the following code prints all three lines — `Last refrain`, `He's a pain`, and `Has no brain`:

```
switch (verse) {
case 3:
    out.print("Last refrain, ");
    out.println("last refrain,");
case 2:
    out.print("He's a pain, ");
    out.println("he's a pain,");
case 1:
    out.print("Has no brain, ");
    out.println("has no brain,");
}
```

For the full story, see Chapter 5.

Comparing Values with a Double Equal Sign

When you compare two values with one another, you use a double equal sign. The line

```
if (inputNumber == randomNumber)
```

is correct, but the line

```
if (inputNumber = randomNumber)
```

is not correct. For a full report, see Chapter 5.

Adding Components to a GUI

Here's a constructor for a Java frame:

```
public SimpleFrame() {
    JButton button = new JButton("Thank you...");
    setTitle("...Katie Mohr and Paul Levesque");
    setLayout(new FlowLayout());
    add(button);
    button.addActionListener(this);
    setSize(300, 100);
    setVisible(true);
}
```

Whatever you do, don't forget the call to the `add` method. Without this call, you go to all the work of creating a button, but the button doesn't show up on your frame. For an introduction to such issues, see Chapter 9.

Adding Listeners to Handle Events

Look again at the previous section's code to construct a `SimpleFrame`. If you forget the call to `addActionListener`, nothing happens when you click the button. Clicking the button harder a second time doesn't help. For the rundown on listeners, see Chapter 16.

Defining the Required Constructors

When you define a constructor with parameters, as in

```
public Temperature(double number)
```

then the computer no longer creates a default parameterless constructor for you. In other words, you can no longer call

```
Temperature roomTemp = new Temperature();
```

unless you explicitly define your own parameterless `Temperature` constructor. For all the gory details on constructors, see Chapter 9.

Fixing Non-Static References

If you try to compile the following code, you get an error message:

```
class WillNotWork {
    String greeting = "Hello";

    public static void main(String args[]) {
        System.out.println(greeting);
    }
}
```

You get an error message because `main` is static, but `greeting` isn't static. For the complete guide to finding and fixing this problem, see Chapter 10.

Staying within Bounds in an Array

When you declare an array with ten components, the components have indices 0 through 9. In other words, if you declare

```
int guests[] = new int[10];
```

then you can refer to the `guests` array's components by writing `guests[0]`, `guests[1]`, and so on, all the way up to `guests[9]`. You can't write `guests[10]`, because the `guests` array has no component with index 10.

For the latest gossip on arrays, see Chapter 11.

Anticipating Null Pointers

This book's examples aren't prone to throwing the NullPointerException, but in real-life Java programming, you see that exception all the time. A NullPointer Exception comes about when you call a method that's supposed to return an object, but instead the method returns nothing. Here's a cheap example:

```
import static java.lang.System.out;
import java.io.File;

class ListMyFiles {

    public static void main(String args[]) {
        File myFile = new File("/Users");
        String dir[] = myFile.list();

        for (String fileName : dir) {
            out.println(fileName);
        }
    }
}
```

This program displays a list of all files in the Users directory.

But what happens if you change /Users to something else — something that doesn't represent the name of a directory?

```
File myFile = new File("&*%$!!");
```

Then the new File call returns null (a special Java word meaning *nothing*), so the variable myFile has nothing in it. Later in the code, the variable dir refers to nothing, and the attempt to loop through all the dir values fails miserably. You get a big NullPointerException, and the program comes crashing down around you.

To avoid this kind of calamity, check Java's API documentation. If you're calling a method that can return null, add exception-handling code to your program.

For the story on handling exceptions, see Chapter 13. For some advice on reading the API documentation, see Chapter 3 and this book's website (www.allmycode.com/JavaForDummies).

Helping Java Find Its Files

You're compiling Java code, minding your own business, when the computer gives you a `NoClassDefFoundError`. All kinds of things can be going wrong, but chances are good that the computer can't find a particular Java file. To fix this, you must align all the planets correctly:

- Your project directory has to contain all the Java files whose names are used in your code.
- If you use named packages, your project directory has to have appropriately named subdirectories.
- If you're running code from your computer's command line, your `CLASSPATH` environment variable must be set properly.

For specific guidelines, see Chapter 14 and this book's website (`www.allmycode.com/JavaForDummies`).

» Finding resources from Oracle

» Reading more about Java

Chapter 19
Ten Websites for Java

No wonder the web is popular: It's both useful and fun. This chapter proves that fact by listing ten useful and fun websites. Each website has resources to help you use Java more effectively. And as far as I know, none of these sites uses adware, pop-ups, or other grotesque things.

This Book's Website

For all matters related to the technical content of this book, visit `www.allmycode.com/JavaForDummies`.

For business issues (for example, "How can I purchase 100 more copies of *Java For Dummies*?"), visit `www.dummies.com`.

The Horse's Mouth

The official Oracle website for Java is `www.oracle.com/technetwork/java`.

Check the official Java API documentation at `http://docs.oracle.com/javase/8/docs/api`.

Consumers of Java technology should visit www.java.com.

Programmers and developers interested in sharing Java technology can go to https://community.oracle.com/community/java.

Finding News, Reviews, and Sample Code

For articles by the experts, visit InfoQ at www.infoq.com and TheServerSide at www.theserverside.com. You always find good reading at these two sites.

Got a Technical Question?

If you're stuck and need help, search for answers and post questions at Stack Overflow (stackoverflow.com).

You can also post questions on the Beginning Java Forum at JavaRanch where the forum's motto is "No question too simple or small . . ." (coderanch.com/f/33/java).

And don't forget. If you have questions about anything you read in this book, send email to me at JavaForDummies@allmycode.com, post a question on www.facebook.com/allmycode, or tweet to the Burd with @allmycode.

Index

Special Characters

A

B

D

E

F

G

H

I

J

K

L

N

O

P

Q

R

S

T

U

V

W

Y

About the Author

Barry Burd received a Master of Science degree in computer science at Rutgers University and a PhD in mathematics at the University of Illinois. As a teaching assistant in Champaign-Urbana, Illinois, he was elected five times to the university-wide List of Teachers Ranked as Excellent by Their Students.

Since 1980, Dr. Burd has been a professor in the Department of Mathematics and Computer Science at Drew University in Madison, New Jersey. He has lectured at conferences in the United States, Europe, Australia, and Asia. He hosts podcasts and videos about software and other technology topics. He is the author of many articles and books, including *Beginning Programming with Java For Dummies, Java Programming for Android Developers For Dummies,* and *Android Application Development All-in-One For Dummies,* all from Wiley.

Dr. Burd lives in Madison, New Jersey, with his wife of n years, where n > 35. In his spare time, he enjoys being a workaholic.

Dedication

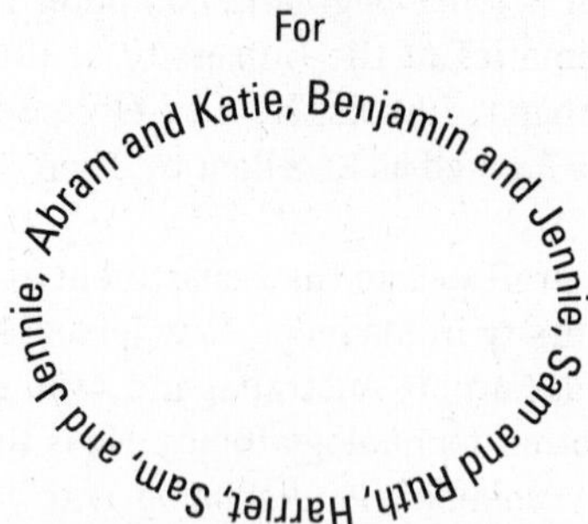
For
Abram and Katie, Benjamin and Jennie, Sam and Ruth, Harriet, Sam, and Jennie,

Author's Acknowledgments

I heartily and sincerely thank Paul Levesque for his work on so many of my books in this series.

Thanks also to Katie Mohr for her hard work and support in so many ways.

Thanks to Chad Darby and Becky Whitney for their efforts in editing this book.

Thanks to the staff at John Wiley & Sons, Inc. for helping to bring this book to bookshelves.

Thanks to Jeanne Boyarsky, Frank Greco, Chandra Guntur, and Michael Redlich for their advice on technical matters.

And a special thanks to Richard Bonacci and Cameron McKenzie for their long-term help and support.

Publisher's Acknowledgments

Acquisitions Editor: Katie Mohr
Senior Project Editor: Paul Levesque
Copy Editor: Becky Whitney
Technical Editor: Chad Darby

Editorial Assistant: Serena Novosel
Sr. Editorial Assistant: Cherie Case
Production Editor: Siddique Shaik
Cover Image: © Melpomene/Shutterstock